PROSTATE BIOPSY INTERPRETATION

Third Edition

Biopsy Interpretation Series

BIOPSY INTERPRETATION SERIES

Series Editor: Jonathan I. Epstein, M.D.

Prostate Biopsy Interpretation, Third Edition
Jonathan I. Epstein and Ximing J. Yang, 2002, 320 pages

Interpretation of Breast Biopsies, Fourth Edition
Darryl Carter, 2002

PROSTATE BIOPSY INTERPRETATION

Third Edition

Biopsy Interpretation Series

Jonathan I. Epstein, M.D.

Professor of Pathology, Urology, and Oncology
The Reinhard Professor of Urologic Pathology
Johns Hopkins Medical Institutions
Baltimore, Maryland

Ximing J. Yang, M.D., Ph.D.

Assistant Professor of Pathology and Surgery
University of Chicago
Chicago, Illinois

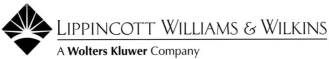

LIPPINCOTT WILLIAMS & WILKINS
A **Wolters Kluwer** Company
Philadelphia · Baltimore · New York · London
Buenos Aires · Hong Kong · Sydney · Tokyo

Acquisitions Editor: Ruth W. Weinberg
Developmental Editor: Michelle M. LaPlante
Production Editor: Frank Aversa
Manufacturing Manager: Ben Rivera
Compositor: Lippincott Williams & Wilkins, Desktop Division
Printer: Maple Press

© **2002 by LIPPINCOTT WILLIAMS & WILKINS**
530 Walnut Street
Philadelphia, PA 19106 USA
LWW.com

Printed in the USA

Library of Congress Cataloging-in-Publication Data

Epstein, Jonathan I.
    Prostate biopsy interpretation / Jonathan I. Epstein, Ximing J. Yang.—3rd ed.
      p. ;cm. — (Biopsy interpretation series)
    Includes bibliographical references and index.
    ISBN 0-7817-3287-5
      1. Prostate—Cancer—Cytodiagnosis. 2. Prostate—Needle biopsy. 3.
Prostate—Diseases—Cytodiagnosis. I. Yang, Ximing J. II. Title. III. Series
      [DNLM: 1. Prostatic Neoplasms—diagnosis. 2. Biopsy, Needle. 3. Prostatic
Diseases—diagnosis. WJ 752 E64p 2002]
    RC280.P7 E58 2002
    616.99′463—dc21   2002016159

10 9 8 7 6 5 4 3 2 1

To my wonderful wife, Bonnie, and my two precious children, David and Jeremy.

Jonathan I. Epstein

To my loving wife, and my wonderful children, Julie and Jason.

Ximing J. Yang

Contents

Preface

This third edition of *Prostate Biopsy Interpretation* represents more than just a revision. Rather, chapters of the book have been totally reorganized and rewritten to reflect rapidly changing knowledge relating to prostate pathology and its clinical correlates. New chapters have been added on subjects such as clinical findings leading to prostate biopsy; biopsy technique and sampling; reporting cancer and its influence on prognosis and treatment; and findings atypical or suspicious for carcinoma. The major new addition to this book is the CD-ROM, containing over 1,700 color images.

Whereas in a textbook, one has only the room to show one or two images of a given entity, the CD-ROM allows the luxury of illustrating at various magnifications numerous examples of each entity. With prostate cancer and its mimickers, where there are many different morphological patterns and variants, it is especially useful to have the opportunity to show multiple images. Illustrating these lesions in color at different magnifications also more closely approximates the experience of looking through a microscope. This will result in a greater degree of diagnostic confidence and skill for the reader when confronted with a difficult prostatic lesion. The ability to use the CD-ROM in a "quiz mode" to review random cases without knowing the answer is an additional benefit that will help pathologists review prostate pathology, either for their own educational benefit or in preparation for board examinations.

Prostate Biopsy Interpretation and the accompanying CD-ROM focus on practical, need-to-know information regarding the diagnosis and prognosis of prostate cancer obtained on biopsy. Although there has been much progress regarding molecular knowledge of prostate cancer, recent studies have not yet yielded information that is ready to be adopted for clinical practice. Consequently, these areas are not covered in this edition. We look forward to future editions when such information can provide use to practicing pathologists.

Jonathan I. Epstein, M.D.
Ximing J. Yang, M.D., Ph.D.

Preface to the First Edition

Within the last few years there has been much change in both our knowledge and our concepts concerning many prostatic entities. The advances in surgical and radiological techniques have led to an increased number of prostate biopsies being performed, and recent pathological techniques have facilitated our evaluation of prostate biopsy material.

New surgical techniques have been developed to enable radical prostatectomy to be performed with minimal morbidity, leading to more aggressive diagnosis and treatment of prostatic carcinoma. Even small, low-grade, incidentally discovered adenocarcinomas of the prostate found in relatively young men may now be treated aggressively because of the lower morbidity and the recently recognized increased risk of long-term progression. The increasing use of transrectal ultrasound and the recent development of biopsy guns that generate thin-core biopsy material with minimal morbidity have resulted in, and will continue to result in, increased numbers of core needle biopsy specimens to evaluate.

Currently, there are only a few general urologic pathology books, and they tend to summarize previous data, often without critically analyzing controversial topics. Furthermore, because of the general nature of these books, only a few photographs are present, and they do not provide the practicing pathologist sufficient help when confronted with diagnostically difficult lesions.

I am very fortunate to practice in an institution at which a wealth of prostate specimens is available for study. More than 600 biopsies (needle and transurethral resection specimens) and almost 200 radical prostatectomies are performed at our institution each year. This book contains an extensive number of photographs culled from these procedures, which will help pathologists in their day-to-day practice with difficult and unusual lesions, as well as common problems encountered in prostate pathology. These include:

1. the distinction between allergic, infectious, posttransurethral resection, and nonspecific granulomatous prostatitis;
2. differentiation of low-grade adenocarcinoma from adenosis and basal cell hyperplasia;
3. a practical approach to the Gleason grading system on biopsy material correlation with radical prostatectomy findings, and influence of grade on therapeutic decisions;

4. use of immunohistochemical techniques, such as prostate-specific antigen, prostate-specific acid phosphatase, and basal-cell-specific antibodies, in the diagnosis of prostate cancer, along with their limitations and potential pitfalls;
5. diagnosis of limited cancer on needle biopsy specimens; and
6. illustrations of rare and recently described entities, such as postoperative spindle cell nodules involving the prostate, cystosarcoma phyllodes of the prostate, adenoid cystic carcinoma of the prostate, and clear cell cribiforming hyperplasia of the prostate.

Commonly encountered problems such as cautery artifact on transurethral resection material, crush artifact on needle biopsy specimens, and the distinction between high-grade transitional cell carcinoma and poorly differentiated adenocarcinoma are all dealt with from the experience of a practicing pathologist who deals with these issues on a day-to-day basis. Furthermore, difficult cases have been selected to include those cases in which the patient underwent radical surgery based on the diagnosis, such that the diagnosis of carcinoma was verified.

In addition to thoroughly illustrating diagnostically difficult and unusual lesions, as well as addressing practical problems in the interpretation of prostate biopsies, the text discusses controversial and confusing topics encountered in prostate pathology. These topics include:

1. classification and prognosis of stage A (incidentally discovered) prostatic carcinoma;
2. intraductal dysplasia of the prostate, its association with cancer, its distinction from other entities not significantly linked with carcinoma, and the significance of finding dysplasia alone on biopsy material;
3. current thoughts on unusual variants of prostate cancer, such as prostatic duct carcinoma (endometrioid carcinoma), colloid carcinoma of the prostate, and carcinomas with neuroendocrine differentiation (small cell carcinoma, carcinoid); and
4. transitional cell carcinoma involving the prostate as it relates to conservative therapy for early bladder cancer, significance of *in situ* transitional cell carcinoma involving the prostate, and significance in identification of prostatic stromal invasion by transitional cell carcinoma.

This book will be of interest to all pathologists who evaluate biopsy material from the prostate. In addition, the discussion of the various clinicopathological features concerning each lesion will be a useful reference to pathologists in general.

Jonathan I. Epstein
1989

Acknowledgments

For her expeditious typing and help in preparation of the manuscript, we are greatly indebted to Ms. Joanne Schlimm. We are also grateful to Raymond Lund and Norman Barker for the excellent quality of the photomicrographs in this book.

Jonathan I. Epstein, M.D.
Ximing J. Yang, M.D., Ph.D.

PROSTATE BIOPSY INTERPRETATION

Third Edition

Biopsy Interpretation Series

1

Clinical Correlates
with Biopsy

Serum Prostate-Specific Antigen,
Digital Rectal Examination,
Transrectal Ultrasound

Needle biopsies of the prostate are performed either because of an abnormal rectal exam, elevated serum prostate-specific antigen (PSA) level, or an abnormal transrectal ultrasound (TRUS); some men are screened because of a strong family history of prostate cancer.

DIGITAL RECTAL EXAMINATION

Asymmetry, induration, and discrete hard nodules are findings on digital rectal examination (DRE) that are suspicious for cancer. The positive predictive value of core needle biopsy of the prostate varies depending on the degree of the palpable abnormality of the prostate, with marked induration or a nodule more likely representing carcinoma than mild induration.

The positive predictive value of an abnormal DRE is only 22% to 36% (1). A more serious limitation of DRE is its low sensitivity (i.e., missing cancer). One-half of cancers removed by radical prostatectomy at our institution are nonpalpable (stage T1c). Although some of these tumors are small, 51% are >0.5 cc and located in the peripheral zone, so that one would have expected them to be palpable. Another 15% to 25% of stage T1c prostate cancers are located in the transition zone (anteriorly) where they are not palpable due to their location (2,3). There is poor interobserver reproducibility even among urologists as to what is an abnormal DRE (4).

TRANSRECTAL ULTRASOUND

The majority of prostate cancers appear on TRUS as hypoechoic relative to the normal peripheral zone, although tumors may also be hyperechoic or isoechoic. Despite initial studies claiming a great value of this test for the detection of prostate cancer, subsequent reports have noted poor sensitivity and specificity limiting its usefulness (5,6). Cancer is as likely to be found in areas that are normal by TRUS as they are to be detected in radiographically abnormal areas. Currently, the major role of TRUS is to direct the needle biopsies of the prostate in either a sextant or alternative (see Chapter 2) distribution. Another function of TRUS is to estimate the size of the prostate that can be used to calculate PSA density (see below). Even this role of TRUS is limited as there is not a great correlation between prostate volume estimated by TRUS and actual prostate volume (7). In part, limitations of TRUS relate to differences in the equipment used and that the exam is heavily operator dependent.

PROSTATE SPECIFIC ANTIGEN

PSA is synthesized in the ductal epithelium and prostatic acini. It is found in normal, hyperplastic, and malignant prostate tissue (8). PSA is secreted into the lumina of the prostatic ducts to become a component of the seminal plasma. It reaches the serum by diffusion from the luminal cells through the epithelial basement membrane and stroma where it can pass through the capillary basement membranes. PSA is a serine protease of the human glandular kallikrein family. In the seminal fluid are gel-forming proteins which function to trap spermatozoa at ejaculation. PSA functions to liquefy the coagulum and break down the seminal clot through proteolysis of the gel-forming proteins into smaller more soluble fragments thus releasing the spermatozoa.

Total Serum PSA: Numerous studies have shown that patients with prostate cancer have, in general, elevated serum PSA levels relative to men without prostate cancer. In contrast to many other laboratory tests, the "normal value" for serum PSA is not a straightforward issue. In general, serum PSA levels above 4 ng/ml are considered to be abnormal. When serum PSA concentrations are 4 to 10 ng/ml the incidence of cancer detection on prostate biopsy in men with a normal DRE is approximately 25%. In men with serum PSA levels of 4 to 10 and an abnormal DRE, approximately 50% of men have cancer on biopsy. With serum PSA levels over 10, the incidence of prostate cancer on biopsy increases to 30% to 40% and 70% in men with normal and abnormal DRE, respectively. However, about 20% of men diagnosed with prostate cancers have PSA levels <4.0 ng/ml. The reason why serum PSA levels are not diagnostic of prostate cancer is that benign prostate tissue also produces serum PSA. Other factors such as prostatitis, infarct, instrumentation of the prostate, and ejaculation also increase serum PSA levels. Routine DRE and TRUS do not appear to elevate serum PSA levels, although vigorous prostatic massages and prostate needle biopsies do.

Following an inciting event, it is recommended that one waits 4 to 6 weeks before using PSA levels to guide clinical decision making. Finasteride, used to treat benign prostatic hyperplasia and hair loss, lowers serum PSA levels on average by approximately 50%. In an attempt to improve the utility of serum PSA tests to detect prostate cancer, while minimizing biopsies performed on men who do not have prostate cancer, variations of the PSA test have been developed.

PSA Density: As noted earlier, benign prostate tissue also contributes to serum PSA levels although not to the same extent as does cancer. Men with enlarged hyperplastic prostate glands will have higher total serum PSA levels than men with small glands. The measurement of serum PSA density factors out the contribution of benign prostatic tissue to serum PSA levels. Serum PSA density reflects the PSA produced per gram of prostate tissue. It is calculated by dividing the total serum PSA level by the estimated gland volume (usually determined by TRUS measurements), with an upper normal value of approximately 0.15. There are conflicting studies as to the advantage of PSA density over that of total serum PSA to detect prostate cancer. Furthermore, the measurement of prostatic volume by TRUS does not correlate particularly well with actual prostatic volume.

Age-Specific PSA Reference Ranges: As men age, their prostates tend to enlarge with benign prostatic hyperplasia. One would then anticipate that overall older men would have higher serum PSA levels than younger men. Derived from measurements of serum PSA levels in a large group of men of varying ages without prostate cancer, the recommended age-specific upper reference ranges for serum PSA are 2.5 ng/ml for men 40 to 49 years of age, 3.5 ng/ml for men 50 to 59 years, 4.5 ng/ml for men 60 to 69 years, and 6.5 ng/ml for men 70 to 79 years. The net effect of using such age-specific PSA reference ranges is that there will be a greater number of biopsies performed in younger men with relatively low serum PSA levels and less biopsies performed in older men with serum PSA levels slightly above the "normal cutoff" of 4.0 ng/ml.

PSA Velocity (Rate of Change of PSA): PSA velocity is based on data from the Baltimore Longitudinal Study of Aging. This is a long-term prospective aging study by the National Institute of Aging where a large group of male subjects return every 2 years for several days of evaluation, including serum PSA tests. Those men who eventually were diagnosed as having prostate cancer had an increased rate of rise in PSA as compared to men who did not have prostate cancer. The rate of change in PSA that best distinguished between men with and without prostate cancer was 0.75 ng/ml per year. Whereas 72% of men with prostate cancer had a PSA velocity of 0.75 ng/ml per year or more, only 5% of men without prostate cancer had a PSA velocity above this cutoff. In order for this test to be valid, it requires that there be at least three PSA measurements available over a period of 1.5 to 2 years. That is because there is substantial short-term variability (up to 20%) between repeat PSA measurements. In a man who has a significant rise in serum PSA levels even though the latest serum PSA test may be below the normal cutoff (<4 ng/ml), this finding is abnormal and should prompt a workup.

Molecular Forms of PSA: In the early 1990s, it was discovered that there are several different molecular forms of PSA in the serum. Most of the measurable serum PSA is bound to the serine protease inhibitor alpha-1 antichymotrypsin (ACT). A smaller fraction (1% to 30%) of the measurable serum PSA is free or noncomplexed PSA. In addition, a minority of PSA is complexed to alpha-2 macroglobulin; because it totally encapsulates the PSA molecule, this component cannot be measured by routine immunoassays. The total serum PSA measured, therefore, reflects both free PSA and PSA complexed to ACT. It has been demonstrated that the percent of free PSA can improve the specificity of PSA testing for prostate cancer. In general, men with higher percent free PSA levels in the serum are less likely to have cancer than men with lower percent free PSA values. The exact cutoff as to an abnormal percent free PSA is a complicated issue and depends on total serum PSA levels, age, and prostate size. As yet, there is no consensus for strict cutoff levels for biopsy using the different free PSA assays available. When percent free PSA is higher than 25%, this indicates a lower risk of cancer as compared to percent free PSA values of less than 10%, which is worrisome for cancer. Some authorities recommend using this test for men with a normal DRE and serum PSA values of between 4 and 10 ng/ml in deciding whether to perform a repeat biopsy following an initial negative biopsy.

PSA: Relation to Posttherapy Follow-up Biopsies: Serum PSA tests may also be used to monitor various treatments of prostate cancer in deciding whether posttherapy biopsies are needed. Following radical prostatectomy, the serum PSA should drop to undetectable levels. Elevated serum PSA levels following radical prostatectomy (>0.2 ng/ml) indicate recurrent or persistent disease. Similarly, following radiotherapy for prostate cancer serum, PSA values will decrease to a nadir although not to the same extent as those following radical prostatectomy. Three subsequent rises in serum PSA values after radiotherapy indicates treatment failure. Although these serum tests indicate failure, many clinicians still perform biopsies to verify recurrent cancer.

COMBINED USE OF TESTS

The likelihood of diagnosing carcinoma on needle biopsy in the face of an abnormal test result (positive predictive value) varies among studies depending on the patient population. Studies by Catalona et al. (9), analyzing a screening population, and Cooner et al. (10), evaluating patients in a urological practice, calculated the positive predictive values of prostate biopsy based on PSA, DRE, and ultrasound (Tables 1.1 and 1.2). In general, the combination of abnormal DRE, TRUS, and PSA tests increases the risk of cancer on biopsy more than an isolated abnormal test.

TABLE 1.1. *Positive predictive value (percent of subjects with cancer if detection method is suspicious)*

Digital rectal examination	Transrectal ultrasound	PSA (ng/ml)	Pos. predictive value (%)	No. ca./no. biopsies
—	—	More than 4.0	31.5	216/686
—	—	4.1 to 9.9	26.1	143/548
—	—	10.0 or more	52.9	73/138
Pos.	—	—	21.4	146/683
Pos.	—	4.0 or less	10.0	48/481
Pos.	—	More than 4.0	48.5	98/202
Pos.	—	4.1 to 9.9	40.8	60/147
Pos.	—	10.0 or more	69.1	38/55
Neg.	—	4.0 or less	•	•
Neg.	—	More than 4.0	24.4	118/484
Neg.	—	4.1 to 9.9	20.7	83/401
Neg.	—	10.0 or more	42.2	35/83
Pos.	Pos.	4.0 or less	13.8	32/232
Pos.	Pos.	More than 4.0	54.7	64/117
Pos.	Pos.	4.1 to 9.9	48.8	40/92
Pos.	Pos.	10.0 or more	68.6	24/35
Pos.	Neg.	4.0 or less	6.9	16/233
Pos.	Neg.	More than 4.0	41.3	26/63
Pos.	Neg.	4.1 to 9.9	35.3	18/51
Pos.	Neg.	10.0 or more	66.7	8/12
Neg.	Pos.	4.0 or less	•	•
Neg.	Pos.	More than 4.0	29.8	57/191
Neg.	Pos.	4.1 to 9.9	25.3	39/154
Neg.	Pos.	10.0 or more	48.6	18/37
Neg.	Neg.	4.0 or less	•	•
Neg.	Neg.	More than 4.0	20.7	57/276
Neg.	Neg.	4.1 to 9.9	17.9	42/234
Neg.	Neg.	10.0 or more	35.7	15/42

Reprinted with permission from Catalona et al. (9).
Pos., suspicious for cancer; Neg., not suspicious for cancer; •, no biopsies in this category.

TABLE 1.2. *Examinations and biopsies with digital rectal examination and prostate-specific antigen correlation in 1,807 patients*

Category	Total pts.	No. pts. biopsied (%)	No. pos. biopsies (%)[a]
All pts.	1,807	835 (46.2)	263 (14.6)
Digital rectal examination			
Pos.	565	470 (83.2)	203 (35.9)
Neg.	1,242	365 (29.4)	60 (4.8)
Prostate-specific antigen:			
+	366	209 (57.1)	74 (20.2)
++	236	227 (96.2)	137 (58.1)
+/++	602	436 (72.4)	211 (35)
−	1,205	399 (33.1)	52 (4.3)
Digital rectal examination/ prostate-specific antigen			
Pos./+	136	129 (94.9)	58 (42.6)
Pos./++	147	146 (99.3)	112 (76.2)
Pos./+/++	283	275 (97.2)	170 (60.1)
Pos./−	282	195 (69.1)	33 (11.7)
Neg./+	230	80 (34.8)	16 (7.0)
Neg./++	89	81 (91.0)	25 (28.1)
Neg./+/++	319	161 (50.5)	41 (12.9)
Neg./−	923	204 (22.1)	19 (2.1)

Reprinted with permission from Cooner et al. (10).
[a]Cancer detection rate (number of positive biopsies/total number of patients)
Prostate-specific antigen: −, 4.0 ng/ml or less; +, 4.1 to 10.0 ng/ml; ++, greater than 10.0 ng/ml; +/++, greater than 4.0 ng/ml.

REFERENCES

1. Scardino PT, Weaver R, Hudson MA. Early detection of prostate cancer. *Hum Pathol* 1992;23: 211–222.
2. Epstein JI, Walsh PC, CarMichael M, et al. Pathological and clinical findings to predict tumor extent of non-palpable (stage T1c) prostate cancer. *JAMA* 1994;271:368–374.
3. Carter HB, Sauvageot J, Walsh PC, et al. Prospective evaluation of men with stage T1C adenocarcinoma of the prostate. *J Urol* 1997;157:2206–2209.
4. Angulo JC, Montie JE, Bukowsy T, et al. Interobserver consistency of digital rectal examination in clinical staging of localized prostatic carcinoma. *Urol Oncol* 1995;1:199–205.
5. Carter HB, Hamper UM, Sheth S, et al. Evaluation of transrectal ultrasound in the early detection of prostate cancer. *J Urol* 1989;142:1008–1010.
6. Coffield KS, Speights VO, Brawn PN, et al. Ultrasound detection of prostate cancer in postmortem specimens with histological correlation. *J Urol* 1992;147:822–826.
7. Matthews GJ, Motta J, Fracchia JA. The accuracy of transrectal ultrasound prostate volume estimation: clinical correlations. *J Clin Ultrasound* 1996;24:501–505.
8. Polascik TJ, Oesterling JE, Partin AW. Prostate specific antigen: a decade of discovery—what have we learned and where are we going. *J Urol* 1999;162:293–306.
9. Catalona WJ, Richie JP, Ahmann FR, et al. Comparison of digital rectal examination and serum prostate specific antigen in the early detection of prostate cancer: results of a multicenter clinical trial of 6,630 men. *J Urol* 1994;151:1283–1290.
10. Cooner WH, Mosley BR, Rutherford CL, et al. Prostate cancer detection in a clinical urological practice by ultrasonography, digital rectal examination and prostate specific antigen. *J Urol* 1990;143: 1146–1154.

2

Needle Biopsy Technique, Tissue Sampling, and Processing of Needle Biopsy and Transurethral Resection Specimens

NEEDLE BIOPSY TECHNIQUE

Currently, the standard method used to diagnose prostate cancer is that of ultrasound-guided systematic sextant biopsy (1). Routine sextant biopsies sample the parasagittal midlobe region of the prostate despite the recognition that many prostate cancers arise posterolaterally (2). In recent years, studies have suggested alternative needle biopsy sampling techniques to increase prostate cancer detection.

Three general modifications of the sextant biopsy technique have been proposed: (a) addition of transition zone biopsies; (b) addition of biopsies for enlarged prostates; and (c) modifying the location of the nontransition zone biopsies. Investigations of nonpalpable (stage T1c) prostate cancer note that 15% to 22% of tumors are located anteriorly within the transition zone (3,4). However, most studies demonstrate a low incidence of cancer found solely in the transition zone biopsy (5,6). A recognized use of transition zone biopsies is when findings are very suspicious for cancer, yet the initial biopsy is benign.

Modifications of routine sextant biopsies have also been proposed based on the size of the prostate gland. Several studies have shown that with larger prostates there is decreased detection of prostate cancer (7–11). However, it is unknown if extra biopsies performed will enhance the detection of prostate cancer. Another issue that has recently been brought forward is that tumors detected in large prostate glands have a better outcome than those found in smaller prostates (12). It remains to be studied whether increased sampling to detect tumors in large prostates may result in a relative increase in the detection of more indolent tumors.

The addition of midline peripheral zone needle biopsies is not supported by most studies including ours (13–15). Most studies, however, have concentrated on the utility of more posterolaterally guided biopsies (13–18). If one were to only perform six needle biopsies of the prostate, then these biopsies should be aimed more towards the posterolateral aspect of the gland. However, combining both routine sextant and posterolateral needle biopsies maximizes the detection of cancer. The importance of posterolateral biopsies is even more dramatized by the preponderance of significant cancers that would be missed by not sampling the posterolateral region (15). At our institution, urologists currently perform routine sampling of both the sextant and posterolateral aspects of the gland with 12 cores sampled per patient.

NEEDLE BIOPSY PROCESSING—FIXATIVE

Although the most common fixative used for prostate needle biopsy is formalin, other fixatives, such as Bouins or Hollandes solutions, are also used to provide enhanced nuclear detail. The disadvantage of these fixatives is that one can see visible nucleoli even in benign glands, such that the significance of finding nucleoli in atypical glands suspicious for carcinoma is not as powerful as when more prominent nucleoli are seen in formalin-fixed tissue. When using fixatives such as Bouins, one must judge what are prominent nucleoli relative to the nucleoli seen in adjacent benign glands. If one does not see nucleoli in the majority of prostate cancers sampled on needle biopsy, it is not necessary to switch from formalin to these other alternative fixatives. Rather, careful attention to microtomy and staining can improve the situation; sections that are too thick or overstained result in hyperchromatic nuclei without visible nucleoli.

NEEDLE BIOPSY PROCESSING—NUMBER OF LEVELS

We evaluated 439 consecutive sextant prostate biopsies to determine if clinically relevant diagnostic information would be lost with less than three levels per tissue core (19). Consecutive 18-gauge sextant biopsies were reviewed for cases containing Gleason grade 3+4=7 adenocarcinoma or perineural invasion by carcinoma. Misdiagnosis of clinically relevant features on prostate biopsy can be minimized with histologic review of three levels per tissue core.

NEEDLE BIOPSY PROCESSING—INTERVENING UNSTAINED SLIDES

Immunohistochemistry stains for high molecular weight cytokeratin may demonstrate the presence or absence of basal cells in a small focus of atypical glands helping to establish a benign or malignant diagnosis, receptively. From 1/94 to present, we have generated intervening unstained slides on all prostate needle biopsies for potential immunohistochemistry stains for high molecular weight cytokeratin, since lesions may not survive deeper sectioning into the block. Of 1,105 prostate needle biopsy cases seen at Hopkins from 1/94 to 12/96, immunohistochemistry staining for high molecular weight cytokeratin was initially done on 94 (8.5%). To see if lesions would still have been present for evaluation if we did not have intervening slides, we repeated the immunohistochemistry stains for high molecular weight cytokeratin off of the paraffin blocks in 81 cases where material was available for study (20). Care was taken to not trim the blocks. In 52 cases, the original high molecular weight cytokeratin helped to establish a diagnosis: In 31 of these cases, the lesion was not present on repeat immunohistochemistry stains from the block. Of these 31 cases, the original high molecular weight cytokeratin from intervening unstained slides helped to establish a cancer (n=23) or benign (n=8) diagnosis. The use of intervening unstained slides was critical to establish a diagnosis in 31/1,105 (2.8%) of prostate needle biopsies. Each laboratory must decide whether these data justify the cost of preparing extra unstained slides.

SAMPLING OF TRANSURETHRAL RESECTION SPECIMENS

In order to minimize undersampling of a high-grade cancer component, tissue should be evenly placed within cassettes, such that there is no overlapping of transurethral resection of the prostate (TURP) chips (21).

1. Initially, submit eight cassettes of tissue in a random fashion. Submission of eight cassettes will identify almost all stage T1b cancers (high-volume or high-grade) (see Chapter 8) and approximately 90% of stage T1a tumors (low-volume and not high-grade) (see Chapter 8) (22–25). Submit the specimen in its entirety if it requires nine cassettes or less.

2. In younger men (<65 years of age), submission of all the tissue may be justified to identify all stage T1a lesions, since studies have shown these men are at increased risk of progression with long-term follow-up and they may be given the option of definitive therapy at some institutions.

3. When stage T1b carcinoma is found on the initial eight slides, it is not necessary to submit additional tissue. We have demonstrated that review of additional material, beyond that of the initial eight cassettes, will not change the stage based on the percent of tumor involvement (21). Although the percent of tumor changed in some cases, the magnitude of the change was never sufficient to change a lesion from <5% (T1a) to >5% (T1b) or vice versa. This finding is expected because the tissue is randomly submitted, and examination of eight cassettes should be representative of the percent of tumor involvement for the entire specimen. If a lesion is classified as stage T1b based on the presence of high-grade tumor, examination of any remaining tissue will also not downstage the cancer even if lower grade tumor is present on the additional tissue examined.

4. When stage T1a carcinoma is found on the initial eight slides reviewed, the remaining tissue should be submitted for review (21). The rationale for submitting the remaining tissue for stage T1a lesions is as follows. There is a small potential of upstaging based on finding high-grade cancer in the additionally submitted tissue. The decision to submit the remaining tissue should not be burdensome because it occurs in only approximately 1.5% of TURP specimens: Approximately 10% to 15% of TURPs have cancer and only 15% of these cases are stage T1a lesions requiring more than nine cassettes

for complete submission. In the few cases with excessive amounts of tissue, it is not unreasonable to submit a maximum total of 16 cassettes, since the potential for upstaging based on grade is relatively small.

REFERENCES

1. Hodge KK, McNeal JE, Terris MK, et al. Random–systematic versus directed ultrasound guided transrectal core biopsies of the prostate. *J Urol* 1989;142:71–74.
2. Stamey TA, McNeal JE, Freiha FS, et al. Morphometric and clinical studies on 68 consecutive radical prostatectomies. *J Urol* 1988;139:1235–1241.
3. Epstein JI, Walsh PC, CarMichael M, et al. Pathological and clinical findings to predict tumor extent of non-palpable (stage T1c) prostate cancer. *JAMA* 1994;271:368–374.
4. Carter HB, Sauvageot J, Walsh PC, et al. Prospective evaluation of men with stage T1C adenocarcinoma of the prostate. *J Urol* 1997;157:2206–2209.
5. Bazinet M, Karakiewicz PI, Aprikian AG, et al. Value of systematic transition zone biopsies in the early detection of prostate cancer. *J Urol* 1996;155:605–606.
6. Fleshner NE, Fair WR. Indications for transition zone biopsy in the detection of prostate Cancer. *J Urol* 1997;57:556–558.
7. Epstein JI, Walsh PC, Sauvageot J, et al. Use of repeat sextant and transition zone biopsies for assessing extent of prostate cancer. *J Urol* 1997;158:1886–1890.
8. Karakiewicz PI, Bazinet M, Aprikian AG, et al. Outcome of sextant biopsy according to gland volume. *Urology* 1997;49:55–59.
9. Uzzo RG, Wei JT, Wladbaum RS, et al. The influence of prostate size on cancer detection. *Urology* 1995;46:831–836.
10. Naughton CK, Smith DS, Humphrey PA, et al. Clinical and pathologic tumor characteristics of prostate cancer as a function of the number of biopsy cores: a retrospective study. *Urology* 1998;52:808–813.
11. Epstein JI, Walsh PC, Carter HB. The significance of prior negative needle biopsies in men subsequently diagnosed with prostate cancer. *J Urol* 1992;162:1649–1652.
12. D'Amico AV, Whittington R, Malkowicz SB, et al. A prostate gland volume of more that 75 cm³ predicts for a favorable outcome after radical prostatectomy for localized prostate cancer. *Urology* 1998; 52:631–636.
13. Eskew LA, Bare RL, McCullough DL. Systemic 5 region prostate biopsy is superior to sextant method for diagnosing carcinoma of the prostate. *J Urol* 1997;157:199–202.
14. Terris MK, Wallen EM, Stamey TA. Comparison of mid-lobe versus lateral systemic sextant biopsies of the detection of prostate cancer. *Urol Int* 1997;59:239–242.
15. Epstein JI, Walsh PC, Lecksell K, et al. The importance of posterolateral needle biopsies in the detection of prostate cancer. *Urology* 2001;57:1112–1116.
16. Norberg M, Egevad L, Holmberg L, et al. The sextant protocol for ultrasound-guided core biopsies of the prostate underestimates the presence of cancer. *Urology* 1997;50:562–566.
17. Eskew LA, Bare RL, McCullough DL. Systemic 5 region prostate biopsy is superior to sextant method for diagnosing carcinoma of the prostate. *J Urol* 1997;157:199–202.
18. Chang JJ, Shinohara K, Bhargava V, et al. Prospective evaluation of lateral biopsies of the peripheral zone for prostate cancer detection. *J Urol* 1998;160:2111–2114.
19. Brat DJ, Wills ML, Lecksell KL, et al. How often are diagnostic features missed with less extensive histological sampling of prostate needle biopsies? *Am J Surg Path* 1999;23:257–262.
20. Green R, Epstein JI. Use of intervening unstained slides for immunohistochemical (IHC) for high molecular weight cytokeratin (HMWCK) on prostate needle biopsies. *Am J Surg Pathol* 1999;23:567–570.
21. McDowell PR, Fox W, Epstein JI. Is submission of remaining tissue necessary when incidental carcinoma of the prostate is found on transurethral resection? *Hum Pathol* 1994;25:493–497.
22. Murphy WM, Dean PJ, Brasfield JA, et al. Incidental carcinoma of the prostate. How much sampling is adequate? *Am J Surg Pathol* 1986;10:170–174.
23. Newman AJ, Graham MA, Carlton CE, et al. Incidental carcinoma of the prostate at the time of transurethral resection: importance of evaluating every chip. *J Urol* 1982;128:948–950.
24. Rohr LR. Incidental adenocarcinoma in transurethral resections of the prostate: partial versus complete microscopic examination. *Am J Surg Pathol* 1987;11:53–58.
25. Vollmer RT. Prostate cancer and chip specimens: complete versus partial sampling. *Hum Pathol* 1986;17:285–290.

3

Gross Anatomy and Normal Histology

GROSS ANATOMY

The prostate weighs approximately 30 to 40 grams in adult men without prominent benign prostatic hyperplasia (BPH). It has the shape of an inverted cone with the base located proximally at the bladder neck and the apex distally at the urogenital diaphragm. The prostatic urethra runs through the center of the gland with a 35° anterior bend at the verumontanum (1). Posteriorly, a thin, filmy layer of connective tissue known as Denonvillier's fascia separates the prostate and seminal vesicles from the rectum.

Initially, the prostate was thought to be composed of distinct anatomic lobes. Today's anatomic theories divide the prostate into inner and outer regions, although right and left lobes are still referred to based on palpation of a midline furrow. The inner is affected predominantly by BPH, and the outer has a predilection for carcinoma, although some carcinomas occur centrally and BPH nodules may be seen peripherally (2). The prostate is divided into four zones: (a) anterior fibromuscular stroma; (b) central zone; (c) peripheral zone; and (d) pre-prostatic region which encompasses the periurethral ducts and the larger transition zone (1) (Color Plate 1).

The anterior fibromuscular stroma, which occupies approximately one-third of the prostate, contains very few glands and consists of smooth muscle tissue and dense fibrous tissue. The central zone forms a cone-shaped volume surrounding the ejaculatory ducts with its apex at the verumontanum and its base at the bladder neck. The peripheral zone is the largest zone and contains 75% of the glandular tissue of the prostate. The peripheral zone is distal to the central zone, and corresponds to a horseshoe-shaped structure extending posteriorly, posterolaterally, and laterally around the inner aspect of the prostate. The most critical area of the preprostatic region is the transition zone which is most affected by hyperplasia. The rationale for separating the outer aspect of the prostate into central and peripheral zones is in part based on both histological differences and differences in the diseases affecting these two areas.

From a diagnostic standpoint, central zone histology may mimic high-grade prostatic intraepithelial neoplasia (PIN) (see Chapter 5). The peripheral zone is much more frequently affected by carcinoma. The central zone is an uncommon site for origin of carcinoma, although it may be secondarily invaded by large peripheral zone tumors. Despite these differences, experts in the field still find difficulties in distinguishing between the central and peripheral zones and often will combine them into one zone when investigating various aspects of prostatic disease. From this standpoint, McNeal's more complicated scheme is often simplified into a two zone concept, corresponding to the inner (transition zone) and outer (peripheral and central zones) sections of the prostate (1).

HISTOLOGY

Rather than provide a complete description of the histology of the prostate, this section will only emphasize those aspects that affect interpretation of prostate biopsy material. The discussion of some topics of prostate histology (i.e., neuroendocrine differentiation) will be deferred to sections of the book dealing with pathology related to these topics. The prostate consists of epithelial and stromal cells. The epithelial cells are arranged in glands consisting of ducts, which branch out from the urethra and terminate into acini. Distinction between a prostatic duct and acinus primarily is based on its architecture as determined on low magnification. Ducts consist of elongated tubular structures with branching as opposed to acini, which are more rounded structures grouped in lobular units. Smaller ducts cut on cross section are indistinguishable from acini.

Epithelial cells in the prostate are (a) transitional (urothelial) cells; (b) secretory cells; (c) basal cells; and (d) neuroendocrine cells. The proximal portions of the prostatic ducts are lined by transitional epithelium similar to the urethra. In distal portions of the prostatic ducts as well as in scattered prostatic acini, there may be alternating areas of cuboidal and columnar epithelium admixed with transitional epithelium. When transitional epithelium is seen within the more peripheral prostatic ducts and acini, it is referred to as transitional cell metaplasia (Fig. 3.1, efig 1-2;3). Transitional cell metaplasia may be a misnomer in that there is no evidence that this process results from metaplasia of a different epithelial cell type. It may be seen in infants and neonates throughout the prostate (author's personal observations). The transitional epithelium is composed of spindle-shaped epithelial cells, with occasional nuclear grooves, which are often oriented with their long axes parallel to the basement membrane. Transitional epithelium may undermine the cuboidal pale staining prostatic glandular epithelium.

Columnar secretory epithelial cells are tall with pale to clear cytoplasm (efig 4;5). These cells are terminally differentiated and stain positively with prostate-

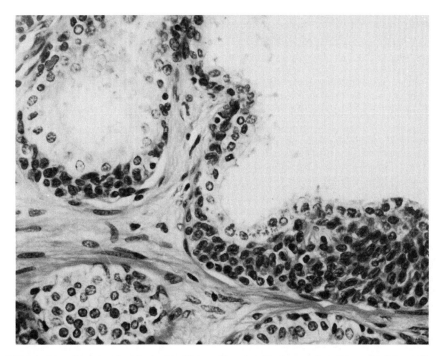

FIG 3.1. Transitional-cell metaplasia with transitional epithelium undermining glandular epithelium. ×355.

specific antigen (PSA), and prostate-specific acid phosphatase (PSAP). Secretory cells lack immunoreactivity with antibodies to high molecular weight cytokeratin (3). Corpora amylacea are seen in approximately 25% of prostate glands in men aged 20 to 40 years, whereas they are rare in carcinomas (4–6). Corpora amylacea are round laminated hyaline eosinophilic structures that may become calcified (efig 6). Although lipofuscin was initially thought to be diagnostic of seminal vesicle epithelium, it may be seen in approximately 50% of cases of benign prostate glands in hematoxylin and eosin (H&E) stained sections, and in almost all cases when studied by special stains such as Fontana-Masson (7). On H&E stained sections, these granules may be either yellow-brown or pale gray-brown with a dark blue rim (efig 7;8;9;10;11-12).

Basal cells lie beneath the secretory cells (efig 13). Basal cell nuclei are cigar-shaped or resemble those of fibroblasts and are oriented parallel to the basement membrane (Fig. 3.2). The cells may be inconspicuous in benign glands and may be difficult to distinguish from surrounding fibroblasts. It is important to recognize basal cells and differentiate them from fibroblasts or an artifactual two-cell layer in cancer, since basal cells are absent in adenocarcinoma of the prostate and may be identified in conditions that mimic prostate cancer (8–9). Whereas

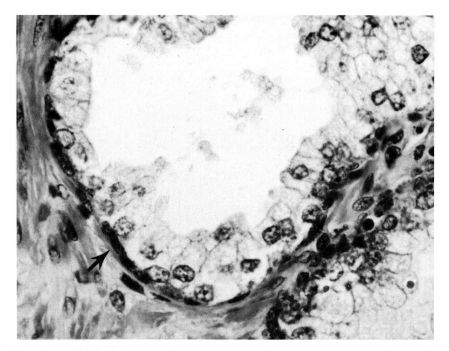

FIG. 3.2. Benign prostate gland with basal layer consisting of hyperchromatic oval nuclei situated beneath the secretory cell layer and parallel to the basement membrane *(arrow).* ×575.

fibroblasts have extremely hyperchromatic and pointed nuclei, basal cells may be recognizable by their more ovoid nuclei with lighter chromatin resembling those of smooth muscle cells. In some institutions' material, basal cell nuclei are more blue-gray and may be surrounded by a halo, whereas secretory cell nuclei appear reddish violet (efig 14). Basal cells may show prominent nucleoli, mimicking high-grade PIN (see Chapter 5). Basal cells also may be identified by their immunohistochemical reaction with antibodies to high molecular weight cytokeratin (3). Basal cells in hyperplastic glands usually are uniformly labeled with these antibodies, although an occasional gland stains discontinuously or even not at all. Basal cells are less differentiated than secretory cells and are almost devoid of secretory products such as PSA and PSAP (efig 15) (10). Basal cells are not myoepithelial cells and do not react with antibodies to muscle-specific actin or S-100, and ultrastructural studies reveal a lack of contractile elements (11–12). It is thought that the basal cells are the stem cell population of the secretory cells; the largest proportion of proliferating cells in the prostate is basal cells (13).

The fourth group of prostatic epithelial cells is those with neuroendocrine differentiation. The prostate contains the largest number of endocrine-paracrine cells of any genitourinary organ (see Chapter 12).

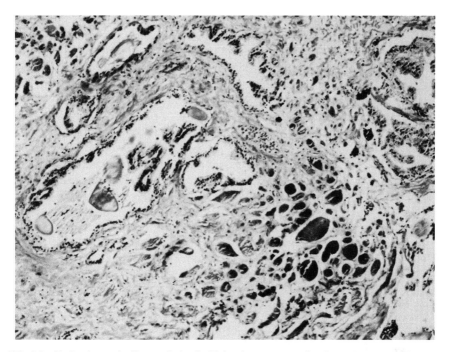

FIG. 3.3. Skeletal muscle fibers admixed with benign prostate glands on transurethral resection. ×75.

Stromal cells are skeletal and smooth muscle cells, fibroblasts, nerves, and endothelial cells. In the most distal (apical) portion of the prostate gland, skeletal muscle of the urogenital diaphragm extends into the prostate (14,15). Though mostly exterior to the gland, skeletal muscle fibers do not uncommonly extend into the peripheral portion of the prostate gland, especially apically and anteriorly (Fig. 3.3, efig 16,17). The finding of skeletal muscle fibers on transurethral resection does not result in an increase in incontinence (16). In the normal prostate, one can also find small nerve bundles. Occasionally, ganglion cells and paraganglia may be seen in the prostate, although they are more commonly identified exterior to the gland (see Chapter 7). Cowper's gland may also occasionally be seen on needle biopsy (see Chapter 7).

BENIGN PROSTATIC HYPERTROPHY

BPH, also referred to as nodular hyperplasia, is the most common urologic disease to affect men. Clinically, hyperplasia is classified into lateral enlargement, middle lobe enlargement, and posterior lobe hyperplasia. Typical hyperplasia of tissue lateral to the urethra is designated as lateral lobe enlargement. Middle lobe enlargement refers to a nodule arising at the bladder neck, which may then project into the bladder, creating a ball-valve obstruction. In posterior lobe hyperplasia there is a bar of tissue, termed the median bar, that arises in the posterior aspect of the urethra. Because of the strategic location of middle or posterior lobe enlargement, relatively small prostates may be associated with marked urinary obstructive symptoms (17).

Franks described five histologic subtypes of prostatic hyperplasia based on their differing epithelial and stromal components (18). The smallest nodules are predominantly stromal, often composed of loose mesenchyma containing prominent small round vessels (efig 18,19). In a needle biopsy specimen, these vessels help differentiate between a mesenchymal tumor and a stromal nodule (Fig. 3.4, efig 20). These nodules are located in the periurethral submucosa and seldom reach large size except near the bladder neck, where they may protrude into the bladder lumen as a solitary midline mass.

Occasionally, there are small pure stromal nodules composed almost entirely of smooth muscle (19). Some of these lesions have been reported as leiomyomas of the prostate (efig 21-24). However, the diagnosis of prostatic leiomyoma should be restricted to only large symptomatic masses of smooth muscle. The issue of distinguishing atypical stromal hyperplasia from stromal neoplasms of the prostate is discussed in Chapter 16.

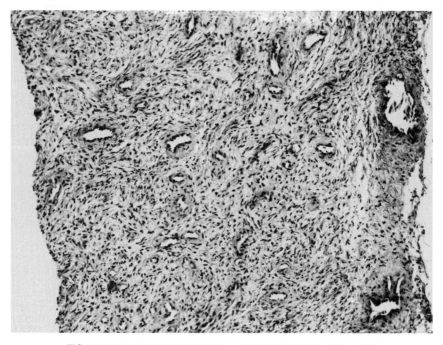

FIG. 3.4. Needle biopsy consisting solely of prostatic stroma. ×155.

The largest and most numerous hyperplastic nodules are almost always laterally situated and tend to occur in the periurethral zone near the proximal end of the verumontanum (1). The glandular component is made up of small and large acini, some showing papillary infoldings and projections containing central fibrovascular cores. The stroma consists of smooth muscle and fibrous tissue, which can occasionally display nuclear palisading mimicking a neural tumor (efig 25-26). Within hyperplastic areas there often is an infiltrate of lymphocytes and plasma cells around the glands. Usually, these are not associated with any infection nor with symptoms of prostatitis (20,21). In more limited hyperplasia, tissue removed by TURP contains a higher percentage component of bladder neck and anterior fibromuscular tissue (22). In larger specimens, usually obtained by enucleation, nodules become a more dominant feature.

In many cases, the histologic diagnosis of nodular hyperplasia does not relate to specific histologic findings but rather to the clinical findings of an enlarged prostate resulting in obstructive symptoms. The presence of papillary infoldings, although more prominent in hyperplasia, is not specific. Only the histologic identification of nodules is diagnostic for hyperplasia. By definition, TURP specimens may be diagnosed as hyperplasia, since surgery has been performed for urinary obstructive symptoms. Needle biopsy specimens should not be diagnosed as showing hyperplasia. First, many needle biopsy specimens do not even sample the transition zone. Secondly, histologic findings on needle biopsy, with the exception of stromal nodules, do not correlate with size of the prostate or urinary obstructive symptoms (23). Finally, signing out a specimen as "BPH" may falsely reassure the urologist that he has sampled the palpable or hypoechoic lesion of concern. Benign needle biopsy specimens of the prostate should be diagnosed as "benign prostate tissue" not as "BPH."

REFERENCES

1. McNeal JE. Normal and pathologic anatomy of prostate. *Urology* 1981;17(suppl):11–16.
2. Oyen RH, Van de Voorde WM, Van Poppel HP, et al. Benign hyperplastic nodules that originate in the peripheral zone of the prostate gland. *Radiology* 1993;189:707–711.
3. Hedrick L, Epstein JI. Use of keratin 903 as an adjunct in the diagnosis of prostate carcinoma. *Am J Surg Pathol* 1989;13:389–396.
4. Humphrey PA, Vollmer RT. Corpora amylacea in adenocarcinoma of the prostate: prevalence in 100 prostatectomies and clinicopathologic correlations. *Surg Pathol* 1990;3:133–141.
5. Andrews GS. The histology of the human foetal and prepubertal prostates. *J Anat* 1951;85:44–54.
6. Moore RA. The evolution and involution of the prostate gland. *J Urol* 1948;60:599–603.
7. Brennick JB, O'Connell JX, Dickersin GR, et al. Lipofuscin pigmentation (so-called "melanosis") of the prostate. *Am J Surg Pathol* 1994;18:446–454.
8. Totten RS, Heinemann NW, Hudson PB, et al. Microscopic differential diagnosis of latent carcinoma of prostate. *Arch Pathol* 1953;55:131–141.
9. Brandes D, Kirchein D, Scott WW. Ultrastructure of the human prostate. Normal and neoplastic. *Lab Invest* 1964;13:1541–1560.
10. Warhol MJ, Longtine JA. The ultrastructural localization of prostatic specific antigen and prostatic acid phosphatase in hyperplastic and neoplastic human prostates. *J Urol* 1985;134:607–613.

11. Srigley JR, Dardick I, Hartwick RWJ, et al. Basal epithelial cells of human prostate gland are not myoepithelial cells: a comparative immunohistochemical and ultrastructural study with the human salivary gland. *Am J Pathol* 1990;126:957–966.
12. Howat AJ, Mills PM, Lyons TJ, et al. Absence of S-100 protein in prostatic glands. *Histopathol* 1988; 13:468–470.
13. Bonkhoff H, Stein U, Remberger K. The proliferative function of basal cells in the normal and hyperplastic human prostate. *Prostate* 1991;24:114–118.
14. Kost LV, Evans GW. Occurrence and significance of striated muscle within the prostate. *J Urol* 1964; 92:703–704.
15. Manley CB Jr. The striated muscle of the prostate. *J Urol* 1966;95:234–240.
16. Graversen PH, England DM, Madsen PO, et al. Significance of striated muscle in curettings of the prostate. *J Urol* 1988;139:751–753.
17. Bartsch G, Muller HR, Oberholzer M, et al. Light microscopic stereological analysis of the normal human prostate and of benign prostatic hyperplasia. *J Urol* 1979;122:487–491.
18. Franks LM. Benign nodular hyperplasia of the prostate: a review. *Ann R Coll Surg* 1954;14:92–106.
19. Moore RA. Benign hypertrophy of the prostate: a morphologic study. *J Urol* 1943;50:680–710.
20. Kohnen PW, Drach GW. Patterns of inflammation in prostatic hyperplasia: a histologic and bacteriologic study. *J Urol* 1979;121:755–760.
21. Nielsen ML, Asnaes S, Hattel T. Inflammatory changes in the noninfected prostate gland. A clinical, microbiological and histological investigation. *J Urol* 1973;110:423–426.
22. McNeal J. Pathology of benign prostatic hyperplasia: Insight into etiology. *Urologic Clin N Amer* 1990;17:477–486.
23. Viglione M, Epstein JI. Should benign prostatic hypertrophy be diagnosed on needle biopsy? *Mod Pathol* 2001;14:127A.

4

Inflammatory Conditions

ACUTE AND CHRONIC PROSTATIC INFLAMMATION

Although acute and chronic prostatitis are common diseases in urologic practice, they are usually diagnosed clinically and treated with antibiotics such that the histologic examination of specimens removed for symptomatic prostatitis is uncommon. Acute bacterial prostatitis consists of sheets of neutrophils within and around acini, intraductal desquamated cellular debris, stromal edema, and hyperemia. With the onset of effective antibiotics, symptomatic prostatic abscess formation is now infrequently seen (1–4). Prostatic abscesses most commonly arise in individuals with preexisting bladder outlet obstruction secondary to a lower urinary tract infection, usually due to coliform organisms. Much less frequently, prostatic abscesses result by dissemination from an extraurinary source of infection, the most common being staphylococcal infections of the skin. Prostatic abscess may also arise as a complication of biopsy or instrumentation. Other risk factors include immunosuppression, diabetes, internal prosthesis, chronic renal failure, indwelling catheters, and chronic prostatitis.

Histologically, symptomatic chronic prostatitis cannot be distinguished from the chronic inflammation that is commonly seen in specimens removed for benign prostatic hyperplasia. Chronic inflammation typically involves the prostate in a periglandular distribution and contains an admixture of plasma cells (efig 27-28). Several studies have shown that in many prostatic specimens with prominent chronic inflammation, organisms cannot be cultured (5,6). Also, in prostatic specimens with positive cultures there is frequently an absence of prominent inflammation within the tissue (7). It is preferable to diagnose inflamed prostate specimens as showing "acute or chronic inflammation" as opposed to "acute or chronic prostatitis" (efig 29).

Clinical prostatitis may give rise to elevated serum prostate-specific antigen (PSA) elevations (8). There are conflicting studies as to whether histologic evidence of either acute or chronic inflammation on biopsy correlates with an increase in total serum PSA levels (9–13). We comment on the histologic presence of chronic inflammation only when it is prominent, as it is fairly ubiquitous.

Regardless of the extent of acute inflammation, we note this finding in our report. Acute and chronic inflammation may result in both architectural and cytologic abnormalities that may be confused with carcinoma (Figs. 4.1 and 4.2) (see Chapter 10).

MALAKOPLAKIA

As in the bladder, the majority of men with prostatic malakoplakia have urinary tract infections, most frequently with *E. coli* (14–16). Malakoplakia may clinically mimic cancer, resulting in prostatic induration and a hypoechoic lesion seen on transrectal ultrasound. Histologically, the lesions are indistinguishable from those occurring in other sites.

GRANULOMATOUS PROSTATITIS

Granulomatous prostatitis is subclassified into infectious granulomas, non-specific granulomatous prostatitis, postbiopsy resection granulomas, and systemic granulomatous prostatitis (17,18). In a series of 200 cases of granulomatous prostatitis, nonspecific granulomatous prostatitis (138 cases) and

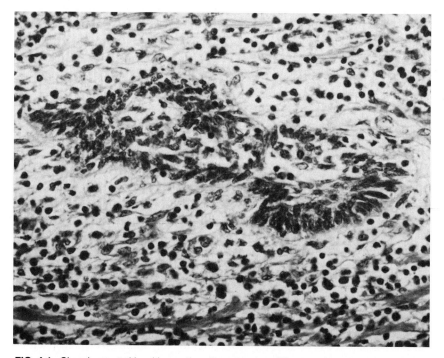

FIG. 4.1. Chronic prostatitis with reactive changes resembling transitional-cell metaplasia.

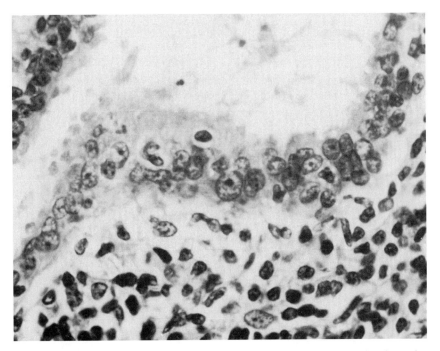

FIG. 4.2. Chronic prostatitis resulting in a reactive nuclear atypia and occasional prominent nucleoli. ×720.

postbiopsy granulomas (49 cases) were the most common. Infectious granulomatous prostatitis occurred in only seven cases, with the remaining six due to systemic granulomatous disorders (18).

Mycotic Prostatitis

Fungal infections of the prostate usually occur in immunocompromised hosts with disseminated mycoses (19). Blastomycosis, coccidiomycosis, and cryptococcosis are the most common diseases (efig 30). Cases have also been reported of histoplasmosis, paracoccidiomycosis, aspergillosis, and candidiasis of the prostate. The histology in these cases is identical to that seen in nonprostatic sites.

Mycobacterial Prostatitis

Mycobacterial prostatitis may occur in patients with systemic tuberculosis, but today it is more commonly seen as a complication of Bacillus Calmette-Guerin (BCG) immunotherapy for superficial bladder carcinoma.

The incidence of prostatic involvement in systemic tuberculosis ranges from 3% to 12%; in over 90% of these cases there is coexisting pulmonary tuberculosis. In patients with urogenital tuberculosis, the prostate is involved in 75% to 95% of the cases (20,21). However, in only 7% to 13% of cases of urogenital tuberculosis is the prostate the sole organ involved. Most cases of tuberculous prostatitis appear to arise from hematogenous dissemination rather than contact with infected urine. Atypical mycobacterial infections of the prostate are exceedingly rare (22,23).

Following BCG immunotherapy for superficial bladder carcinoma, patients may have fever, mild hematuria, and urinary frequency. Approximately 40% of these men have an abnormal digital rectal exam, and 55% have ultrasonographic abnormalities of the prostate (24–26). These lesions may further mimic carcinoma by elevating serum PSA levels. Following BCG, biopsies show caseating or noncaseating granulomas in 22% of cases and acid-fast stains are positive in approximately 50% of these cases. Histologically, the findings in BCG prostatitis are indistinguishable from those of tuberculous prostatitis occurring as a result of systemic infection. Small noncaseating granulomas are found in the periglandular stroma, as seen in early hematoge-

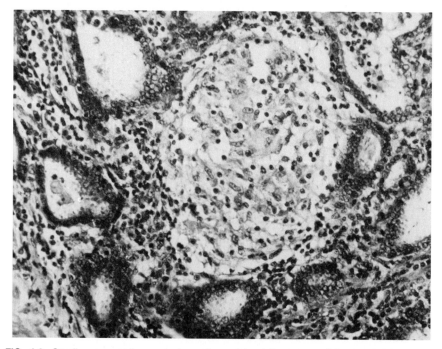

FIG. 4.3. Small noncaseating granuloma in periglandular stroma following BCG therapy. ×265.

nous dissemination of systemic tuberculosis (Fig. 4.3, efig 31,32). As these granulomas enlarge, they may eventually destroy glands (efig 33). There also may be large granulomas with caseous necrosis, consisting of grumous fine granular debris, as opposed to coagulative necrosis seen in postbiopsy resection granulomas (efig 34-37). Large caseating granulomas predominate within the peripheral zone of the prostate, although the transition zone or central zone may also be involved (Fig. 4.4). In addition to the more peripherally located caseating and noncaseating granulomas, there are almost always small suburethral granulomas (Fig. 4.5). In some instances, the suburethral granulomas are well-formed and discrete, and in other cases more ill-defined granulomatous inflammation is seen. Regardless of the histologic pattern of BCG-related granulomatous prostatitis or the presence of acid-fast bacilli on special stains, patients are usually asymptomatic and require no specific therapy (24,25). It is not necessary in a man with a history of BCG therapy to perform stains for acid-fast organisms to evaluate prostatic granulomas; it is debatable whether stains for fungi should be done for completeness. Rarely, patients develop disseminated infection with BCG, accompanied by systemic signs and symptoms.

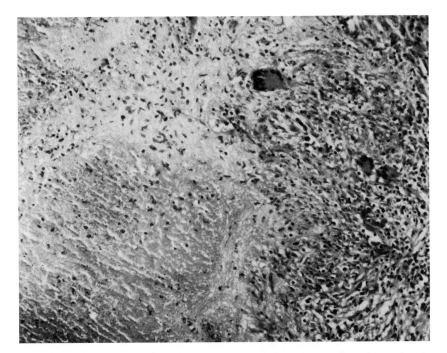

FIG. 4.4. Caseating necrosis with surrounding multinucleated giant cells and granulomatous inflammation following BCG therapy. ×160.

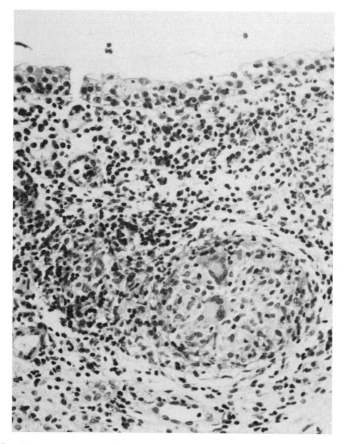

FIG. 4.5. Small noncaseating granuloma beneath prostatic urethral surface following BCG therapy. ×265.

Nonspecific Granulomatous Prostatitis

The most commonly diagnosed granulomatous process within the prostate is nonspecific granulomatous prostatitis. In a study of 25,387 benign prostate specimens, the incidence of nonspecific granulomatous prostatitis was 0.5% (18). Lesions occurred over broad ages ranging from 18 to 86 years of age with a mean and median age of 62 years. Common symptoms included irritative voiding symptoms (50%), fever (46%), chills (44%), and obstructive voiding symptoms (32%). In 82% of men, there was pyuria and in 46% there was hematuria. Seventy-one percent of men experienced a urinary tract infection at an average of 4 weeks prior to diagnosis. In 59% of the men, the rectal exam revealed an indurated prostate suspicious for adenocarcinoma. The etiology of this lesion is thought to be a reaction to bacterial toxins, cell debris, and secretions spilling into the stroma from blocked ducts.

Nonspecific granulomatous prostatitis mimics prostate carcinoma on rectal exam and ultrasound, and can result in an elevated serum PSA level. At the same time, the pathologist could be confronted with a biopsy where the histology may closely mimic carcinoma (see Chapter 7).

The earliest lesion in nonspecific granulomatous prostatitis consists of dilated ducts and acini filled with neutrophils, debris, foamy histiocytes, and desquamated epithelial cells (Fig. 4.6, efig 38-39). Rupture of these ducts and acini results in a localized granulomatous and chronic inflammatory reaction (Fig. 4.7, efig 43). Extension of the infiltrate into surrounding ductal and acinar units gives rise to the characteristic lobular dense infiltrate of lymphocytes, plasma cells, and histiocytes typical of more advanced nonspecific granulomatous prostatitis (Figs. 4.8 and 4.9, efig 44,45). Many of the histiocytes have foamy cytoplasm and some are multinucleated. Neutrophils and eosinophils make up a smaller component of the inflammatory infiltrate. Often within the center of these large inflammatory nodules are dilated and partially effaced acini. Older lesions of nonspecific granulomatous prostatitis show a more prominent fibrous component (efig 46).

In most cases, there is little histologic similarity between nonspecific granulomatous prostatitis and infectious granulomatous inflammation of the prostate, and special stains for organisms need not be performed. In general, the lesions

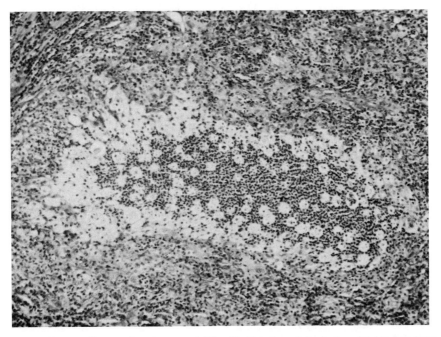

FIG. 4.6. Nonspecific granulomatous prostatitis with dilated prostatic duct containing numerous neutrophils and foamy histiocytes. ×115.

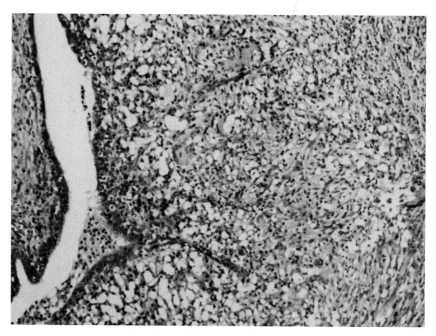

FIG. 4.7. Early lesion of nonspecific granulomatous prostatitis shows partially ruptured duct with surrounding granulomatous inflammation. ×145.

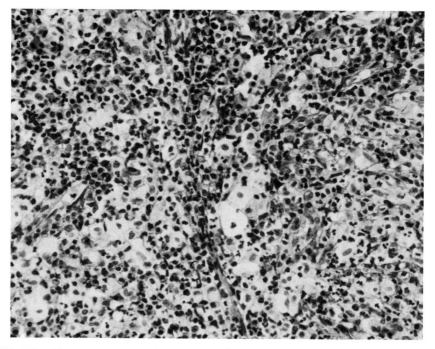

FIG. 4.8. Infiltrate of nonspecific granulomatous prostatitis consisting of foamy histiocytes, neutrophils, lymphocytes, plasma cells, and some eosinophils. ×300.

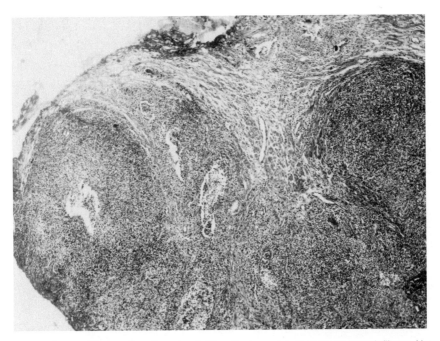

FIG. 4.9. Nonspecific granulomatous prostatitis with dense lobular inflammatory infiltrate. Note partially destroyed acinus within center of one of the lobules of inflammation *(left)*. ×50.

of nonspecific granulomatous prostatitis are not as granulomatous as those due to infection, and are composed of a more mixed inflammatory infiltrate. Though discrete small granulomas can be seen in nonspecific granulomatous prostatitis, they are invariably seen with the early lesion surrounding a ruptured dilated duct or acinus. In contrast, early infectious noncaseating granulomas surround intact acini. Although small abscesses may be present at the center of nodules of nonspecific granulomatous prostatitis, caseous necrosis is absent. In some instances, nonspecific granulomatous prostatitis may resemble an infectious granulomatous process, justifying the performance of special stains for organisms (Fig. 4.10, efig 47,48).

Recognition that nonspecific granulomatous prostatitis may contain abundant eosinophils should prevent a misdiagnosis of allergic granulomatous prostatitis. The eosinophils reflect a subacute inflammatory reaction rather than an allergic disorder. Allergic symptoms are absent and only rarely do these men have hypereosinophilia.

Nonspecific granulomatous prostatitis is treated with warm sitz baths, fluids, and antibiotics if a urinary tract infection is documented. Most patients' symptoms resolve within a few months although slightly over 50% of men have a persistent abnormal rectal exam 2 to 8 years following diagnosis.

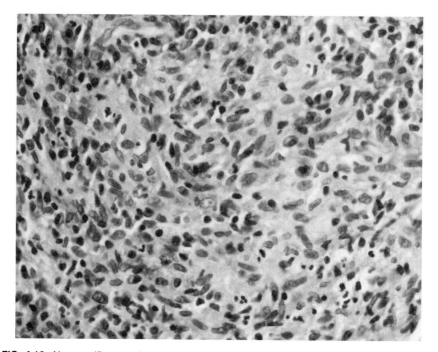

FIG. 4.10. Nonspecific granulomatous prostatitis resembling infectious granulomatous prostatitis.

Postbiopsy Granulomas

Prostatic granulomas are frequent sequelae after transurethral resection (17,27). The posttransurethral resection interval with which these granulomas may be identified ranges from 9 days to 52 months. Although it is much more common to have a granulomatous reaction following transurethral resection, similar linear granulomas may rarely develop following needle biopsy (efig 49-50).

Postbiopsy granulomas are composed of a central region of fibrinoid necrosis surrounded by palisading epithelioid histiocytes (Color Plate 2, efig 51,52). In contrast to infectious granulomas, the necrosis in postbiopsy granulomas often contains ghost-like structures of vessels, acini, and stroma (Color Plate 3, efig 53). Though these lesions can assume a multitude of shapes, some of the more common shapes observed are those of wedge-shaped granulomas, ovoid granulomas, and long tortuous granulomas dissecting through the tissue (Fig. 4.11). The irregularity of their shapes also distinguishes these granulomas from infectious granulomas. Following transurethral resection of the prostate (TURP), nonspecific foreign body giant cell granulomas are frequently seen in addition to the characteristic necrobi-

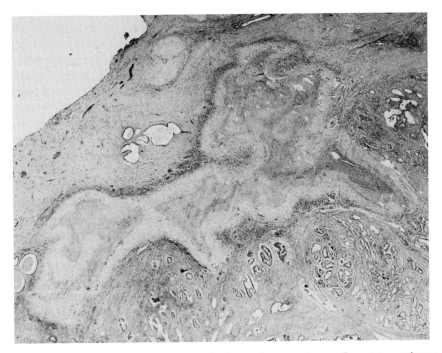

FIG. 4.11. Irregular elongated posttransurethral resection granuloma adjacent to carcinoma *(lower right corner).* ×16.

otic granulomas (efig 54). Postbiopsy granulomas also rarely occur following a needle biopsy.

In cases where the prior transurethral resection occurred within the last month, abundant eosinophils may be identified. Prior to the recognition of this disorder, postbiopsy granulomas with numerous eosinophils had been reported in the literature as allergic granulomatous prostatitis. In contrast to allergic granulomatous prostatitis, the eosinophils are localized around postbiopsy granulomas rather than diffusely infiltrating the stroma. Inflammation surrounding postbiopsy granulomas where there is a longer interval from the prior transurethral resection is usually minimal consisting predominantly of lymphocytes and plasma cells with scattered eosinophils.

The postbiopsy granuloma appears to be a reaction to altered epithelium and stroma from the trauma of previous cautery. The recognition of similar postbiopsy granulomas in other sites following cautery, argues against the process resulting solely from altered epithelium or secretions unique to the prostate. The lesion is so characteristic and distinct from infectious granulomas, so that stains for organisms are usually not necessary. Postbiopsy granulomas are asymptomatic, incidental findings requiring no treatment.

Systemic Granulomatous Prostatitis

This category encompasses cases with tissue eosinophilia such as allergic granulomatous prostatitis and Churg-Strauss syndrome, as well as those without eosinophilia such as Wegener's granulomatous prostatitis (18,28). Allergic granulomatous prostatitis as part of a more generalized allergic reaction is an exceedingly rare condition (17,18,29). Of the 12 patients with allergic granulomatous prostatitis reported in the literature, all have had either asthma or evidence of systemic allergic reaction at the time of diagnosis of their prostatic lesions. Furthermore, the majority of the effected individuals had increased blood eosinophil counts. In some instances, the severity of the asthmatic symptoms fluctuated synchronously with the severity of the urinary obstructive symptoms. In a few cases the condition was systemic with granulomas found in other organs, and in one instance the systemic granulomatous process contributed to a patient's death. Because allergic granulomatous prostatitis may be systemic in nature requiring prompt aggressive treatment with steroids, it is important to distinguish the rare allergic granulomatous prostatitis from the more common postbiopsy granulomas with eosinophils.

Histologically, allergic granulomatous prostatitis consists of multiple small, ovoid granulomas surrounded by numerous eosinophils (Color Plate 4, efig 55,56). The regularity of the size and shape of these granulomas, the eosinophilic necrosis within the granulomas, and the extensive infiltration of eosinophils throughout the stroma, not just surrounding the granulomas, separate this entity from that of postbiopsy granulomas with eosinophils (Color Plate 5, efig 57-59). Rarely following a recent prior transurethral resection, the granulomas may resemble those seen in allergic granulomatous prostatitis. In these instances the history of a recent prior-transurethral resection as well as the localization of eosinophils around the granulomas rather than diffusely infiltrating the stroma, distinguish postbiopsy granulomas from allergic granulomatous prostatitis. Nonspecific granulomatous prostatitis with numerous eosinophils must also be distinguished from allergic granulomatous prostatitis.

MISCELLANEOUS INFECTIONS

Rare cases of cytomegalovirus and herpes zoster involving the prostate have been reported (30,31). Other prostatic infections, some of which are more commonly seen in developing countries, are exceedingly rare in North America and Europe. These include schistosomiasis, amoebic prostatitis, syphilis, actinomycosis, echinococcosis, and brucellosis (32–37).

REFERENCES

1. Meares EM Jr. Prostatitis and related disorders. In: Walsh PC, Retik AB, Stamey TA, Baugham ED Jr eds. *Campbell's Urology,* 6th ed. Philadelphia: W.B. Saunders; 1992;807–822.
2. Granados EA, Riley G, Salvador J, et al. Prostatic abscess: diagnosis and treatment. *J Urol* 1992; 148:80–82.

3. Sohlberg OE, Chetner M, Ploch N, et al. Prostatic abscess after transrectal ultrasound guided biopsy. *J Urol* 1991;146:420–422.
4. Mamo GJ, Rivero MA, Jacobs SC. Cryptococcal prostatic abscess associated with the acquired immunodeficiency syndrome. *J Urol* 1992;148:889–890.
5. Gorlick JI, Senterfit LB, Vaughan ED Jr. Quantitative bacterial tissue cultures from 209 prostatectomy specimens: findings and implications. *J Urol* 1988;139:57–60.
6. Kohnen PW, Drach GW. Patterns of inflammation in prostatic hyperplasia: a histologic and bacteriologic study. *J Urol* 1979;121:755–760.
7. Nielsen ML, Asnaes S, Hattel T. Inflammatory changes in the non-infected prostate gland. A clinical, microbiological and histological investigation. *J Urol* 1973;110: 423–426.
8. Neal DE, Clejan S, Sarma D, et al. Prostate specific antigen and prostatitis. Effect of prostatitis on serum PSA in the human and nonhuman primate. *Prostate* 1982;20:105–111.
9. Hasui Y, Marutsuka K, Asada Y, et al. Relationship between serum prostate specific antigen and histological prostatitis in patients with benign prostatic hyperplasia. *Prostate* 1994;25:91–96.
10. Ornstein DK, Smith DS, Humphrey PA, et al. The effect of prostate volume, age, total prostate specific antigen level and acute inflammation on the percentage of free serum prostate specific antigen levels in men without clinically detectable prostate cancer. *J Urol* 1998;159:1234–1237.
11. Jung K, Meyer A, Lein M, et al. Ratio of free-to-total prostate specific antigen in serum cannot distinguish patients with prostate cancer from those with chronic inflammation of the prostate. *J Urol* 1998;159:1595–1598.
12. Okada K, Kojima M, Naya Y, et al. Correlation of histological inflammation in needle biopsy specimens with serum prostate-specific antigen levels in men with negative biopsy for prostate cancer. *Urology* 2000;55:892–898.
13. Nadler RB, Humphrey PA, Smith DS, et al. Effect of inflammation and benign prostatic hyperplasia on elevated serum prostate specific antigen levels. *J Urol* 1995;154:407–413.
14. Koga S, Arakaki Y, Matsuoka M, et al. Malakoplakia of prostate. *Urology* 1986; 37:160–161.
15. Sujka SK, Nalin BT, Asirwatham JE. Prostatic malakoplakia associated with prostatic adenocarcinoma and multiple prostatic abscesses. *Urology* 1989;34:159–161.
16. Sarma HN, Ramesh K, al Fituri O, et al. Malakoplakia of the prostate gland—a report of two cases and review of the literature. *Scand J Urol Nephrol* 1996; 30:155–157.
17. Epstein JI, Hutchins GM. Granulomatous prostatitis. Distinction among allergic, non-specific, and post-transurethral resection lesions. *Hum Pathol* 1984;15:818–825.
18. Stillwell TJ, Engen DE, Farrow GM. The clinical spectrum of granulomatous prostatitis: A report of 200 cases. *J Urol* 1987;138:320–323.
19. Wise GJ, Silver DA. Fungal infections of the genitourinary system. *J Urol* 1993;149:1377–1388.
20. Auerbach O. Tuberculosis of the genital system. *Q Bull Sea View Hosp* 1942;7:188–207.
21. Moore RA. Tuberculosis of the prostate gland. *J Urol* 1937;37:372–384.
22. Mikolich DJ, Metes SM. Granulomatous prostatitis due to mycobacterium avium complex. *Clin Infect Dis* 1992;14:589–591.
23. Lee LW, Burgher LW, Price EB, et al. Granulomatous prostatitis: association with isolation of mycobacterium kansasii and mycobacterium fortuitum. *JAMA* 1987;237:2408–2409.
24. Oates RD, Stilmant MM, Freedlund MC, et al. Granulomatous prostatitis following bacillus Calmette-Guerin immunotherapy of bladder cancer. *J Urol* 1988;140:751–754.
25. Mukamel E, Konichezky M, Engelstein D, et al. Clinical and pathological findings in prostates following intravesicle bacillus Calmette-Guerin installation. *J Urol* 1990;144:1399–1400.
26. Miyashita H, Troncoso P, Babaian RJ. BCG-induced granulomatous prostatitis: a comparative ultrasound and pathologic study. *Urology* 1992;39:364–367.
27. Mies C, Balogh K, Stadecker M. Palisading prostate granulomas following surgery. *Am J Surg Pathol* 1984;8:217–221.
28. Bray VJ, Hasbergen JA. Prostatic involvement in Wegener's granulomatosis. *Am J Kidney Dis* 1991; 17:578–580.
29. Kelalis PP, Harrison EG Jr., Greene LF. Allergic granulomas of the prostate in asthmatics. *JAMA* 1964;180:963–967.
30. Benson PJ, Smith CS. Cytomegaloprostatitis. *Urology* 1992;30:165-167.
31. Clason AE, McGeorge A, Garland C, et al. Urinary retention and granulomatous prostatitis following herpes zoster infection: a report of 2 cases with a review of the literature. *Brit J Urol* 1982;54:166–169.
32. Zaher MF, El-deeb A. Bilharziasis of the prostate: its relation to bladder neck obstruction and its management. *J Urol* 1971;106:257–261.

33. Goff DA, Davidson RA. Amebic prostatitis. *South Med J* 1984;77:1053–1054.
34. Thompson L. Syphilis of the prostate. *Am J Syph* 1920;4:323–341.
35. DeSouza E, Katz DA, Dwarzack DL, Long G. Actinomycosis of the prostate. *J Urol* 1985;133: 290–291.
36. Houston W. Primary hydatid cyst of the prostate gland. *J Urol* 1975;113:732–733.
37. Kelalis PP, Greene LF, Weed LA. Brucellosis of the urogenital tract: a mimic of tuberculosis. *J Urol* 1962;88:347–353.

5

Prostatic Intraepithelial Neoplasia and Its Mimickers

This lesion was first described in the 1960s by McNeal (1), and more precisely characterized in 1986 by McNeal and Bostwick at which time the entity was called intraductal dysplasia; currently it is referred to as prostatic intraepithelial neoplasia (PIN) (2–4). PIN consists of architecturally benign prostatic acini or ducts lined by cytologically atypical cells. PIN was initially subcategorized into three grades. PIN 1 was characterized by increased nuclear size with increased variability of nuclear size, along with irregular focal crowding and multilayering. In PIN 2, there were similar features to PIN 1 with the additional finding of hyperchromatism and occasional small prominent nucleoli. The hallmark of PIN 3 was the finding of numerous large prominent nucleoli. High-grade PIN encompasses both PIN 2 and PIN 3, and low-grade PIN is equivalent to PIN 1. The distinction between low- and high-grade PIN is the finding of prominent nucleoli in high-grade PIN. Uncommonly, the diagnosis of high-grade PIN will be made in the absence of prominent nucleoli if there is significant nuclear pleomorphism.

HISTOLOGIC APPEARANCE OF PIN

Low-grade PIN consists of preexisting benign prostate glands with minimal epithelial proliferation in terms of nuclear stratification, where nuclei are minimally enlarged without prominent nucleoli.

Although high-grade PIN is characterized by nuclear atypia, there is often accompanying architectural abnormalities. At low magnification, glands that are separated by a modest amount of stroma and have a normal overall architectural pattern characterize high-grade PIN. These glands resemble benign glands in that they are large, branch, and have papillary and undulating luminal surfaces. At low magnification, glands with high-grade PIN have a basophilic appearance (Fig. 5.1, efig 60,61). This basophilic appearance is due to a combination of features including enlarged nuclei, hyperchromatism, overlapping nuclei, and epithelial hyperplasia (Fig. 5.2, efig 62). The earliest form of high-grade PIN is characterized by

33

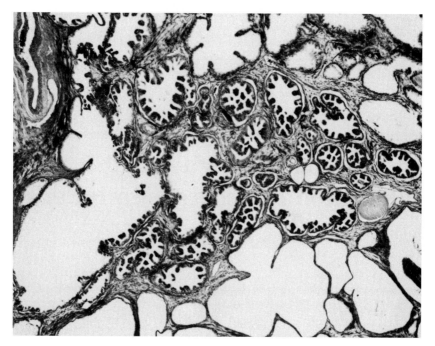

FIG. 5.1. High-grade PIN with preservation of normal architectural pattern of the prostate. Basophilic appearance of high-grade PIN is the result of piling up of the nuclei, high nuclear-to-cytoplasm ratio, hyperchromatism, and amphophilic cytoplasm.

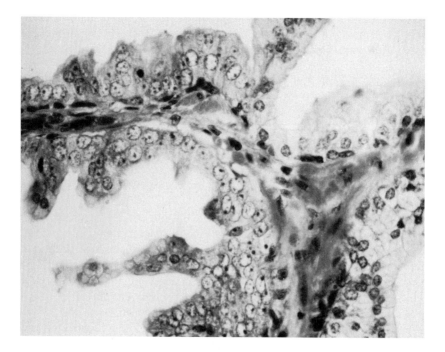

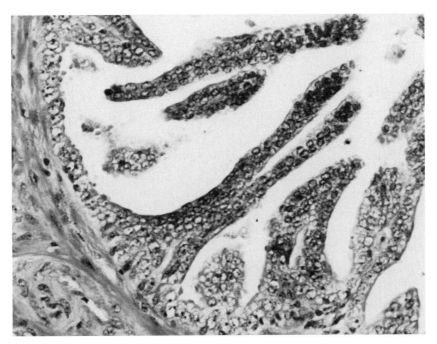

FIG. 5.3. Prominent, tall papillary tufts within high-grade PIN. Nuclei appear more benign toward the luminal surface of the papillary projections. Note large nuclei with multiple, frequent nucleoli diagnostic of high-grade PIN toward the edge of the gland up against the basement membrane.

nuclear atypia without significant epithelial hyperplasia. The basal cell layer may or not be visible and the demarcation between atypical and normal nuclei is frequently abrupt. With more pronounced forms of high-grade PIN, nuclei become more piled up and develop micropapillary projections. These micropapillary projections are similar to those seen with micropapillary intraductal carcinoma of the breast, in that they are composed of tall epithelial buds lacking fibrovascular cores (Fig. 5.3). An interesting phenomenon in high-grade PIN is that nuclei towards the center of the gland tend to have a more bland cytologic appearance, as compared to the nuclei peripherally located up against the basement membrane (Fig. 5.3, efig 61). The grade of PIN is assigned based on assessment of the nuclei peripherally located up against the basement membrane. With further epithelial hyperplasia, more complex architectural patterns appear such as Roman bridge and cribriform formation (Figs. 5.4–5.6). The various patterns of PIN have been designated as flat

FIG. 5.2. High magnification of high-grade PIN showing large vesicular nuclei with prominent nucleoli that have lost their basal orientation and have become crowded and overlapping. Note within a single gland the abrupt transition between benign-appearing nuclei and PIN nuclei. Flat PIN is noted in the gland on the top with tufting pattern in the gland seen in the lower left.

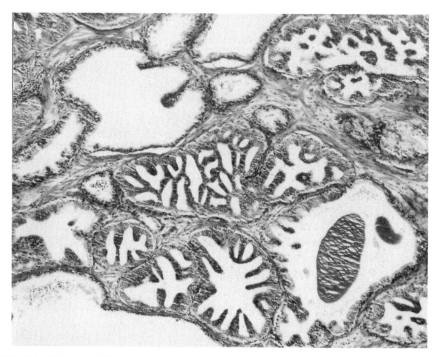

FIG. 5.4. High-grade PIN with spectrum of architectural atypia ranging from micropapillary tufts to Roman bridge formation to cribriform glands.

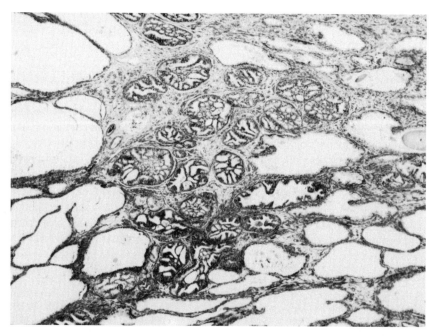

FIG. 5.5. Numerous cribriform glands fitting into the normal prostatic architecture without identifiable small glands of infiltrating cancer.

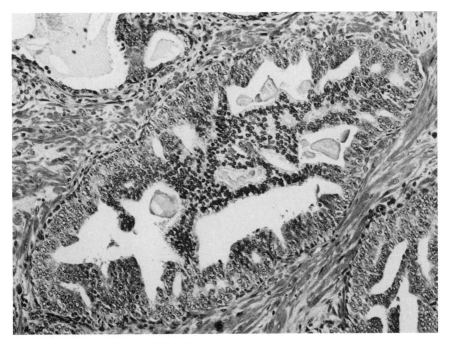

FIG. 5.6. Higher magnification of Fig. 4.5 showing cribriform gland formation with maturation of nuclei toward the center and a lack of recognizable infiltrating component.

(efig 63-64;65;66-67;68-69), tufting (efig 70-71;72-73;74-75), micropapillary (efig 76-77;78-81;82), and cribriform (efig 83-84;85-87;88-89) (5). Unusual subtypes of high-grade PIN include PIN with signet-ring features, small cell neuroendocrine PIN, PIN with mucinous features (efig 90-91;92-94), foamy PIN (efig 95-97;98-99;100-102), and PIN with inverted nuclei (efig 103;104)(6-7). High-grade PIN may also show focal necrosis (efig 105-106).

RELATIONSHIP OF PIN TO CANCER

Comparing prostates with carcinoma to those without carcinoma, there is an increase in the size and number of high-grade PIN foci, in addition to an increased incidence of higher grade PIN (8). Also, with increasing amounts of high-grade PIN there are a greater number of multifocal carcinomas. This observation follows if high-grade PIN is a precursor to some carcinomas, since with more precursor lesion one would expect that there would be more early carcinomas. The finding of zones of high-grade PIN from which there appears to be budding off glands of carcinoma is further histologic evidence that high-grade PIN is a precursor to some prostate carcinomas (Fig. 5.7, efig 107-108;109-110). McNeal has designated these foci as "transitive glands," although most other investigators prefer the term "high-grade PIN with

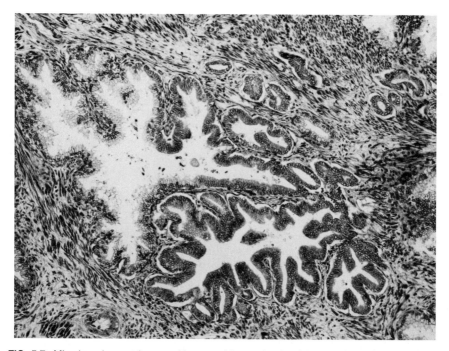

FIG. 5.7. Microinvasive carcinoma with several large glands of high-grade PIN and adjacent small focus of cytologically similar glands of infiltrating carcinoma *(upper right)*. Note in one PIN gland abrupt transition between normal and atypical epithelium.

microinvasive carcinoma"(9). Several studies have also noted an increase of high-grade PIN in the peripheral zone of the prostate, corresponding to the site of origin for most adenocarcinomas of the prostate (8). This increase in high-grade PIN in the peripheral zone compared to the transition zone persists even when taking into account the greater size of the peripheral zone. All these findings would be expected if high-grade PIN is a precursor lesion to carcinoma of the prostate.

There is a growing body of data demonstrating that the expression of various biomarkers in high-grade PIN are either: (a) the same in high-grade PIN and carcinoma, as opposed to benign prostate tissue; or (b) intermediate between benign prostate tissue and carcinoma (8,10).

It has been shown that high-grade PIN is more closely related to peripheral, as opposed to transition zone cancers (8). Intermediate- or high-grade cancers are also more likely to be associated with high-grade PIN, compared to low-grade cancer. This weaker association of high-grade PIN to low-grade transition zone carcinomas is also supported by the histologic differences of high-grade PIN and transition zone carcinomas. Centrally located low-grade adenocarcinomas tend to have bland cytologic features often lacking nuclear enlargement or nucleoli in contrast to high-grade PIN. Peripherally located intermediate grade carcinomas often have identical cytologic features to those of high-grade PIN.

MIMICKERS OF PIN

PIN on one hand must be distinguished from several benign entities, and on the other must be differentiated from variants of infiltrating carcinoma.

Central Zone Histology

Glands within the central zone up at the base of the prostate are complex and large with numerous papillary infoldings, and often are lined by tall-pseudostratified epithelium with eosinophilic cytoplasm (efig 111-112;113-114;115-116;117;118;119-120). Occasionally, a prominent basal cell layer surrounds these glands. Often glands with this histology will be seen at the end of the core and may be associated with thick muscle bundles typical of bladder neck. We have seen numerous cases on needle biopsy of central zone glands that have been overdiagnosed as high-grade PIN (11). Roman bridge and cribriform patterns may be present where the nuclei stream parallel to the glandular bridges, in contrast to the more rigid bridges seen in PIN (Figs. 5.8 and 5.9). These benign central zone epithelial proliferations are primarily distinguished from PIN by their lack of cytologic atypia.

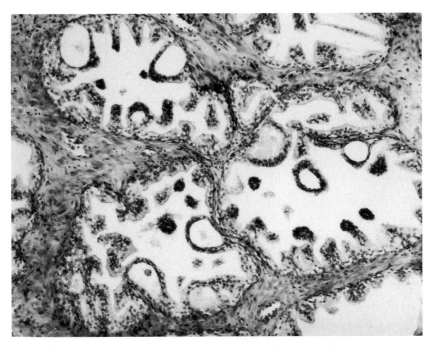

FIG. 5.8. Benign Roman bridge formation seen at the base of the prostate.

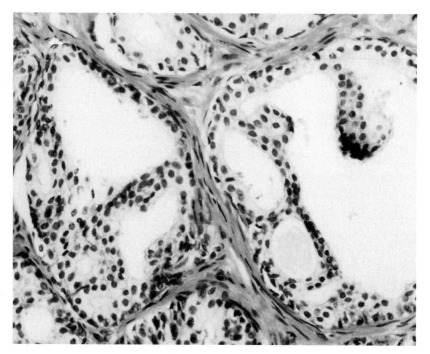

FIG. 5.9. Benign cribriform formation seen at the base of the prostate. Note benign cytology.

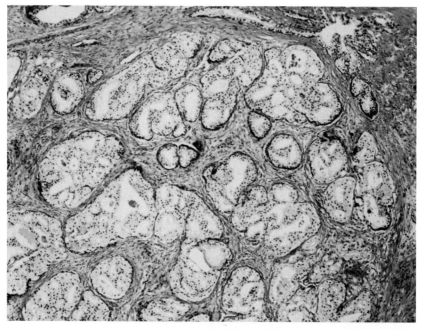

FIG. 5.10. Clear-cell cribriform hyperplasia composed of a circumscribed nest of glands with clear cells growing in a prominent cribriform pattern.

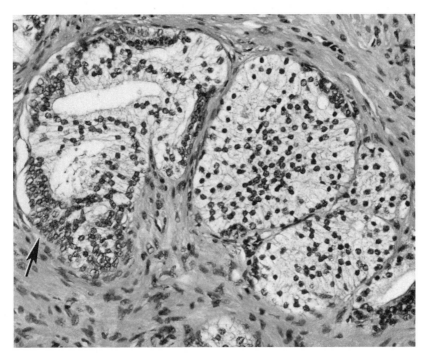

FIG. 5.11. Clear-cell cribriform hyperplasia. Note that some glands may be cut tangentially where cribriform pattern is not apparent. Also note knot of basal cells polarized at one edge of a cribriform gland *(arrow)*. Basal cells may not be apparent around all cribriform nests.

Clear Cell Cribriform Hyperplasia

Clear cell cribriform hyperplasia consists of crowded cribriform glands with clear cytoplasm sometimes growing as a nodule and in other instances more diffusely (Figs. 5.10–5.12, efig 121-122;123-124)(12). The key distinguishing feature of clear cell cribriform hyperplasia from PIN is the lack of nuclear atypia. Furthermore, within a nodule of clear cell cribriform hyperplasia, at least some of the cribriform glands show a strikingly evident basal cell layer, which is unique for this entity (Fig. 5.13). Immunostaining with antibodies to high molecular weight cytokeratin cannot distinguish between the two entities, since both have a patchy basal cell layer.

Basal Cell Hyperplasia

Otherwise typical basal cell hyperplasia may show prominent nucleoli along with mitotic activity (13,14) (Color Plate 6, efig 125-126). Because of the prominent nucleoli, these lesions may be mistaken for high-grade PIN. Although occasionally the distinction between these two entities may be difficult, usually they are

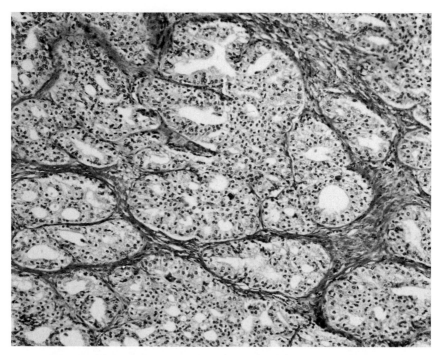

FIG. 5.12 Clear-cell cribriform hyperplasia with crowded cribriform glands.

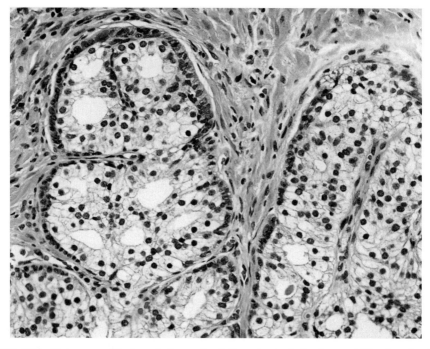

FIG. 5.13. Higher magnification of clear-cell cribriform hyperplasia shows striking basal cell layer and benign cytology in contrast to high-grade PIN.

TABLE 5.1. *Differential diagnosis: high-grade PIN and basal cell hyperplasia with nucleoli*

Basal cell hyperplasia with nucleoli	High-grade PIN
Proliferation of small glands	Architecturally benign (large glands without crowding)
Occasional solid nests	Glands with well-formed lumina
Basal cells with atypical nuclei (blue) undermine secretory cells with benign nuclei (red/violet)	No two distinct cell population
Basal cell nuclei stream parallel to basement membrane	Atypical cells oriented perpendicular to basement membrane
Atypical nuclei positive for high molecular weight cytokeratin	Atypical nuclei negative for high molecular weight cytokeratin, with underlying flattened benign-appearing cells positive

distinct (Table 5.1). There is a proliferation of small round crowded glands in basal cell hyperplasia, whereas in PIN the atypical nuclei fill preexisting larger benign glands that are separated from each other by a greater amount of stroma (efig 127-128;129-131). The nuclei in basal cell hyperplasia tend to be round and at times form small solid basaloid nests. In contrast, the nuclei in PIN tend to be more pseudostratified and columnar and do not occlude the glandular lumina. Within areas of basal cell hyperplasia, atypical basal cells can be seen undermining the overlying benign appearing secretory cells (Fig. 5.14, efig 132-134). The basal cells in

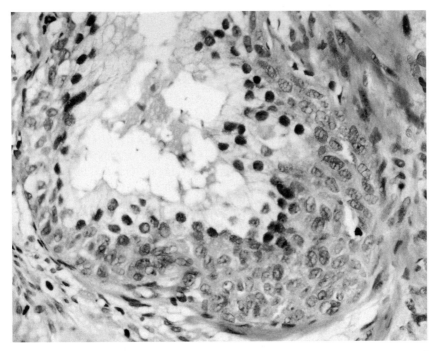

FIG. 5.14. Cytologically atypical basal cell hyperplasia with undermining of secretory cells. (From Epstein and Armas, ref. 14, with permission.)

these foci tend to have a streaming morphology parallel to the basement membrane. PIN has full thickness cytologic atypia with the nuclei oriented perpendicular to the basement membrane. An additional difference between the two entities is that most cases of basal cell hyperplasia are found in TURP specimens, indicating growth in the transition zone, in contrast to PIN's preferential location in the periphery of the prostate. Occasionally, when there are only a few glands to evaluate, such as on needle biopsy, immunohistochemical stains are needed to distinguish the two. Basal cell hyperplasia, when studied with antibodies to high molecular weight cytokeratin, reveal immunoreactivity in the multilayered atypical basal cell nuclei (15) (Color Plate 7, efig 135-137). In PIN, the high molecular weight cytokeratin labels only the flattened cytologically benign basal cell layer beneath negatively stained atypical cells of PIN (Color Plate 8). The basal cells in benign glands, even when not proliferative, can also have prominent nucleoli and be mistaken for high-grade PIN (Color Plate 9, efig 138;139-140;141-142;143). In some institutions' material, basal cell nuclei have a blue-gray appearance, in contrast to the red-violet hue of secretory cell nuclei. Basal cell hyperplasia may also be cribriform further mimicking high-grade PIN (efig 144;145) (Also see Chapter 7). Whereas cribriform PIN glands represent a single glandular unit with punched out lumina, many of the glands within a focus of cribriform basal cell hyperplasia appeared as fused individual basal cell hyperplasia glands. The use of cytokeratin 34βE12 can help in difficult cases. In cribriform basal cell hyperplasia, high molecular weight cytokeratin shows multilayered staining of the basal cells in some of the glands and a continuous layer of immunoreactivity. Cribriform PIN demonstrates an interrupted immunoreactive single cell layer of basal cells. Occasionally, basal cell hyperplasia occurs in larger preexisting benign glands; in contrast to high-grade PIN, these cells have scant cytoplasm with round nuclei (efig 146-149).

Cribriform Acinar Adenocarcinoma

In some cases, it is impossible to distinguish a focus of cribriform PIN from cribriform Gleason pattern 3 adenocarcinoma. The finding of cribriform glands with this morphology infiltrating out of the prostate demonstrates that this pattern does not always represent PIN. Although the distinction between cribriform Gleason pattern 3 and cribriform PIN may be difficult, from a diagnostic standpoint, this is usually not critical. Almost always when there are atypical cribriform glands, they are accompanied by small atypical infiltrating glands where the diagnosis of infiltrating tumor can be made (Fig. 5.15). Only when cribriform glands are so large and/or back-to-back that they are inconsistent with cribriform PIN should infiltrating cribriform carcinoma be diagnosed on H&E stained sections in the absence of small atypical infiltrating glands. Immunohistochemistry with antibodies to high molecular weight keratin can be used in difficult cases to differentiate these two entities. In the setting of numerous atypical cribriform glands, a negative reaction in all of the glands is diagnostic of carcinoma; positive staining, even if patchy, verifies the lesion as cribriform PIN (Color Plate 10, Figs. 5.16 and 5.17, efig 150-153;154-156;157-158;159-160). If presented with only a few cribriform glands,

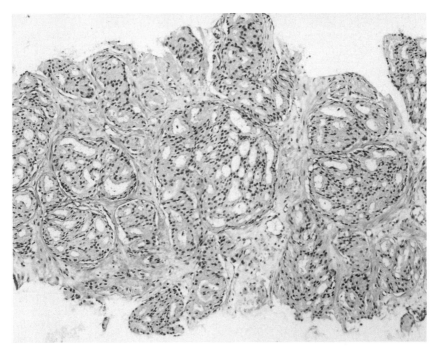

FIG. 5.15. Infiltrating adenocarcinoma in which cribriform glands are accompanied by small infiltrating glands of adenocarcinoma. Whether the cribriform glands represent high-grade PIN or infiltrating carcinoma is not critical in these instances.

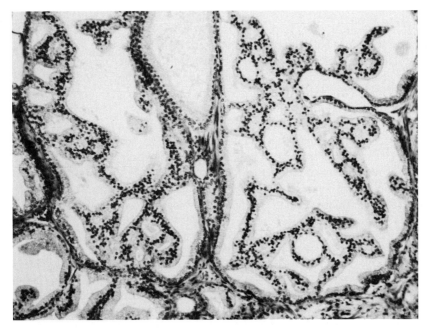

FIG. 5.16. Infiltrating adenocarcinoma composed of back-to-back cribriform glands.

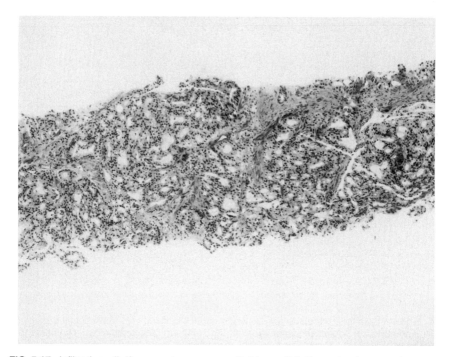

FIG. 5.17. Infiltrating cribriform carcinoma on needle biopsy. Cribriform glands are too large and irregular to be high-grade PIN.

negative staining is not diagnostic of carcinoma. This results from the patchy nature with which high molecular weight keratin labels PIN, and the recognition that even benign glands may occasionally not be labeled with antibodies to high molecular weight keratin (15). When there are only one or a few small cribriform glands on needle biopsy without small glands of infiltrating carcinoma, these cases in general are not diagnostic of infiltrating carcinoma. Instead, the diagnosis is "Focus of atypical cribriform glands" with a comment that "The distinction between cribriform PIN and cribriform carcinoma can not be made with certainty, and repeat biopsy is recommended (efig 161-163;164-165;166-167)." We have reported that this finding is associated with a higher association of cancer on repeat biopsy (50%) than the finding of high-grade PIN on biopsy (16) (see Chapter 10 for differential diagnosis of atypical cribriform glands from carcinoma).

Ductal Adenocarcinoma

A more difficult distinction is between cribriform PIN and the rarer ductal adenocarcinoma of the prostate (see Chapter 11) (Table 5.2) (17–19). Ductal adenocarcinomas are aggressive tumors, often of advanced pathological stage, and associated with a poor prognosis. Their distinction from cribriform PIN is critical. There are several features that distinguish these two lesions. Ductal adenocarcinomas are often centrally located in the periurethral region and sampled on TURP (Fig. 5.18,

TABLE 5.2. *Differential diagnosis: high-grade PIN and ductal adenocarcinoma*

High-grade PIN	Ductal adenocarcinoma
Uncommon in transition zone	Transition zone is a frequent site
Micropapillary projections without fibrovascular cores	True papillary fronds with fibrovascular cores
Architecturally benign (normal-sized glands, evenly spaced)	May be back-to-back glands and/or much larger glands than typical benign glands
At most, only focal necrosis	May have extensive comedonecrosis
Uncommon to see detached fragments on needle biopsy	Common to see detached cribriform and/or papillary fragments on biopsy
Patchy basal cell layer or rare glands may be negative	Patchy basal cell layer or many glands may be negative

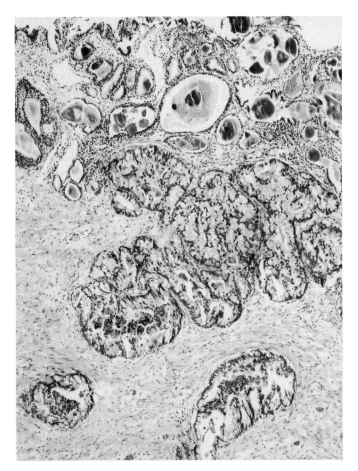

FIG. 5.18. Ductal adenocarcinoma of TURP beneath urothelial surface *(top)*.

efig 168-169). PIN is uncommonly found within the periurethral region and infrequently seen on TURP. Ductal adenocarcinomas often contain true papillary fronds with well-established fibrovascular cores, whereas PIN more frequently reveals micropapillary fronds with tall columns of epithelium without fibrovascular stalks (efig 170-172). Ductal adenocarcinomas frequently contain comedonecrosis, which may be extensive (efig 173). PIN usually lacks comedonecrosis, and when present is focal. Finally, ductal adenocarcinomas may consist of very large and/or back-to-back glands, whereas glands involved by PIN are of the size and distribution of benign glands (efig 174-176). The use of high molecular weight cytokeratin in this differential diagnosis is problematical, as both high-grade PIN and ductal adenocarcinoma may display a patchy basal cell layer. However, absence of a basal cell layer in numerous glands rules out PIN (efig 177).

DIAGNOSIS OF PIN ON BIOPSY MATERIAL

Low-Grade PIN

Low-grade PIN should not be documented as a finding in pathology reports for several reasons. First, there is a lack of reproducibility in its diagnosis even by uropathologists. In a study of interobserver reproducibility of PIN on needle biopsy, no specimens were uniformly interpreted by a panel of expert consultants as representing low-grade PIN (20). McNeal's quotation summarizes his consideration of low-grade PIN: "There is not a sharp line of demarcation between grade 1 dysplasia and mild degrees of deviation from normal histology"(21). More importantly, the finding of low-grade PIN on needle biopsy does not confer an increased likelihood of finding prostate cancer in a given individual on subsequent biopsy. Men with serum PSA levels of 4 to 10 ng/mL and an initial benign prostate biopsy have a 19% likelihood of finding prostate cancer on repeat biopsy (22). When low-grade PIN is identified on needle biopsy, the risk of detecting carcinoma on a subsequent set of biopsies ranges from 13% to

TABLE 5.3. *PIN on needle biopsy: subsequent risk of carcinoma*

	Low-grade PIN	High-grade PIN	PSA*	DRE*	TRUS*
Brawer (23)	18%		—	—	—
O'Dowd (45)		27%	—	—	—
Langer (34)		27%	No	No	No
Kronz (48)		31%	—	—	—
Davidson (44)		35%	Yes	No	No
Raviv (26)	13%	48%	Yes	Yes	Yes
Weinstein (47)		53%	No	No	No
Keetch (25,46)	24%	58%	No	—	Yes
Aboseif (24)	17%	79%	—	—	—

*Correlation of serum PSA levels, DRE (digital rectal examination), and TRUS (transrectal ultrasound) findings with subsequent risk of carcinoma.

24%, with an average of 18% (23–26) (Table 5.3). Consequently, the risk of cancer with low-grade PIN on biopsy is the same as with totally benign tissue on biopsy. The diagnosis of low-grade PIN on a needle biopsy pathology report may lead to multiple potentially unnecessary repeat biopsies, incurring economic expense and potential morbidity. In the uncommon needle biopsy specimens that are reported as borderline between low- and high-grade PIN, the surgeon and patient must decide how aggressively to pursue repeat biopsy based on other clinical findings.

High-Grade PIN: Incidence

The finding of high-grade PIN on needle biopsy is important because of the increased risk of adenocarcinoma conferred by this diagnosis. The incidences of high-grade PIN on biopsy range from 1.5% to 24% (27-41) (Table 5.4). The median incidence of high-grade PIN on biopsy based on these studies and at our institution is approximately 5% to 6% (41).

There are several likely reasons for the observed variation in the incidence of high-grade PIN in large biopsy series. The most likely is interobserver variability in making the distinction between low- and high-grade PIN. High-grade PIN is distinguished primarily by the finding of prominent nucleoli. This is a subjective finding, and pathologists with a lower threshold for interpreting nucleoli as "prominent" will diagnose high-grade PIN more frequently. It is also unknown whether only very rare prominent nucleoli justify a diagnosis of high-grade PIN. Especially in the United States, where medicolegal issues are of enormous concern, some pathologists may diagnose PIN as high-grade in equivocal cases to mitigate potential liability should adenocarcinoma be found on subsequent biopsy.

TABLE 5.4. *Incidence of high-grade PIN on needle biopsy*

Hoedemaeker (30)	0.7%
Cheville (29)	1.5%
Novis (36)	3.9%
Renshaw (38)	4.0%
Orozco (37)	4.0%
Horninger (31)	4.7%
Langer (34)	4.8%
Mettlin (35)	5.2%
Sakr (40)	5.4%
Wills (41)	5.5%
Reyes (39)	7.4%
Alsikafi (27)	6.8%
Hu (32)	8.0%
Bostwick (community hospital) (28)	9.5%
Bostwick (28)	16.5%
Kim (33)	24%

Initial studies analyzing the relative risk of finding cancer after a diagnosis of high-grade PIN on needle biopsy were obtained using formalin as a fixative. Alternative fixatives are in increasingly wide use, some of which enhance nuclear detail and nucleolar prominence. The reported incidence of high-grade PIN may vary between studies due to differences in the fixatives employed. Whether the diagnosis of high-grade PIN on biopsies processed with these different fixatives has the same risk of associated carcinoma as studies that have used formalin fixed tissue remains unknown.

Differences in prostate biopsy sampling techniques are another potential explanation for variations in the reported incidence of high-grade PIN on biopsy. Obtaining more needle biopsy cores in each patient presumably optimizes sampling of the prostate and leads to an increased likelihood of identifying high-grade PIN (42). There are also potential differences amongst patient populations that could account for variations in the incidence of high-grade PIN detected on needle biopsy, as it has been demonstrated that African-Americans with serum PSA values of less than 4 ng/ml have a higher incidence than white men (43).

High-Grade PIN: Risk of Cancer

The importance of recognizing high-grade PIN on needle biopsy is its association with carcinoma on repeat biopsy. This risk of carcinoma on subsequent biopsy ranges from 27% to 79% (Table 5.3) (24–26,34,44–48). The largest studies published to date on this issue reports a 23% to 35% risk of cancer on subsequent biopsy (44,45,48). If cancer is not found on the first two follow-up biopsies, we have recently shown that it will unlikely be found.

One of the only studies to look at the risk of cancer in men with multiple follow-up biopsies demonstrated that cases where the predominant pattern of PIN was flat/tufting was associated with only a 17% risk of cancer on repeat biopsy (48). In contrast, when the predominant PIN pattern was micropapillary/cribriform the risk of a subsequent cancer diagnosis was 40% and 71%, respectively, depending on whether one or more than one core was involved with PIN. If this data is confirmed, it may be that flat/tufting high-grade PIN occupying one core, which is the most common form of high-grade PIN seen on biopsy, need not be aggressively pursued with rebiopsy. Currently, we are recording the pattern of high-grade PIN and the number of involved cores both to provide information to the clinician and to further study this issue. Although there is growing skepticism as to the significance of high-grade PIN on needle biopsy, until there is a consensus as to the risk of cancer following its diagnosis, it is still probably prudent for all men with high-grade PIN on biopsy to have a repeat biopsy. However, it should be recognized that there is a potential for this recommendation to be modified as new data emerges.

No consensus exists regarding the results of digital-rectal exam or transrectal ultrasound findings in enhancing the prediction of which men with a finding of high-grade PIN will have carcinoma on repeat biopsy (Table 5.3). It is not surprising that ultrasound does not discriminate between cases with only PIN from those with PIN and carcinoma since it has been demonstrated that high-grade PIN may appear indistinguishable from cancer as a hypoechoic lesion (49). High-grade PIN by itself does not appear to elevate serum PSA levels (50–52). Consequently, one might anticipate that in a man with an elevated serum PSA level and high-grade PIN on biopsy, the elevated serum PSA reflects an unsampled cancer. However, studies have not uniformly demonstrated that serum PSA values predict which men with high-grade PIN on initial biopsy will have cancer on repeat biopsy (Table 5.3).

Several studies have addressed the optimal rebiopsy technique in men with isolated high-grade PIN on initial biopsy. Shepherd and associates found that cancer was ipsilateral and in the same quadrant as the initial high-grade PIN in only 64% and 50% of cases, respectively (46). Langer and associates found that systematic sextant biopsy was as likely to reveal carcinoma as compared to targeting the initial PIN site (34). In another study, Kamoi reported that repeat biopsy only of the initial PIN site would have missed 40% of the carcinomas eventually discovered (53). All these studies concluded that repeat prostate needle biopsy of men with high-grade PIN should include random repeat sextant biopsies of the prostate. The finding of high-grade PIN on needle biopsy thus does not indicate a specific site at risk for synchronous, occult prostate cancer, but instead indicates a higher likelihood of occult carcinoma being found anywhere in the prostate. The timing of repeat biopsy has been a source of some confusion as well, with many surgeons recommending repeat biopsy in 6 months. The source of this recommendation is unclear, and no rationale exists for delaying repeat biopsy in men with isolated high-grade PIN on initial biopsy.

High-Grade PIN: Significance on TURP Material

The significance of finding high-grade PIN on TURP is more controversial. Whereas two studies have found that high-grade PIN on TURP places an individual at higher risk for the subsequent detection of cancer (54,55), a long-term study from Norway demonstrated no association between the presence of high-grade PIN on TURP and the incidence of subsequent cancer (56). In a younger man with high-grade PIN on TURP, we would recommend that needle biopsies be performed to rule out a peripheral zone cancer. In an older man without elevated serum PSA levels, clinical follow-up is probably sufficient. When high-grade PIN is found on TURP, some pathologists recommend sectioning deeper into the corresponding block and most pathologists recommend processing the entire specimen (54).

Histology of PIN on Biopsy

Figures 5.19 and 5.20 demonstrate typical examples of high-grade PIN on biopsy; low-grade PIN may look similar at low power, but lacks prominent

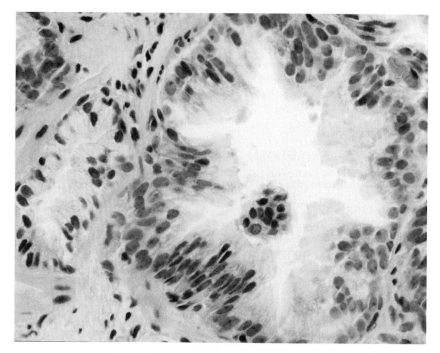

FIG. 5.19. High-grade PIN on needle biopsy.

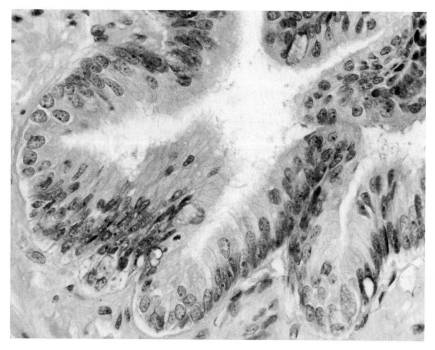

FIG. 5.20. High-grade PIN on needle biopsy.

nucleoli (efig 178-179;180-181;182-183;184;185-186;187;188-189;190;191-192;193-198;199-201;202-203;204-205). Large glands that are architecturally benign with papillary infolding and branching, yet are very basophilic at low power, characterize high-grade PIN. This basophilia is due to a combination of nuclear enlargement, hyperchromasia, stratification, and cytoplasmic amphophilia. If architecturally benign glands do not stand out at lower magnification due to their basophilia, we usually do not analyze them at higher magnification for the presence of prominent nucleoli. At higher magnification, nuclei are enlarged with prominent nucleoli. Occasionally, there are cases of high-grade PIN despite the lack of prominent nucleoli, based on marked pleomorphism, prominent nuclear enlargement, and hyperchromasia (20) (Fig. 5.21, efig 206-207;208-209). With the exception of those unusual cases with significant pleomorphism, if one has to hunt at high magnification for a rare cell with prominent nucleoli then we do not recommend diagnosing high-grade PIN. These cases could be diagnosed as low-grade PIN, but for the reasons described previously we do not use this diagnosis (Fig. 5.22, efig 178-179; 180-181;210;211-212). The most common issue that may lead in some cases to discrepant diagnoses between low- and high-grade PIN is in the definition of "prominent," when describing nucleolar enlargement and visibility. Occasionally, there will be cases borderline between low- and high-grade PIN, which

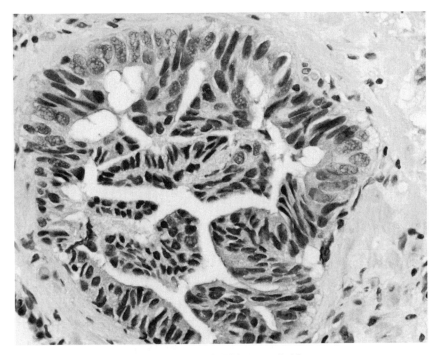

FIG. 5.21. High-grade PIN on needle biopsy.

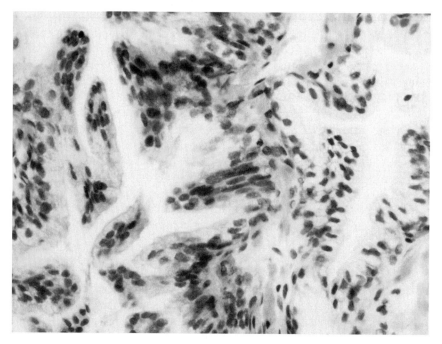

FIG. 5.22. Glands consistent with low-grade PIN *(left)* in contrast to benign glands *(right)*.

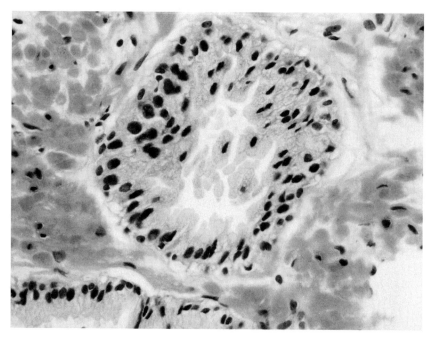

FIG. 5.23 Borderline lesion between low- and high-grade PIN on needle biopsy.

may be reported as such on the pathology report (Fig. 5.23, efig 213-215;216-217;218;219-220).

Cases of high-grade PIN associated with only a few adjacent small atypical glands may also be controversial as to whether coexistent infiltrating cancer is present. In cases with a few small atypical glands adjacent to high-grade PIN, the issue is whether the small glands represent outpouchings or tangential sections off the adjacent PIN gland or represent microinvasive cancer PINATYP (Fig. 5.24, efig 221-222;223;224-225;226;227;228-229;230-232;233)(57). When the small atypical glands are too numerous and too crowded to be outpouchings or tangential sections off of PIN glands, then infiltrating cancer can be diagnosed (Fig. 5.25, efig 234-235;236-237;238-239;240;241-242). The threshold for diagnosing infiltrating cancer in these cases varies among pathologists. Immunohistochemical stains usually do not aid in the distinction between high-grade PIN and high-grade PIN with microinvasive cancer. High-grade PIN shows a discontinuous basal cell layer when labeled with antibodies to high molecular weight keratin, and even entirely benign glands may not always be labeled with this antibody. Consequently, the lack of immunohistochemical staining with antibodies to high molecular weight keratin in only a few cribriform or small glands is not diagnostic of infiltrating cancer. Some cases may have the appearance of PINATYP yet will be entirely negative for high molecular weight cytokeratin; these foci may be diagnostic of cancer if there are many glands that are not immunoreactive (Color Plate

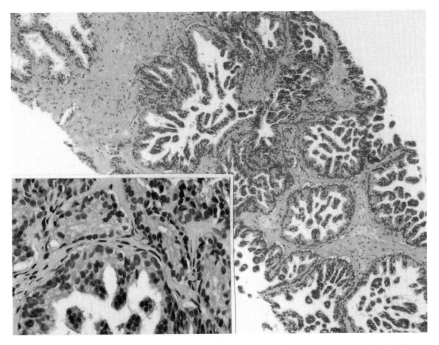

FIG. 5.24. High-grade PIN with inset showing several adjacent atypical small glands.

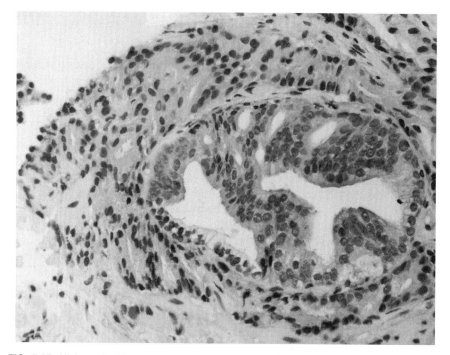

FIG. 5.25. High-grade PIN surrounded by fused small glands diagnostic of infiltrating carcinoma.

10) (efig 243-245;246-247). One may also see classic PIN where some of the glands show the expected patchy basal cell layer and a few identical glands are negative for high molecular weight keratin; these cases we would still diagnose as high-grade PIN (efig 248-249). It illustrates how one has to be cautious diagnosing cancer based on only a few glands that are negative for high molecular weight keratin. Rarely, we have seen cases where the differential diagnosis was PINATYP and PIN with cancer, where the presence of sperm within the small atypical glands helped to rule out invasive cancer; only glands in continuity with the main prostatic ducts, such as PIN, would occasionally contain sperm (efig 250-251). Other biomarkers, such as ploidy, also do not discriminate between high-grade PIN and infiltrating cancer (58-62).

PIN VERSUS CARCINOMA IN SITU

Based on much of the data, high-grade PIN appears to be a precursor to some forms of carcinoma of the prostate. For these reasons, some individuals feel that all examples of high-grade PIN should be termed "carcinoma in-situ." The one piece of evidence that we have for premalignant lesions in other organs which is lacking in the prostate, is the natural history of high-grade PIN. In the cervix, for example, cases of high-grade intraepithelial neoplasia have been followed and a higher than expected number of these lesions develop into infiltrating carcinoma at the site of the precursor lesion over a defined period of time. With the prostate, there is currently no such capability of monitoring a PIN focus to determine whether (a) there isn't already infiltrating carcinoma at that site or (b) when infiltrating carcinoma evolves has it done so in the immediate vicinity of the PIN focus. Because we do not know when high-grade PIN is found on biopsy material what percentage of patients develops infiltrating carcinoma over a given follow-up interval, most authorities do not use the term "carcinoma in situ of the prostate." The term "carcinoma in situ of the prostate" has implications that these lesions will develop into infiltrating carcinoma at a sufficiently high frequency that may lead some aggressive clinicians to treat these lesions in a radical fashion. Given the controversy as to whether infiltrating adenocarcinoma of the prostate should always be treated aggressively, it is doubtful that these potential precursor lesions should be treated by aggressive therapy until their natural history is better understood.

Only when the cribriform glands are so extensive and/or irregular in their outline can infiltrating cancer be diagnosed with confidence on needle biopsy (Fig. 5.26). In recent years, some authors have proposed that certain cribriform patterns

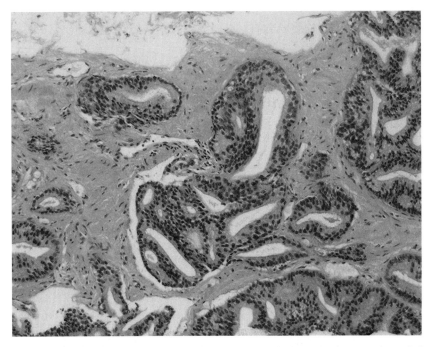

FIG. 5.26. Infiltrating cribriform prostate cancer where the cribriform glands are too crowded to represent high-grade PIN.

of high-grade PIN should be considered as "intraductal carcinoma of the prostate." McNeal describes three patterns of "intraductal carcinoma" (63,64). The first is where "The epithelium exhibits a *trabecular pattern;* narrow strands, often only two cell layers thick, spanned the lumen without stromal support, intersecting randomly to form a lacework of very orderly structure." Within this trabecular pattern, the nuclei within the center of the cribriform glands often showed a more benign appearance than those more peripherally located. In the second pattern, "the classic *cribriform* pattern, multiple small, round to elongated lumens perforated a central compartment cell mass which typically comprised more than half of the luminal space." The third pattern is a "*solid* pattern throughout the central compartment, without clear differentiation between the central area and the perimeter cells." In a subgroup of this pattern, prominent coagulation necrosis (comedonecrosis) was present. McNeal distinguished what he calls "cribriform intraductal carcinoma" from Gleason pattern 4 invasive carcinoma by "the presence of residual segments of the basal cell layer and by the fact the size, contour, and branching pattern of the normal duct architecture were usually identifiable." In their study on radical prostatectomy specimens, they found that the presence and extent of "intraductal carcinoma" correlated with postprostatectomy progression of cancer. The second and third patterns of "intraductal carcinoma" were associated with a higher risk of relapse following radical prostatectomy than the trabecular pattern. Using the same definition, Rubin et al. found that "intraductal carcinoma" was also associated with a high risk of PSA failure following radical prostatectomy (65). However, "intraductal cribriform carcinoma" was closely correlated with tumor volume and once tumor volume was accounted for, the presence of "intraductal carcinoma" was not correlated with PSA failure. The authors concluded that the close association between high tumor volume and "intraductal carcinoma" supports the theory that "intraductal carcinoma" is a late event in tumor progression more compatible with intraductal spread of tumor than with PIN. Wilcox et al. also studied this issue showing that patients with "intraductal carcinoma" have a higher Gleason score and total volume and were more likely to show seminal vesicle involvement and disease progression than those patients without "intraductal carcinoma"; intraductal carcinoma was of independent prognostic significance (66). However, the authors concluded that there was significant morphological overlap between high-grade PIN and "intraductal carcinoma" and adenocarcinoma involving secondary ducts. The authors questioned whether reproducible criteria could be developed to distinguish the spread of a cancer within ducts ("intraductal carcinoma") from high-grade PIN. They also demonstrated that cribriform "intraductal cancer" had a better prognosis than cases with the more solid/comedonecrosis pattern of intraductal carcinoma. The authors propose that although there is compelling evidence that both the cribriform and solid pattern of "intraductal carcinoma" should be considered to represent fully manifest carcinoma, criteria have not yet been established with sufficient detail to permit its consistent recognition by pathologists. They still prefer to classify these lesions as high-grade PIN (Fig. 5.27, efig 85-87;252-253;254-255;256-258).

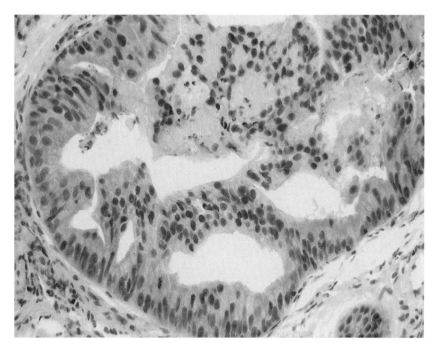

FIG. 5.27. Intraductal carcinoma.

However, the finding of cytologically malignant cells in a duct showing central comedonecrosis they feel warrants the diagnosis of "intraductal carcinoma" even though there may be occasional basal cells identified (Fig. 5.28, efig 259-260;261-263;264-266). There is precedent for this as it has been demonstrated, for example, in prostatic duct adenocarcinoma, that basal cells may be present (67). Many of the lesions described by McNeal as "intraductal carcinoma" we would classify as prostatic duct adenocarcinoma regardless of the presence of basal cells. We agree with Wilcox et al. in that "the finding of solid or cribriform intraductal foci as the only evidence of malignancy on a needle biopsy should not result in definitive therapy, although it might be an indication of an underlying clinically aggressive prostatic carcinoma. We still retain the use of the term high-grade PIN for these two intraductal proliferations." We also agree with them that "intraductal comedonecrosis pattern be considered to represent carcinoma, for both theoretical and practical (treatment) purposes." We diagnose these lesions as "intraductal carcinoma" with a comment that invariably this finding on biopsy is associated with unsampled infiltrating cancer in the prostate. However, it has been my experience as well as those of others, that the chance of encountering the comedonecrosis pattern of intraductal carcinoma as the only evidence of malignancy on a set of needle biopsy specimens is remote. In cases with extensive atypical cribriform glands on biopsy without necrosis, we sign them out as cribriform high-grade PIN, yet

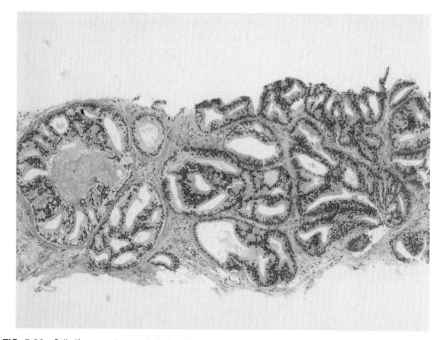

FIG. 5.28. Cribriform and crowded glands with focal comedonecrosis *(left)*. Although most consistent with infiltrating cribriform carcinoma, some pathologists may consider this still to be consistent with high-grade PIN.

emphasize that these lesions are much more frequently associated with cancers than other forms of PIN and strongly recommend repeat biopsy.

PIN—THE UNIVERSAL PRECURSOR TO PROSTATE CANCER?

One might assume that high-grade PIN is the universal precursor lesion to prostatic adenocarcinomas. However, there is some data that raises questions regarding the relationship of PIN to carcinoma. In a study by Sakr et al. from Wayne State University, they noted that the onset of high-grade PIN occurred later than the onset of carcinoma (68). This is at odds to what one would expect if PIN is a precursor lesion to all prostate cancers. Furthermore, 70% of the prostates with early carcinomas lacked any high-grade PIN within the entirely embedded prostate glands. In addition, even in those prostate glands where there existed both early cancer and high-grade PIN, only in 1/3 of the cases was the PIN adjacent to cancer. Other evidence against PIN being a universal precursor to prostatic carcinomas is that transition zone cancers uncommonly show adjacent PIN. It appears that high-grade PIN is a precursor lesion to many peripheral intermediate to high-grade adenocarcinomas of the prostate. However, PIN is not required to be present adjacent to these early carcinomas. Low-grade carcinomas, especially those present within the transition zone are not closely related to high-grade PIN.

REFERENCES

1. McNeal JE. Origin and development of carcinoma in the prostate. *Cancer* 1969;23:24–34.
2. McNeal JE, Bostwick DG. Intraductal dysplasia: a pre-malignant lesion of the prostate. *Hum Pathol* 1986;17:64–71.
3. Bostwick DG, Brawer MK. Prostatic intra-epithelial neoplasia and early invasion in prostate cancer. *Cancer* 1987;59:788–794,.
4. Drago JR, Mostofi FK, Lee F. Introductory remarks and workshop summary. *Urology* 1989;34 (suppl):2–3.
5. Bostwick DG, Amin MB, Dundore P, et al. Architectural patterns of high-grade prostatic intraepithelial neoplasia. *Hum Pathol* 1993;24:298–310.
6. Reyes AO, Swanson PE, Carbone JM, et al. Unusual histologic types of high-grade prostatic intraepithelial neoplasia. *Am J Surg Pathol* 1997;21:1215–1222.
7. Berman DM, Yang J, Epstein JI. Foamy gland high grade prostatic intraepithelial neoplasia. *Am J Surg Pathol* 2000;24:140–144.
8. Haggman MJ, Macoska JA, Wojno KJ, et al. The relationship between prostatic intraepithelial neoplasia and prostate cancer: critical issues. *J Urol* 1997;158:12–22.
9. McNeal JE, Villers A, Redwine EA, et al. Microcarcinoma in the prostate: its association with duct-acinar dysplasia. *Hum Pathol* 1991;22:644–652.
10. Bostwick DG, Pacelli A, Lopez-Beltran A. Molecular biology of prostatic intraepithelial neoplasia. *Prostate* 1996;29:117–134.
11. Srodon M, Epstein JI. Central zone histology of the prostate. *Human Pathol* (in press).
12. Ayala AG, Srigley JR, Ro JY, Abdul-Karim FW, Johnson DE. Clear cell cribriform hyperplasia of prostate: report of 10 cases. *Am J Surg Pathol* 1986;10:665–671.
13. Devaraj LT, Bostwick DG. Atypical basal cell hyperplasia of the prostate: immunophenotypic profile and proposed classification of basal cell proliferations. *Am J Surg Pathol* 1993;17:645–659.
14. Epstein JI, Armas OA. Atypical basal cell hyperplasia of the prostate. *Am J Surg Pathol* 1992;16:1205–1214.
15. Hedrick L, Epstein JI. Use of high molecular weight cytokeratin as an adjunct in the diagnosis of prostate carcinoma. *Am J Surg Pathol* 1989;13:389–396.
16. Kronz JD, Shaikh AA, Epstein JI. Atypical cribriform lesions on prostate biopsy. *Am J Surg Path* 2001;25:147–155.
17. Bostwick DG, Kindrachuk RW, Rouse RV. Prostatic adenocarcinoma with endometrioid features: clinical, pathologic, and ultrastructural findings. *Am J Surg Pathol* 1985;9:595–609.
18. Epstein JI, Woodruff J. Prostatic carcinomas with endometrioid features: a light microscopic and immunohistochemical study of ten cases. *Cancer* 1986;57:111–119.
19. Christensen W, Walsh PC, Epstein JI. Prostatic duct adenocarcinoma: findings at radical prostatectomy. *Cancer* 1991;67:2118–2124.
20. Epstein JI, Grignon DJ, Humphrey PA, et al. Interobserver reproducibility in the diagnosis of prostatic intraepithelial neoplasia. *Am J Surg Pathol* 1995;19:873–886.
21. McNeal JE. Significance of duct-acinar dysplasia in prostatic carcinogenesis. *Urology* (suppl) 1989;34:9–15.
22. Keetch DW, Catalona WJ, Smith DS. Serial prostatic biopsies in men with persistently elevated serum prostate specific antigen values. *J Urol*, 1994;151:1571–1574.
23. Brawer MK, Bigler SA, Sohlberg OE, et al. Significance of prostatic intraepithelial neoplasia on prostate needle biopsy. *Urology* 1991;38:103–107.
24. Aboseif S, Shinohara K, Weidner N, et al. The significance of prostatic intraepithelial neoplasia. *Br J Urol* 1995;76:355–359.
25. Keetch DW, Humphrey PA, Stahl D, et al. Morphometric analysis and clinical follow-up of isolated prostatic intraepithelial neoplasia in needle biopsy of the prostate. *J Urol* 1995;154:347–351
26. Raviv G, Janssen T, Zlotta AR, et al. Prostatic intraepithelial neoplasia: Influence of clinical and pathological data on the detection of prostate cancer. *J Urol* 1996;156:1050–1055.
27. Alsikafi NF, Gerber GS, Yang XJ, et al. High-grade prostatic intraepithelial neoplasia (PIN) with adjacent atypical glands is associated with a higher rate of cancer on subsequent prostatic needle biopsy than high grade PIN alone. *J Urol* 2000;163(suppl):90.
28. Bostwick DG, Qian J, Frankel K. The incidence of high grade prostatic intraepithelial neoplasia in needle biopsies. *J Urol* 1995;154:1791–1794.
29. Cheville JC, Reznicek MJ, Bostwick DG. The focus of "atypical glands, suspicious for malignancy" in prostatic needle biopsy specimens: incidence, histologic features, and clinical follow-up of cases diagnosed in a community practice. *Am J Clin Path* 1997;108:633–640.

30. Hoedemaeker RF, Kranse R, Rietbergen JBW, et al. Evaluation of prostate needle biopsies in a population-based screening study. *Cancer* 1999;85:145–152.
31. Horninger W, Volgger H, Strohmeyer D, et al. Predictive value of percent free prostate specific antigen in high grade prostatic intraepithelial neoplasia: results of the Tyrol prostate specific antigen screening project. *J Urol* 2001;165:1143–145.
32. Hu JC, Palapattu GS, Kattan MW, et al. The association of selected pathological features with prostate cancer in a single-needle biopsy accession. *Hum Pathol* 1998;29:1536–1538.
33. Kim SC, Weiser AC, Nadler RB, et al. The changing incidence of high grade prostatic intraepithelial neoplasia: clinical implications. *J Urol* 2000;163(suppl):279.
34. Langer JE, Rover ES, Coleman BG, et al. Strategy for repeat biopsy of patients with prostatic intraepithelial neoplasia detected by prostate needle biopsy. *J Urol* 1996;155:228–231.
35. Mettlin C, Lee F, Drago J, et al. The American Cancer Society National Cancer Detection Project: findings on the detection of early prostate cancer in 2425 men. *Cancer* 1991;67:2949–2958.
36. Novis DA, Zarbo RJ, Valenstein PA. Diagnostic uncertainty expressed in prostate needle biopsies. A college of American pathologists Q-probes study of 15753 prostate needle biopsies in 332 institutions. *Arch Pathol Lab Med* 1999;123:687–692.
37. Orozco R, O'Dowd G, Kunnel B, et al. Observations on pathology trends in 62, 537 prostate biopsies obtained from urology private practices in the United States. *Urology* 1998;51:186–195.
38. Renshaw AA, Santis WF, Richie JP. Clinicopathological characteristics of prostatic adenocarcinoma in men with atypical prostate needle biopsies. *J Urol* 1998;159:2018–2022.
39. Reyes AO, Humphrey PA. Diagnostic effect of complete histologic sampling of prostate needle biopsy specimens. *Am J Clin Pathol* 1998;109:416–422.
40. Sakr WA, Angelakis K, deGuia K. The prevalence and evolution of isolated high-grade prostatic intraepithelial neoplasia (HGPIN) in African American (AA) and Caucasian (C) men—A study of needle biopsies. *J Urol* 2000;163(suppl):56.
41. Wills ML, Hamper UM, Partin AW, et al. Incidence of high-grade prostatic intraepithelial neoplasia in sextant needle biopsy specimens. *Urology* 1997;49:367–373.
42. Rosser CJ, Broberg J, Case D, et al. Detection of high-grade prostatic intraepithelial neoplasia with the five-region biopsy technique. *Urology* 1999;54:853–856.
43. Bigler SA, Fowler JE, Lynch C, et al. Prospective study of correlations between biopsy-detected high grade prostatic intraepithelial neoplasia, serum prostate specific antigen concentration, and race. *Cancer* 2001;91:1291–1296.
44. Davidson D, Bostwick D, Qian J, et al. Prostatic intraepithelial neoplasia is a risk factor for adenocarcinoma: predictive accuracy in needle biopsies. *J Urol* 1993;154:1295–1299.
45. O'Dowd GJ, Miller MC, Orozco R, et al. Analysis of results within 1 year after a noncancer diagnosis. *Urology* 2000;55:553–559.
46. Shepherd D, Keetch DW, Humphrey PA, et al. Repeat biopsy strategy in men with isolated prostatic intraepithelial neoplasia on prostate needle biopsy. *J Urol* 1996;156:460–463.
47. Weinstein MH, Epstein JI. Significance of high grade prostatic intraepithelial neoplasia (PIN) on needle biopsy. *Hum Pathol* 1993;24:624–629.
48. Kronz JD, Allan CH, Shaikh AA, et al. Predicting cancer following a diagnosis of high grade PIN (HGPIN) on needle biopsy. *Am J Surg Pathol* 2001;25:1079–1085.
49. Hamper UM, Sheth S, Walsh PC, et al. Stage B adenocarcinoma of the prostate: transrectal US and pathologic peripheral zone lesions. *Radiology* 1991;180:101–104.
50. Ronnette BM, CarMichael MJ, Carter HB, et al. Does prostatic intraepithelial neoplasia result in elevated serum prostate specific antigen levels? *J Urol* 1993;150:386–389.
51. Alexander EE, Qian J, Wollan PC, et al. Prostatic intraepithelial neoplasia does not appear to raise serum prostate-specific antigen concentration. *Urology* 1997;47:693–698.
52. Ramos CG, Carvahal GF, Mager DE, et al. The effect of high grade prostatic intraepithelial neoplasia on serum total and percentage of free prostate specific antigen levels. *J Urol* 1999; 162:1587–1590.
53. Kamoi K, Troncoso P, Babaian RJ. Strategy for repeat biopsy in patients with high grade prostatic intraepithelial neoplasia. *J Urol* 2000;163:819–823.
54. Gaudin PB, Sesterhenn IA, Wojno KJ, et al. Incidence and clinical significance of high grade prostatic intraepithelial neoplasia in TURP specimens. *Urology* 1997;49:558–563.
55. Pacelli A, Bostwick DG. Clinical significance of high-grade prostatic intraepithelial neoplasia in transurethral resection specimens. *Urology* 1997;50:355–359.
56. Harvei S, Skjorten FJ, Robsahm TE, et al. Is prostatic intraepithelial neoplasia in the transition/central zone a true precursor of cancer? A long-term retrospective study in Norway. *Br J Cancer* 1998; 78:46–49.

57. Kronz JD, Shaikh AA, Epstein JI. High-grade prostatic intraepithelial neoplasia with adjacent small atypical glands (PINATYP) on prostate biopsy. *Hum Pathol* 2001;32:389–395.
58. Weinberg DS, Weidner N. Concordance of DNA content between prostatic intraepithelial neoplasia and concomitant invasive carcinoma. *Arch Pathol Lab Med* 1993;117:1132–1137.
59. Amin MB, Schultz DS, Zarbo RJ, et al. Computerized static DNA ploidy analysis of prostatic intraepithelial neoplasia. *Arch Pathol Lab Med* 1993;117:794–798.
60. de la Torre M, Haggman M, Brandstedt S, et al. Prostatic intraepithelial neoplasia and invasive carcinoma in total prostatectomy specimens: distribution, volumes, and DNA ploidy. *Br J Urol* 1993;72:207–213.
61. Greene DR, Wheeler TM, Egawa S, et al. A comparison of the morphological features of cancer arising in the transition zone and in the peripheral zone of the prostate. *J Urol* 1991;146:1069–1076.
62. Baretton GB, Vogt T, Blasenbreu S, et al. Comparison of DNA ploidy in prostatic intraepithelial neoplasia and invasive carcinoma of the prostate: an image cytometric study. *Hum Pathol* 1994;25:506–513.
63. McNeal JE, Yemoto CEM. Spread of adenocarcinoma within prostatic ducts and acini. Morphologic and clinical correlations. *Am J Surg Pathol* 1996;20:802–814.
64. Cohen RJ, McNeal JE, Baillie T. Patterns of differentiation and proliferation in intraductal carcinoma of the prostate: significance for cancer progression. *Prostate* 2000;43:11–19.
65. Rubin MA, de La Taille A, Bagiella E, et al. Cribriform carcinoma of the prostate and cribriform prostatic intraepithelial neoplasia: incidence and clinical implications. *Am J Surg Pathol* 1998;22:840–848.
66. Wilcox G, Soh S, Chakraborty S, et al. Patterns of high-grade prostatic intraepithelial neoplasia associated with clinically aggressive prostate cancer. *Hum Pathol* 1998;29:1119–1123.
67. Samaratunga H, Singh M. Distribution pattern of basal cells detected by cytokeratin 34 beta E12 in primary prostatic duct adenocarcinoma. *Am J Surg Pathol* 1997;21:435–440.
68. Sakr WA, Haas GP, Cassin BF, et al. The frequency of carcinoma and intraepithelial neoplasia of the prostate in young male patients. *J Urol* 1993;150:379–385.

6

Diagnosis of Limited Adenocarcinoma of the Prostate

DIAGNOSIS ON NEEDLE BIOPSY

There are two main issues in the diagnosis of limited cancer on needle biopsy of the prostate. The first is the recognition of limited carcinoma and the prevention of false-negative diagnoses, dealt with in this chapter. The second issue concerns lesions mimicking adenocarcinoma of the prostate and the prevention of false-positive diagnoses, which is discussed in Chapter 7.

The underdiagnosis of limited adenocarcinoma of the prostate on needle biopsy is one of the most frequent problems in prostate pathology. It is hard to obtain data on this phenomenon, as most institutions do not want for medicolegal reasons to go back and review old cases for potential missed cases of cancer. Some data come from one of the author's (Epstein) consultation practice, where we looked for lesions on needle biopsy that were missed by the contributor (1). Of 1,840 patients that had all slides submitted in consultation and dotted by the referring pathologist, the following lesions were missed: small atypical glands suspicious for cancer (35 patients; 1.9%); prostatic adenocarcinoma (32 patients; 1.7%); high-grade prostatic intraepithelial neoplasia (PIN) (30 patients; 1.6%); and high-grade PIN with atypical small glands (5 patients; 0.3%). A second study that provides some information on this issue is from one of the author's (Epstein) review of a teaching hospital's prostate biopsies. The review was performed shortly after the initial pathologists rendered their diagnosis so as not to impact patient care (2). Of 387 parts from 224 consecutive prostate needle biopsy cases from a 520-bed urban academic center, 0.5% and 2.3% were diagnosed as cancer on rereview, although they were originally diagnosed as benign and atypical, respectively.

At the edge of most adenocarcinomas, scattered neoplastic glands infiltrate widely between larger benign glands (Fig. 6.1). It is therefore not uncommon to have several needle biopsy cores of prostatic tissue where there are only a few

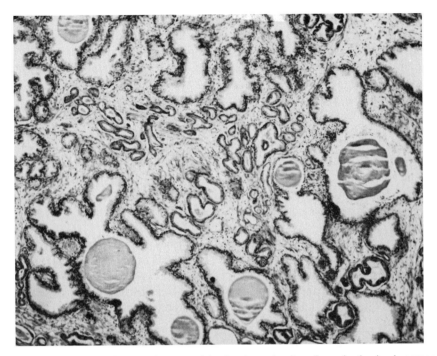

FIG. 6.1. Periphery of adenocarcinoma nodule showing extension of neoplastic glands among larger benign glands. ×55.

malignant glands. The importance of recognizing limited adenocarcinoma of the prostate is that there is often no correlation between the amount of cancer seen on the needle biopsy and the amount of tumor present within the prostate. There may be only a few neoplastic glands in the core biopsy, despite significant tumor within the prostate gland (see Chapter 8).

Not everyone has the same threshold for diagnosing limited adenocarcinoma of the prostate on needle biopsy. Furthermore, everyone's threshold for diagnosing limited adenocarcinoma evolves over time and is influenced both by one's remote and recent experiences. It is expected that not everyone will feel equally comfortable in establishing a definitive diagnosis from some of the photographs of limited adenocarcinoma within this chapter. However, it is important to recognize these foci as atypical and suspicious for carcinoma, so that further workup might lead to a more definitive diagnosis.

It is important when examining needle biopsy specimens to gain an appreciation of what the nonneoplastic prostate looks like. In order to identify limited amounts of cancer on needle biopsy material, one first has to identify the normal nonneoplastic prostate and then look for glands that do not fit in. Although most prostates are relatively similar in their histological appearance, some contain numerous small foci of crowded glands similar to adenosis. In such a case, the diagnosis of cancer based on a small focus of crowded glands with minimal cytologic atypia should be performed with caution. Other men's prostate glands are characterized by widespread atrophy; one should in these cases hesitate to diagnose cancer if the atypical glands have scant cytoplasm.

Evaluating an atypical focus in a needle biopsy of the prostate should be a methodical process. When reviewing needle biopsies, one should develop a mental balance sheet where on one side of the column are features favoring the diagnosis of carcinoma and on the other side of the column are features against the diagnosis of cancer. At the end of evaluating a case, hopefully all of the criteria are listed on one side of the column or the other such that a definitive diagnosis can be made. It will be stressed throughout this chapter that the diagnosis of cancer should be based on a constellation of features rather than relying on any one criterion by itself.

In general, scanning of prostate needle biopsies should be performed at 4× to10× magnification. Reviewing needle biopsies at lower magnifications runs the risk of overlooking limited foci of carcinoma. Evaluation of prostate needle biopsies at higher magnification is also nonproductive as glands with slight nuclear atypia taken out of context of their architectural pattern will often be erroneously confused with adenocarcinoma.

The recognition of limited adenocarcinoma of the prostate is first performed at low magnification. One pattern seen at low magnification that should raise a suspicion of carcinoma is the presence of a focus of crowded glands (efig 267-268;269-270;271-272;273-275). Of six tissue cores sampled by large core needle (14 gauge), the only atypical area was a focus of crowded glands illustrated in Figure 6.2. Towards one edge of the field are a group of benign glands, one containing corpora amylacea, and towards the other at the end of the core, there is a benign atrophic gland. In between these benign glands is the focus of crowded glands.

At higher magnification seen in Figure 6.3, some of the glands are shown to have enlarged prominent nucleoli. Prominent nucleoli, while important in the diagnosis of cancer on needle biopsy, should not be the sole criterion used to establish the diagnosis. Reliance on prominent nucleoli for the diagnosis of prostate cancer will potentially lead both to an underdiagnosis as well as to an overdiagnosis of prostate cancer. The significance of prominent nucleoli must be taken in the context of the architectural pattern and other features present within the case. Although it has been stated that multiple nucleoli, especially those eccentrically located in the nucleus, are diagnostic of cancer, we have not utilized this criteria in our own practice; additional studies have not been performed to validate this criterion (3).

The photomicrograph of Figure 6.3 also illustrates the problem of identifying basal cells by light microscopy. In cases of obvious carcinoma, there may be cells that closely mimic basal cells. These cells when labeled with antibodies to high molecular weight keratin are negative and represent fibroblasts closely apposed to the neoplastic glands. Consequently, in a focus that is con-

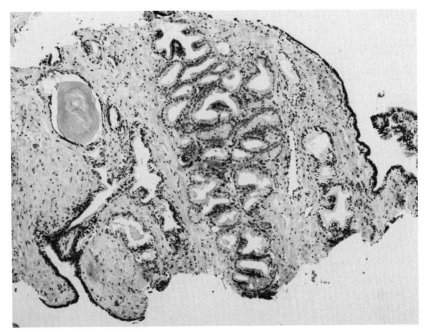

FIG. 6.2. Numerous back-to-back glands of adenocarcinoma of the prostate filling the stroma between atrophic benign glands. ×75.

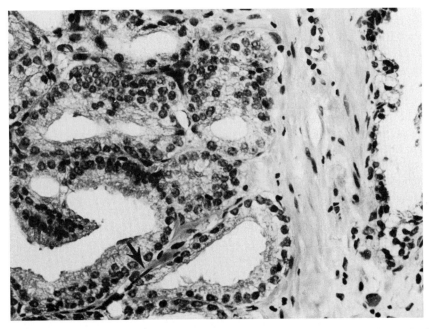

FIG. 6.3. Higher magnification of Figure 6.3 showing increase in nuclear size within neoplastic glands containing abundant cytoplasm, as opposed to the adjacent atrophic benign gland *(right)*. Also note that surrounding several neoplastic glands there are thin hyperchromatic elongated nuclei of fibroblasts that may mimic a basal cell layer *(arrow)*. ×480.

sistent with cancer architecturally and which has other features supportive of the diagnosis of carcinoma at higher power, a search for basal cells by light microscopy may be counter-productive. Because of the difficulty in distinguishing basal cells from fibroblasts as well as the problem with stratification of neoplastic nuclei due to tangential sectioning or thick sections, these authors usually do not search for basal cells in cases that satisfy the criteria for adenocarcinoma of the prostate (efig 276-277;278-279). It is always helpful to first identify glands that you are confident are benign, and then compare these benign glands to the atypical glands which you are considering to diagnose as adenocarcinoma of the prostate. The greater the number of differences between the recognizable benign glands and the atypical glands the more confidently a malignant diagnosis can be established. Figure 6.3 shows that in many adenocarcinomas of the prostate, nuclei are enlarged relative to surrounding benign prostatic nuclei. Often, nuclear enlargement may be present when prominent nucleoli are not (efig 280-281;282-283;284-285;286-287;288-289;290-292). This case was initially seen at a local community hospital where the focus in question was diagnosed as atypical and then sent to another academic center for a second opinion. The academic center diagnosed the case as benign at which point the case was referred to The Johns Hopkins Hospital. We diagnosed this focus as adenocarcinoma of the prostate and the patient underwent a radical prostatectomy shortly thereafter. The radical prostatectomy showed extensive tumor with extraprostatic extension. This case demonstrates the disparities between the amount of tissue that may be sampled by the urologist, the amount of carcinoma that may be present within the needle biopsy, and the extent of tumor in the prostate gland. Nuclear hyperchromatism is another cytologic feature that may help to distinguish cancerous from benign glands (efig 293; 294-295;296-297;298-299;300-301).

The second architectural pattern that is suspicious for adenocarcinoma of the prostate is the presence of small glands situated between larger benign glands (efig 302; 303-304;305). In most adenocarcinomas, the neoplastic glands are smaller than adjacent benign glands. Color plate 11 demonstrates a focus of small glands adjacent to a larger benign gland. Benign glands are recognized by their larger size, papillary infolding, and branching. At higher magnification, the small glands show several features more commonly seen in adenocarcinoma. Nuclei are somewhat enlarged although prominent nucleoli are not particularly visible. Large glands with straight luminal borders is also a feature of cancer, which is also described under the entity of "pseudohyperplastic cancer" (efig 306-307;308-309).

Several of the neoplastic glands in color plate 11 contain prostatic intraluminal crystalloids. Prostatic crystalloids are dense eosinophilic crystal-like structures that appear in various geometric shapes such as rectangular, hexagonal, triangular and rod-like structures (efig 310-312)(4,5). Prostatic crystalloids have been reported in 25% of cancers seen on biopsy material, yet may also be seen in benign prostate acini (6,7). The likelihood of finding crystalloids is dependent on the number of malignant glands present and the grade; crystalloids are inversely correlated with the Gleason grade (7). Crystalloids, although not diagnostic of carcinoma, are more frequently found in cancer than in benign glands. The one condition that mimics cancer where crystalloids are frequently seen is adenosis, which consists of a lobule of pale-staining glands (see Chapter 7). Consequently, if crystalloids are seen in small glands with an infiltrative appearance in between benign glands, where adenosis is not in the differential, they may help to establish a diagnosis of cancer. The finding of prostatic crystalloids in benign glands does not indicate an increased risk of cancer on subsequent biopsy (efig 313)(6).

Also noted in one of the neoplastic glands in Color Plate 11 is a mitotic figure. Mitoses, although not frequent in adenocarcinoma of the prostate, are much more commonly seen in cancer than in benign glands (efig 314-315;316-317). Consequently, this focus is diagnostic of cancer based on its architectural pattern, nuclear enlargement, crystalloids, and a mitotic figure.

An incidental finding in Color Plate 11 is lipofuscin pigment within the adjacent benign prostatic gland (8). It is important not to overdiagnose benign prostate glands with lipofuscin pigment as seminal vesicle. Otherwise, cases such as the one illustrated in Color Plate 11, would be erroneously diagnosed as adenocarcinoma of the prostate invading the seminal vesicles, whereby the patient would be denied potentially curative surgery. Other features differentiating benign prostate glands from seminal vesicle epithelium on needle biopsy are discussed in Chapter 7. The lack of lipofuscin in atypical glands suspicious for cancer, if there is prominent pigment in the surrounding benign glands, may help to establish a definitive diagnosis of cancer; lipofuscin is uncommon in high-grade PIN and rare in cancer (efig 318-320).

The presence of small cancerous glands situated in between benign glands is a manifestation of their infiltrative nature. When small atypical glands are seen on both sides of a benign gland it is even more diagnostic of malignancy (efig 321-323;324-325;326-327).

Although in the past there has been much less consideration paid to cytoplasmic features as compared to nuclear qualities, the nature of the cytoplasm may be critical in the diagnosis of some carcinomas. In some adenocarcinomas of the prostate, the cytoplasm of the malignant glands is more amphophilic than the surrounding benign glands that have pale to clear cytoplasm (Color Plate 12, efig 328-329;330-333;334-335;336-337). In order for this criterion to be helpful, the benign prostate glands must be appropriately stained such that they have a pale to clear appearance. In a study of consult cases, we found that in 32% of the cases this criterion was not applicable since the benign glands also exhibited amphophilic cytoplasm (7). Because we find this feature to be helpful in a large number of cases, one's hematoxylin and eosin (H&E) stains should be adjusted so that the cytoplasm of the benign glands appears pale to clear.

Color Plate 13 demonstrates a subtler example of amphophilic cytoplasm in malignant glands. The benign glands are characterized by larger size, small nuclei, and pale to clear cytoplasm. The other glands are suspicious for cancer based on their small size and minimal nuclear enlargement. However, the feature of note in this particular example is that the cytoplasm in all of the cancerous glands is slightly more amphophilic than the surrounding benign glands.

Another diagnostic criterion is the nature of intraluminal secretions. Blue-tinged mucinous secretions seen on H&E stained sections are mostly observed in carcinomas, and only rarely identified in benign glands (Color Plate 14,efig 338-339;340-342;343-344;345-346;347-348;349-350). The prevalence of these blue-tinged secretions is in part influenced by the nature of the H&E stain. In some institutions' referral material, this feature appears to be fairly prevalent, whereas in other institutions, it is uncommonly seen. Some laboratory's H&E stains are too basophilic, where even benign glands contain blue-tinged mucinous secretions. When normal colonic glands that are present on most prostate biopsies show an intense blue appearance, pathologists have to be cautious in placing too much weight on blue-tinged mucin in prostate glands as a diagnostic criterion for cancer. Although initial reports suggested that acid mucin stains could distinguish malignant from benign glands, subsequent articles demonstrated that acid mucin is variably present in mimickers of carcinoma such as adenosis and atrophic glands (9,10). Color Plate 15 shows a subtler example of blue-tinged mucinous secretions in adenocarcinoma where there are wispy, stringy, faint blue secretions. This figure also demonstrates another type of intraluminal secretion that may aid in the diagnosis of limited cancer. Whereas corpora amylacea are prominent in benign glands and rarely seen in cancer, pink amorphous acellular secretions seen in Color Plate 16 are identified in approximately half of cancers on needle biopsy and only occasionally seen in benign glands (efig 351-352;353-354;355;356-357;358) (7,11). These secretions are amorphous as contrasted to corpora amylacea, which are well-circumscribed round to oval structures with concentric lamellar rings. Both pink and blue secretions often coexist in the same glands (efig 359-360;361-363;364-365;366-367;368;369). As with all of the criteria mentioned to this point, this feature is not specific for carcinoma. Rather, the presence of intraluminal secretions should be taken in context of the architectural pattern, and the nuclear and cytoplasmic features.

There are three features that have not to date been identified in benign glands, and which are in and of themselves diagnostic of cancer. These are mucinous fibroplasia (collagenous micronodules), glomerulations, and perineural invasion (12,13).

Occasionally, intraluminal mucinous secretions are so extensive that they become focally organized. This lesion, known as either mucinous fibroplasia or collagenous micronodules, is typified by very delicate loose fibrous tissue with an

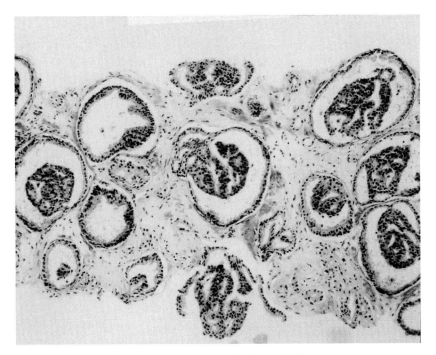

FIG. 6.4. Adenocarcinoma with glomeruloid pattern.

ingrowth of fibroblasts (Color Plate 17, efig 370-371;372-373;374-375;376-378;379-380;381-382;383-384;385-386;387-388;389;390-391). Mucinous secretions can displace the epithelium, resulting in atrophic cytoplasm and small pyknotic nuclei, whereby these foci can be difficult to recognize as cancer (Color Plate 18).

Glomerulations (Fig. 6.4) consists of glands with a cribriform proliferation that is not transluminal (efig 392;393;394;395-396;397-398;399;400). Rather, these cribriform formations are attached to only one edge of the gland resulting in a structure superficially resembling a glomerulus.

Perineural invasion is seen in approximately 20% of needle biopsies of the prostate showing adenocarcinoma (14). In order for perineural invasion to be diagnostic of adenocarcinoma, the glands in question should circumferentially surround the nerve (efig 401;402-403;404;405;406-407). Figure 6.5 shows the only atypical gland in this particular case that is wrapping around a nerve. Occasionally, glands with perineural invasion have a peculiar proclivity to resemble a benign hyperplastic gland. However, despite the benign cytology and papillary infoldings, the fact that this gland is wrapping around the nerve is diagnostic of adenocarcinoma. Perineural invasion must be distinguished from perineural indentation by benign prostate glands (15,16) (efig 408-409;410-411;412;413;

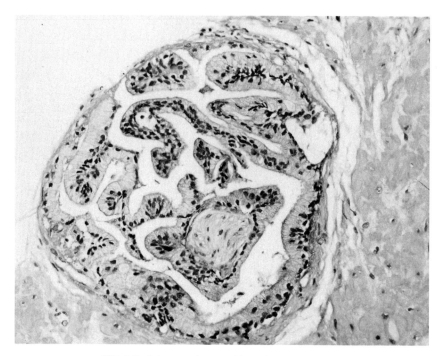

FIG. 6.5. Adenocarcinoma with perineural invasion.

414). As shown in Figure 6.6, benign prostate glands can on occasion indent peripheral nerves. These glands are distinguished from cancer by their benign cytology and atrophic appearance and the fact that these glands are not circumferentially surrounding the nerve.

In a 1995 study, we analyzed 300 consecutive cases sent in for consultation (7). These cases represented relatively limited adenocarcinoma of the prostate on needle biopsy. As shown in Table 6.1 the most frequent findings were nuclear enlargement and prominent nucleoli seen in approximately 75% of the cases. In addition to the 24% of cases with no prominent nucleoli, 25% of cases had only rare prominent nucleoli. In many of these cases, the referring pathologist specifically noted that the lack of prominent nucleoli prevented them from definitively establishing a malignant diagnosis. The lack of prominent nucleoli in many of these cases probably reflected a sampling problem where areas of the tumor with prominent nucleoli were not biopsied. In other cases, overstained sections obscured nuclear detail. The referral nature of this case material further accounted for the high percentage of cases without prominent nucleoli. This study demonstrates that had prominent nucleoli been relied upon to establish a diagnosis of cancer, a significant number of carcinomas would have been underdiagnosed. In some cases without prominent

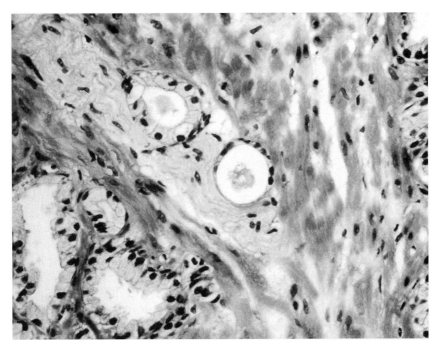

FIG. 6.6. Perineural indentation by benign glands.

nucleoli, nuclear enlargement was readily evident and helped to establish a diagnosis. Pink and blue amorphous secretions were present in approximately half of cases and crystalloids were seen in 25% of cases. Amphophilic cytoplasm was present in 41% of cases, yet was not able to be evaluated in 32%, since the entire section was amphophilic. Mitoses and perineural invasion were present to a somewhat lesser extent (Table 6.2). The finding of only 3% of cases with perineural invasion in this series is attributable to the following: Cases with perineural invasion are more readily diagnosable by pathologists and would not have been sent in for consultation.

TABLE 6.1. *Frequency of diagnostic criteria in limited prostate cancer*

	Nuclear enlargement	Prominent nucleoli	Pink secretions	Blue mucin	Crystalloids
None	23%	24%	47%	66%	75%
Rare	14%	25%	22%	14%	13%
Occasional	26%	30%	19	13%	7%
Diffuse	37%	21%	12%	7%	5%
Total	100%	100%	100%	100%	100%

TABLE 6.2. *Frequency of diagnostic criteria in limited prostate cancer*

	Amphophilic cytoplasm (%)	Mitoses (%)	Perineural invasion (%)
Absent	27	89	97
Present	41	11	3
Unable to evaluate	32	—	—
Total	100	100	100

In the evaluation of an atypical focus, the presence of several of the features can help establish a diagnosis of cancer even when limited tumor is present. In only 2% of the cases of limited tumor sent in for consultation was the diagnosis solely based on the architectural pattern (7). In these cases, when none of the features listed in Table 6.3 are present and the diagnosis is made on the architectural pattern, one should be extremely cautious and only diagnose cancer when the pattern is overtly malignant.

Occasionally, high-grade adenocarcinoma of the prostate may also be difficult to diagnose on needle biopsy. With an increase in the numbers of needle biopsies being performed for early disease detected by screening techniques, we are seeing an increase in the detection of small high-grade adenocarcinomas (17) (efig 415-416). Figure 6.7 demonstrates an area of increased cellularity that was the only atypical focus in this case. Although by itself not diagnostic, the presence of too many cells per unit area where the cells are not obvious inflammatory or stromal cells, raises the question of a poorly differentiated prostate cancer. When labeled with antibodies to prostate-specific antigen (PSA), prostate-specific acid phosphatase (PSAP), and pancytokeratin, these individual cells were shown to be epithelial in nature. Given that there is no benign epithelial process with this pattern, the diagnosis of high-grade adenocarcinoma can be rendered. Figure 6.8 shows

TABLE 6.3. *Features more common in adenocarcinoma as compared to benign glands*

Nuclear
  Prominent nucleoli
  Enlarged nuclei
  Hyperchromatism
  Mitotic figures
Cytoplasmic
  Amphophilia
  Sharp luminal border
  Lack of lipofuscin
Luminal
  Blue-tinged mucinous secretions
  Pink amorphous secretions
  Crystalloids
  Lack of corpora amylacea
Architectural
  Mucinous fibroplasia
  Perineural invasion
  Glomerulations

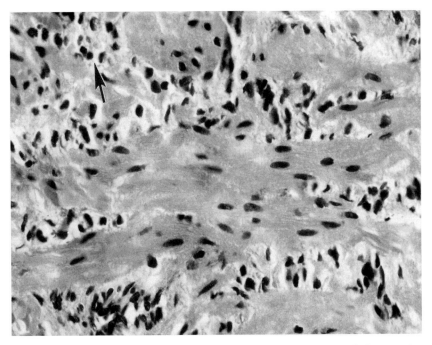

FIG. 6.7. High-grade adenocarcinoma resembling inflammatory cells. Note foci suggestive of glandular differentiation *(arrow)*.

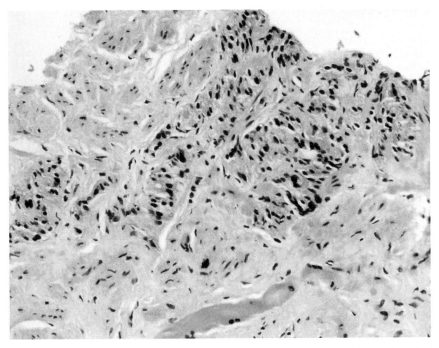

FIG. 6.8. Small focus of high-grade adenocarcinoma on needle biopsy. Nuclei lacked cytologic atypia at higher magnification.

another focus of limited high-grade cancer on needle biopsy. Despite the lack of cytologic atypia, this focus is diagnostic of adenocarcinoma because of the lack of well-formed glands, inconsistent with a benign process. Example of cancers with crush artifact and cancers associated with inflammation are illustrated in Chapter 10.

There are cases that some pathologists may not feel comfortable diagnosing as adenocarcinoma based on the architectural pattern of small glands infiltrating in between larger benign glands if there is a lack of cytologic atypia. In these cases where there are a large number of atypical glands present for evaluation, the use of antibodies to high molecular weight cytokeratin may resolve the diagnosis (efig 417-419;420-422). In some cases, there will be faint staining of cancer glands with antibodies to high molecular weight cytokeratin; this staining is nonspecific if it is not seen in a basal cell distribution and is still supportive of a malignant diagnosis (efig 423-426;427-428). More rarely, one can see occasional cancer cells that are strongly positive for antibodies to high molecular weight cytokeratin, yet as long as these cells are not in a basal cell distribution, these cells represent aberrant expression of the antigen in cancer (efig 429-431). Figure 6.9 demonstrates a case where the referring pathologist was initially uncomfortable in establishing a diagnosis due to the lack of cytologic atypia. Negative staining for high molecular

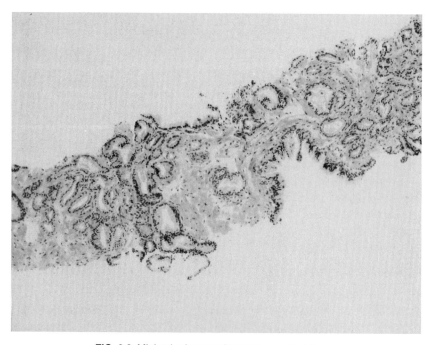

FIG. 6.9 Minimal adenocarcinoma on needle biopsy.

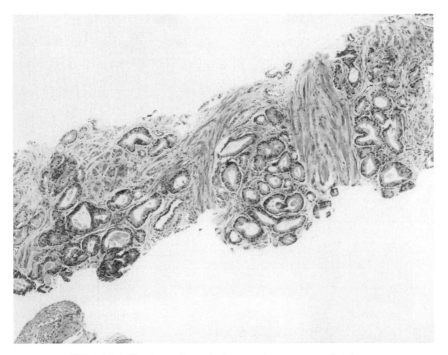

FIG. 6.10. Infiltrative pattern of adenocarcinoma on needle biopsy.

weight cytokeratin in these small glands along with the pattern lead to a definitive diagnosis of malignancy (Color Plate 19). The use of high molecular weight cytokeratin when presented with only a few atypical glands is not as diagnostic, since benign glands may not show uniform positivity with this marker (18). Negative staining for high molecular weight cytokeratin is most diagnostic when more than a few glands are present for evaluation and the morphologic features are very suspicious for carcinoma. Rather than used to establish a diagnosis of cancer, we use the high molecular weight cytokeratin stain to help verify a suspicious focus as cancer (19–24). If we favor a focus as benign and the stain is negative, we will diagnose it as atypical rather than as cancer (see Chapter 10). Figure 6.10 is another example of cancer diagnosable based on an infiltrative pattern with groups of small glands separated by bands of smooth muscle.

CARCINOMAS MIMICKING BENIGN GLANDS

Just as there are benign mimickers of prostate cancer (Chapter 7) , some cancers closely resemble benign prostate glands in their architectural pattern and may not be recognized as malignant.

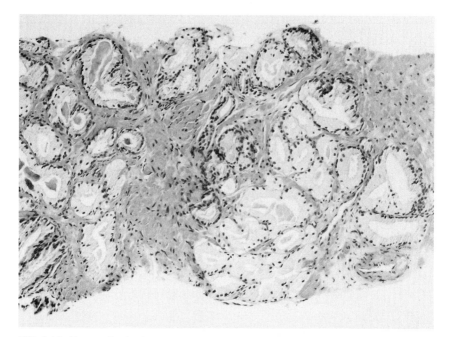

FIG. 6.11. Foamy-gland adenocarcinoma at low power with crowded pale-staining glands.

Foamy gland cancer must be recognized as carcinoma by its abundant foamy cytoplasm, its architectural pattern of crowded and/or infiltrative glands, and frequently present pink acellular secretions (25) (Figs. 6.11 and 6.12, Color Plate 20, efig 432;433-435;436-438;439-441;442-443;444-445;446-448;449-450;451-453;454;455-456;457;458;459-461). Although the cytoplasm has a xanthomatous appearance, it does not contain lipid, but rather empty vacuoles (26). More typical features of adenocarcinoma such as nuclear enlargement and prominent nucleoli are frequently absent, which makes this lesion difficult to recognize as carcinoma. Despite its benign cytology, 96% of the cases when there is an associated nonfoamy cancer it is Gleason score >4, such that foamy gland carcinoma appears best classified as intermediate-grade carcinoma. In foamy gland carcinoma the cytoplasm is copious with nuclei occupying <10% of the cell height. Characteristically, the nuclei in foamy gland carcinoma are small, round, and densely hyperchromatic. The nuclei in foamy gland carcinoma are actually rounder than those of benign prostatic secretory cells.

Atrophic prostate cancers are rare and may be present on needle biopsy, usually unassociated with a prior history of hormonal therapy (27,28). The diagnosis of carcinoma in these cases is made on (a) a truly infiltrative process

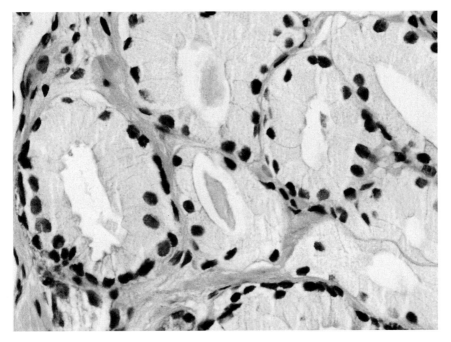

FIG. 6.12. High magnification of foamy-gland carcinoma showing abundant xanthomatous cytoplasm and small, round, benign-appearing nuclei.

with individual small atrophic glands situated between larger benign glands; (b) the concomitant presence of ordinary less atrophic carcinoma; and (c) greater cytologic atypia than is seen in benign atrophy (Fig. 6.13) (efig 462-464;465-466;467-468;469-470;471-473;474-475;476;477-478;479-481;482-283;484-485;486-488;489-491;492-493;494-495;496-498;499-501;502-503; 504-505;506-507).

Pseudohyperplastic prostate cancer is characterized by the presence of larger glands with branching and papillary infolding (29,30) (Figs. 6.14 and 6.15, efig 508-513;514-518;519-523;524-526;527-529;530-532;533-535; 536-540;541-543;544-545;546-549;550-554;555-558;559-561;562-564;565-566;567-570;571-572;573-575;576-580). The recognition of cancer with this pattern is based on the architectural pattern of numerous closely packed glands as well as nuclear features more typical of carcinoma. A variant of pseudohyperplastic adenocarcinoma composed of markedly dilated glands with abundant cytoplasm may be particularly difficult to recognize as malignant. This form of cancer can be recognized by the appearance of numerous large glands that are almost back-to-back with straight even luminal borders, and abundant cytoplasm. Comparably sized benign glands either have papil-

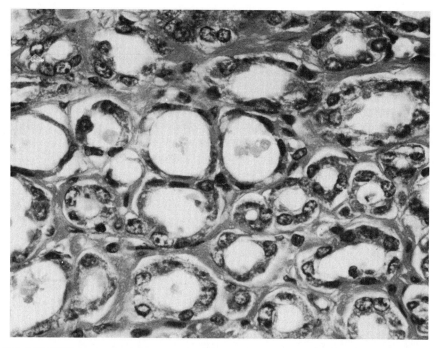

FIG. 6.13. While some glands have an atrophic appearance with bland nuclei, in others, nuclear features are more recognizably malignant with large nuclei and visible nucleoli. ×520.

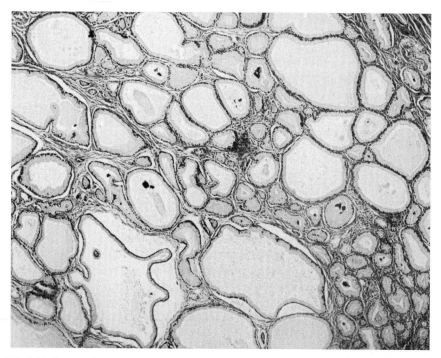

FIG. 6.14. Low-grade carcinoma composed of large, uniform, open pale-staining glands. Note the lace of papillary infolding in the large glands as opposed to benign hyperplastic glands. ×45.

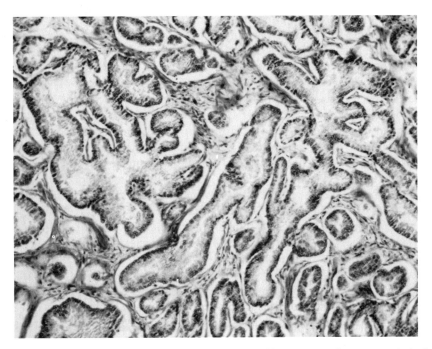

FIG. 6.15. Infiltrating adenocarcinoma with complex branching pattern, a feature more typically seen in benign glands. ×110.

lary infoldings or are atrophic. The presence of cytologic atypia in some of these glands further distinguishes them from benign glands. It is almost always helpful to verify pseudohyperplastic cancer with the use of immuno- histochemistry for high molecular weight cytokeratin. As with foamy gland cancer, pseudohyperplastic cancer, despite its benign appearance, may be associated with intermediate grade cancer and can exhibit aggressive behav- ior (i.e., extraprostatic extension).

DIAGNOSIS ON TRANSURETHRAL RESECTION

Whereas nuclear features play a prominent role in the diagnosis of adenocar- cinoma of the prostate on needle biopsy material, they are often not as helpful in diagnosing low-grade adenocarcinoma on transurethral resection specimens. Often low-grade adenocarcinomas of the prostate lack enlarged nuclei and prominent nucleoli, and mitoses are rarely found (31). Cytoplasmic features are often not very helpful since they are often pale-clear, similar to benign glands. The most useful feature in diagnosing low-grade adenocarcinoma on transurethral resection material is the recognition of cancer's architectural growth pattern as seen at relatively low magnification.

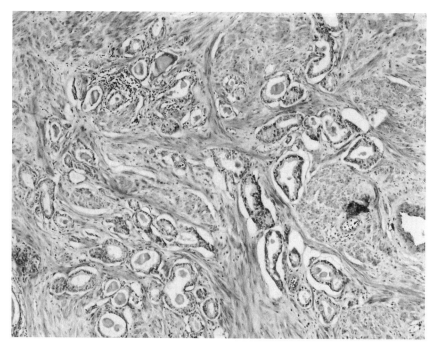

FIG. 6.19. Infiltrative appearance of low-grade adenocarcinoma.

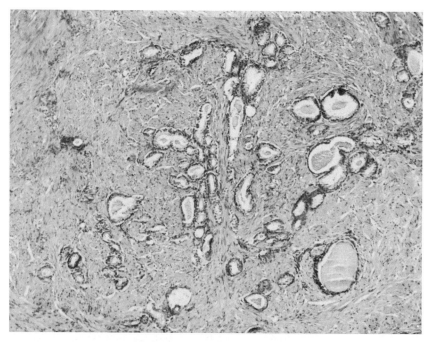

FIG. 6.20. Glands of low-grade adenocarcinoma of the prostate infiltrating in different directions into the prostatic stroma. ×60.

Many of the following illustrated examples are somewhat repetitive in that they demonstrate the same abnormal growth pattern of low-grade prostate carcinoma. This repetition is intentional since it is difficult to convey with words concepts such as "infiltrative," "haphazard," or "growing in an irregular fashion," features which are better depicted by numerous visual examples (efig 581-583;584-585;586-587;588-589;590-591;592-593;594-595; 596;597-599;600-601;602-603;604-605;606-609;610-611;612-613;614).

Benign prostatic glands tend to grow either as circumscribed nodules within benign prostatic hyperplasia or radiate in columns out from the urethra in a linear fashion. In contrast, adenocarcinoma of the prostate grows in a haphazard fashion. Although low-grade carcinoma tends to be fairly well circumscribed, the glands infiltrate for a short distance in different directions out into the prostatic stroma (Figs. 6.16–6.22:, Color Plate 21). Glands oriented perpendicular to each other and glands separated by bundles of smooth muscle are indicative of an infiltrative process. Another feature used to diagnose adenocarcinoma of the prostate is the appearance of glands splitting the muscle fibers in an infiltrative fashion (Fig. 6.23). In Figure 6.24, glands of adenocarcinoma of the prostate infiltrate among and split small bundles of smooth muscle fibers in an irregular fashion. Although this pattern is suggestive of adenocarcinoma, occasionally benign glands can also be seen in between large smooth muscle bundles (Fig. 6.25). Another feature asso-

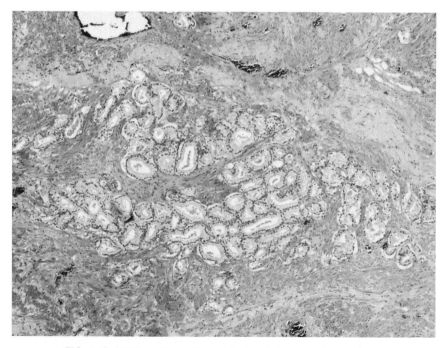

FIG. 6.16. Haphazard growth pattern of low-grade adenocarcinoma.

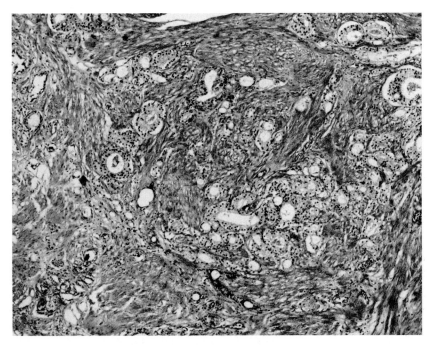

FIG. 6.17. Irregular growth pattern of low-grade prostatic adenocarcinoma (from Kramer and Epstein, ref. 23, with permission). Antibodies to high molecular weight cytokeratin demonstrated a lack of basal cells, verifying the diagnosis.

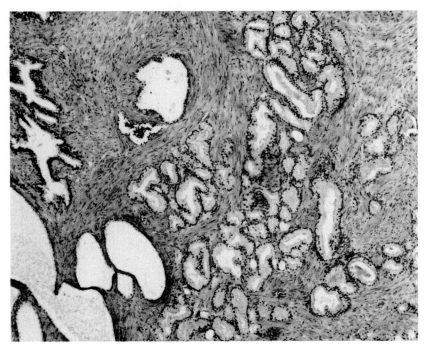

FIG. 6.18. Low-grade adenocarcinoma infiltrating in different directions contrasted with adjacent benign atrophic glands *(left).*

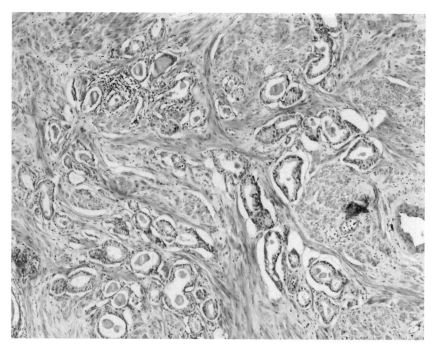

FIG. 6.19. Infiltrative appearance of low-grade adenocarcinoma.

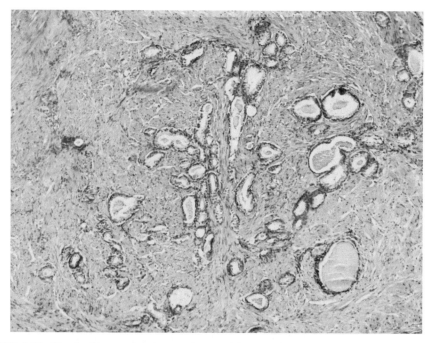

FIG. 6.20. Glands of low-grade adenocarcinoma of the prostate infiltrating in different directions into the prostatic stroma. ×60.

84

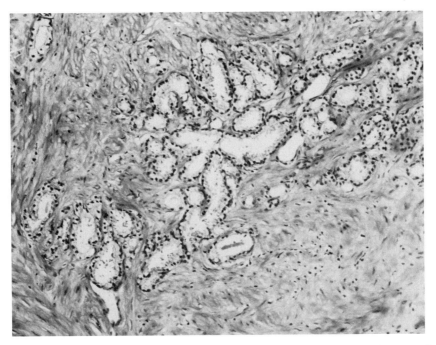

FIG. 6.21. Low-grade adenocarcinoma extending in different directions into the prostatic stroma, lacking the linear circumscribed lobular pattern seen with benign glands. ×125.

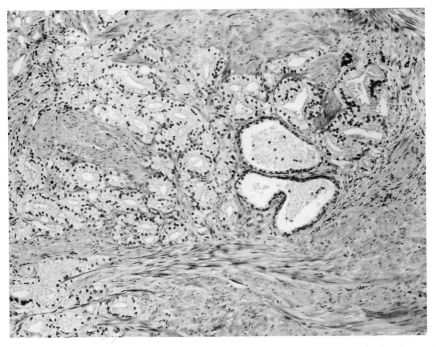

FIG. 6.22. Low-grade adenocarcinoma splitting smooth-muscle bundle. Neoplastic glands stand out in contrast to adjacent larger to benign atrophic glands.

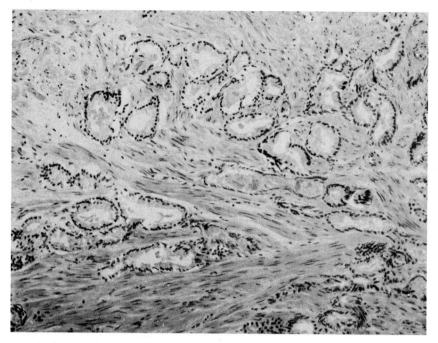

FIG. 6.23. Glands of adenocarcinoma splitting and streaming through the smooth muscle of the prostate. ×115.

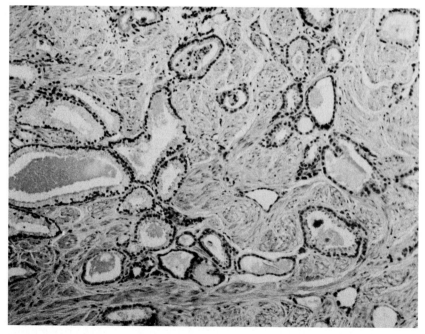

FIG. 6.24. Adenocarcinoma of the prostate infiltrating in and among bundles of smooth muscle. ×115.

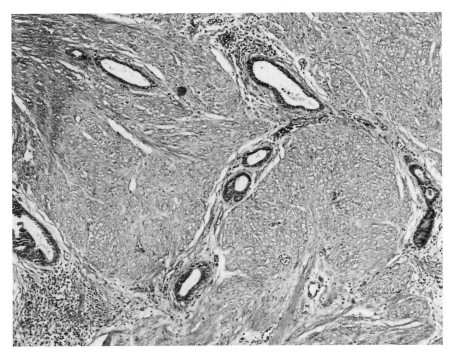

FIG. 6.25. Benign glands situated in between larger smooth-muscle bundles.

ciated with cancer is that some of the vessels among the cancer may show a proliferation of cells resembling glomus cells (32) (efig 615).

In some cases, comparison of the neoplastic glands to the surrounding benign
glands is helpful in that there are certain features that are more frequent in adenocarcinoma as compared to benign glands. These features have been discussed
earlier in the chapter and are listed in Table 6.3. Glands of adenocarcinoma of
the prostate tend to have a discrete crisp, sharp luminal border without undula-
tions or ruffling of the cytoplasm (Fig. 6.14). In contrast, equivalently sized
benign glands have a ragged luminal surface with small papillary infoldings and
a convoluted appearance (Fig. 6.26). The finding of apical snouts is not helpful
in distinguishing benign versus malignant glands as they can be seen in both. As
with all carcinomas, low-grade carcinomas have only a single cell layer without
a basal cell layer. A true basal cell layer must be distinguished from an artifactual two-cell layer in carcinoma due to either tangential sectioning, thick sections, or adjacent fibroblasts.

High molecular weight cytokeratin identification of basal cells is sometimes
more diagnostic on transurethral resection, as there are a greater number of glands
available for evaluation (efig 616-619). Because occasional benign glands fail to
express immunoreactivity with antibodies to high molecular weight cytokeratin,

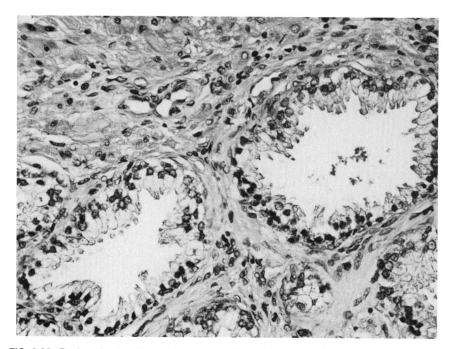

FIG. 6.26. Benign glands with undulation and ruffling of the luminal border, giving it an irregular, convoluted appearance. ×300.

caution must be exercised in interpreting a negative result in a small focus of atypical glands. However, when a large number of glands as seen in Color Plate 21 completely lack immunoreactivity to high molecular weight cytokeratin, that would be highly unusual for a benign condition and is strong supporting evidence for the diagnosis of adenocarcinoma. Cautery can also result in false negative staining for high molecular weight cytokeratin. Before interpreting a negative result of high molecular weight cytokeratin staining as diagnostic of cancer, there should be benign glands on the same chip that are immunoreactive as an internal positive control.

A problem unique to material removed by transurethral resection is cautery artifact (efig 620-621, Color Plate 22). Extensive cautery artifact in a suspicious focus may prevent a definitive diagnosis of carcinoma. However, even in some cases with extensive cautery artifact, the presence of solid sheets of cells with high nuclear to cytoplasmic ratios and hyperchromatism could be nothing else but that of carcinoma (Fig. 6.27). There are also some cases of better differentiated gland forming carcinomas with extensive cautery artifact that, based on a pattern of numerous back-to-back glands, is also diagnostic of carcinoma. The presence of extensive cautery artifact is also one of the few situations where immunohistochemistry for PSA or PSAP may help in establishing the diagnosis of prostatic adenocarcinoma. Occasionally, cellular cauterized hyperchromatic cells are seen encircling a prostatic nerve (Fig. 6.28). Immunohistochemistry

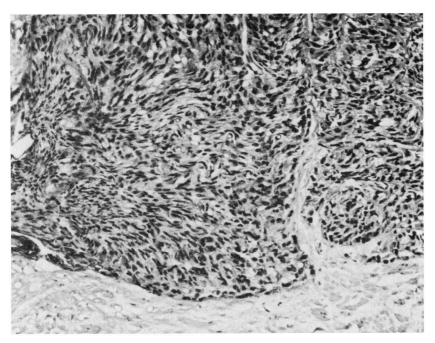

FIG. 6.27. Cauterized sheet of adenocarcinoma. ×165.

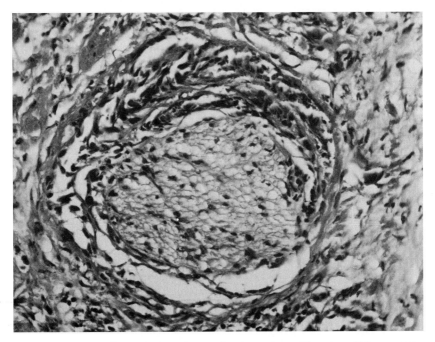

FIG. 6.28 Cauterized carcinoma showing perineural invasion. ×300.

with PSA and PSAP can identify these cells as being of prostatic origin, and thus diagnostic of prostatic carcinoma. PSA and PSAP may also facilitate the diagnosis of prostatic adenocarcinoma in the setting of cauterized high-grade carcinoma composed of infiltrating individual cells. While the finding of individual cells are suspicious for cancer, the lack of good cytologic detail may make it difficult to definitively identify them as epithelial, stromal, or inflammatory. If these individual cells infiltrating throughout the stroma are positive for PSA or PSAP, the diagnosis of infiltrating poorly differentiated adenocarcinoma is established.

REFERENCES

1. Kronz JD, Milord R, Wilentz R, et al. Lesions missed on prostate biopsies by pathologists. *Mod Pathol* 2001;14:114A.
2. Griffiths RC, Epstein JI. Review of prostate needle biopsies by an expert. *Mod Pathol* 2001;14:110A.
3. Helpap B. Observations on the number, size, and location of nucleoli in hyperplastic and neoplastic prostatic diseases. *Histopathology* 1988;13:203–211.
4. Holmes E. Crystalloids of prostatic carcinoma: relationship to Bence-Jones crystals. *Cancer* 1977; 39:2073–2080.
5. Ro JY, Ayala AG, Ordonez NG, Cartwright J, Mackay B. Intraluminal crystalloids in prostatic adenocarcinoma: immunohistochemical, electron microscopic, and x-ray microanalytic studies. *Cancer* 1986;57:2397–2407.
6. Henneberry JM, Kahane H, Epstein JI. The significance of intraluminal crystalloids in prostatic glands on needle biopsy. *Am J Surg Pathol* 1997;21:725–728.
7. Epstein JI. Diagnostic criteria of limited adenocarcinoma of the prostate on needle biopsy. *Hum Pathol* 1995;26:233–239.
8. Brennick JB, O'Connel JX, Dickersin GR, et al. Lipofuscin pigmentation (so-called "melanosis") of the prostate. *Am J Surg Pathol* 1994;18:446–454.
9. Epstein JI, Fynheer J. Acidic mucin in the prostate: Can it differentiate adenosis from adenocarcinoma? *Hum Pathol* 1992;23:1321–1325.
10. Goldstein NS, Qian J, Bostwick DG. Mucin expression in atypical adenomatous hyperplasia if the prostate. *Hum Pathol* 1995;26:887–891.
11. Humphrey PA, Vollmer RT. Corpora amylacea in adenocarcinoma of the prostate: prevalence in 100 prostatectomies and clinicopathologic correlations. *Surg Pathol* 1990;3:133–141.
12. McNeal JE, Alroy J, Villers A, et al. Mucinous differentiation in prostatic adenocarcinoma. *Hum Pathol* 1991;22:979–988.
13. Baisden BL, Kahane H, Epstein JI. Perineural invasion, mucinous fibroplasia and glomerulations: diagnostic features of limited cancer on prostate needle biopsy. *Am J Surg Pathol* 1999;23:918–924.
14. Bastacky SI, Walsh PC, Epstein JI. Relationship between perineural tumor invasion on needle biopsy and radical prostatectomy capsular penetration in clinical stage B adenocarcinoma of the prostate. *Am J Surg Pathol* 1993;17:336–341.
15. Carstens PHB. Perineural glands in normal and hyperplastic prostates. *J Urol* 1980;123:686–688.
16. McIntyre TL, Frazini DA. The presence of benign prostatic glands in perineural spaces. *J Urol* 1986;135:507–509.
17. Yang XJ, Lecksell K, Epstein JI. The significance of small foci of high grade prostate cancer on needle biopsy. *Urology* 1999;54:528–532.
18. Goldstein NS, Underhill J, Roszka J, et al. Cytokeratin 34 beta E-12 immunoreactivity in benign prostatic acini. Quantitation, pattern assessment, and electron microscopic study. *Am J Clin Pathol* 1999; 112:69–74.
19. Wojno KJ, Epstein JI. The utility of basal cell specific anti-cytokeratin antibody (34 beta E12) in the diagnosis of prostate cancer: a review of 228 cases. *Am J Surg Pathol* 1195;19:251–260.
20. Hedrick L, Epstein JI. Use of keratin 903 as an adjunct in the diagnosis of prostate carcinoma. *Am J Surg Pathol* 1989;13:389–396.
21. O'Malley FP, Grignon DJ, Shum DT. Usefulness of immunoperoxidase staining with high-molecu-

lar-weight cytokeratin in the differential diagnosis of small-acinar lesions of the prostate gland. *Virchows Arch A Pathol Anat Histopathol* 1990;417:191–196.

22. Shah IA, Schlageter MO, Stinnett P, et al. Cytokeratin immunohistochemistry as a diagnostic tool for distinguishing malignant from benign epithelial lesions of the prostate. *Mod Pathol* 1991;4:220–224.

23. Brawer MK, Peehl DM, Stamey TA, et al. Keratin immunoreactivity in the benign and neoplastic human prostate. *Cancer Res* 1985;45:3663–3667.

24. Nagle RB, Ahmann FR, McDaniel KM, et al. Cytokeratin characterization of human prostatic carcinoma and its derived cell lines. *Cancer Res* 1987;47:281–286.

25. Nelson RS, Epstein JI. Prostatic carcinoma with abundant xanthomatous cytoplasm: foamy gland carcinoma. *Am J Surg Pathol* 1996;20:419–426.

26. Tran TT, Sengupta E, Yang XJ. Prostatic foamy gland carcinoma with aggressive behavior: Clinicopathologic, immunohistochemical, and ultrastructural analysis. *Am J Surg Pathol* 2001;25:618–623.

27. Cina SJ, Epstein JI. Adenocarcinoma of the prostate with atrophic features. *Am J Surg Pathol* 1997; 21:289–295.

28. Egan AJM, Lopez-Beltran A, Bostwick DG. Prostatic adenocarcinoma with atrophic features: malignancy mimicking a benign process. *Am J Surg Pathol* 1997;21:931–935.

29. Levi AW, Epstein JI. Pseudohyperplastic prostatic adenocarcinoma on needle biopsy and simple prostatectomy. *Am J Surg Pathol* 2000;24:1039–1046.

30. Humphrey PA, Kaleem Z, Swanson PE, et al. Pseudohyperplastic prostatic adenocarcinoma. *Am J Surg Pathol* 1998;22:1239–46.

31. Kramer CE, Epstein JI. Nucleoli in low-grade prostate adenocarcinoma and adenosis. *Hum Pathol* 1993;24:618–623.

32. Garcia FU, Taylor CA, Hou JS. Increased cellularity of tumor-encased native vessels in prostate carcinoma is a marker for tumor progression. *Mod Pathol* 2000;13:717–722.

7

Mimickers of Adenocarcinoma of the Prostate

MIMICKERS OF GLEASON SCORE 2-6 ADENOCARCINOMA

Adenosis

There are several mimickers of Gleason 2–6 adenocarcinoma (Table 7.1. One of the most common lesions that may be confused with carcinoma is adenosis (1–3). The other commonly used term for adenosis is "atypical adenomatous hyperplasia (AAH)." We prefer the term "adenosis," as prefacing "adenomatous hyperplasia" with "atypical" has adverse consequences both in terms of practical patient management and in our theoretical framework of this entity. As outlined below, there are very little data in support of a relation between adenosis and carcinoma. By designating these lesions as "atypical," many patients will be subjected to unnecessary repeat biopsies. Conceptually, as has happened in the past, use of the term "atypical adenomatous hyperplasia" will result in this entity being considered with PIN as precursors to carcinoma of the prostate. Whereas there is strong evidence that prostatic intraepithelial neoplasia (PIN) is a precursor to some prostate cancers, this evidence is lacking in adenosis.

TABLE 7.1. *Benign mimickers of Gleason score 2–6 adenocarcinoma*

Entity	Predominant mode of sampling
Atrophy	TURP = Needle
Cowper's glands	TURP = Needle
Radiation atypia	TURP = Needle
Adenosis	TURP > Needle
Basal cell hyperplasia	TURP > Needle
Nephrogenic adenoma	TURP >> Needle
Seminal vesicles	Needle > TURP
Verumontanum hyperplasia	Needle > TURP
Mesonephric hyperplasia	TURP
Colonic mucosa	Needle

There is a wide spectrum in the literature in terms of the reported incidence of adenosis on transurethral resection of the prostate (TURP), ranging from 2.2% to 19.6% (4,5). The reason for this broad range is different thresholds for diagnosing a focus of crowded glands as adenosis. Included within the lower threshold are prostate specimens with foci of crowded glands, which could be considered a minimal example of adenosis, although they do not closely mimic adenocarcinoma. At the other extreme, seen in 1.6% of benign TURPs performed at The Johns Hopkins Hospital, adenosis closely mimics adenocarcinoma of the prostate. The diagnosis of adenosis should be restricted to cases with a sufficiently atypical growth pattern that one has to seriously consider the diagnosis of low-grade cancer. This gradual spectrum within adenosis from a crowded focus of obviously benign glands to lesions that share similar features, yet more closely resemble cancer, supports the concept that adenosis is a hyperplastic rather than neoplastic lesion. As adenosis preferentially occurs within the transition zone, it is more frequently seen on TURP as an incidental finding than on needle biopsy. However, in approximately 0.8% of needle biopsies, adenosis may be identified. This incidence is infrequent enough that many pathologists do not consider it in the differential diagnosis of small glandular lesions on needle biopsy. However, the frequency of adenosis on needle biopsy is sufficiently high that there is a good chance that one will see this lesion in one's practice with the potential to overdiagnose it as adenocarcinoma.

The distinction of adenosis from low-grade adenocarcinoma is based on architectural and cytologic features (Table 7.2). In order to minimize misdiagnoses, the constellation of histologic features seen in a lesion should outweigh the significance of any one diagnostic feature (efig 622-626;627-631;632-637;638-640;641-645;646-650;651-654;655-659;660-661;662-664;665-667;668-671;672-674;675-676). At scanning magnification, adenosis is characterized by a lobular proliferation of small glands (Figs. 7.1–7.5). In contrast, low-grade car-

TABLE 7.2. *Diagnostic criteria for adenosis*

Adenosis	Low-grade carcinoma
Features seen at low and intermediate magnification	
Lobular growth	May be infiltrative/haphazard
Small crowded glands admixed with larger glands	May be pure population of small crowded glands
Features seen at high magnification	
Huge (>3 micron) nucleoli absent	Occasionally huge nucleoli present
Small glands share cytoplasmic and nuclear features with admixed larger benign glands	Small glands differ from surrounding benign glands in cytoplasmic and/or nuclear features
Pale-clear cytoplasm	May have amphophilic cytoplasm
Blue-tinged mucinous secretions rare	Blue-tinged mucinous secretions common
Corpora amylacea common	Corpora amylacea rare
Occasional glands with basal cells	Basal cells absent
Basal cell–specific antikeratin antibodies label basal cells in some small glands	Small glands are not immunoreactive with basal cell–specific antikeratin antibodies

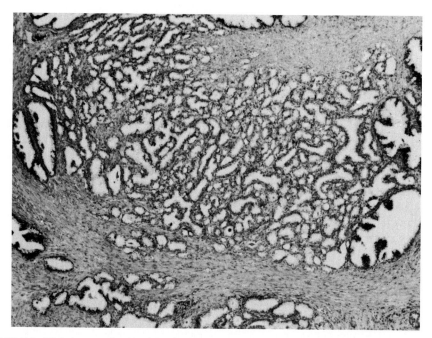

FIG. 7.1. Well-circumscribed nodule of adenosis. Note intermingled among small glands suspicious for carcinoma, larger elongated glands with occasional branching more typical of benign glands, yet similar in their nuclear and cytoplasmic features to the small glands. ×45.

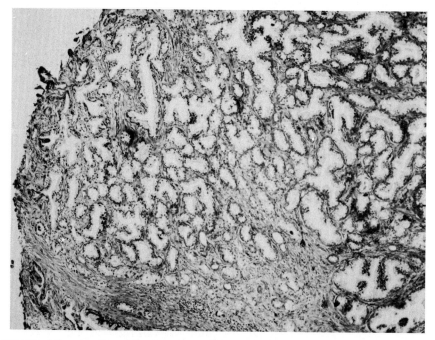

FIG. 7.2. Adenosis with small pale-staining glands suspicious for carcinoma *(left)* merging with larger, more irregular glands that appear benign *(right)*. ×55.

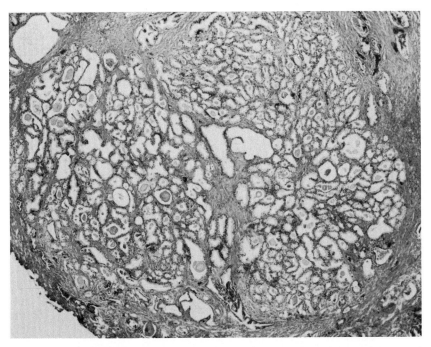

FIG. 7.3. Well-circumscribed nodule of adenosis with scattered, large, benign-appearing glands, in and among similar-appearing smaller glands suspicious for carcinoma. ×35.

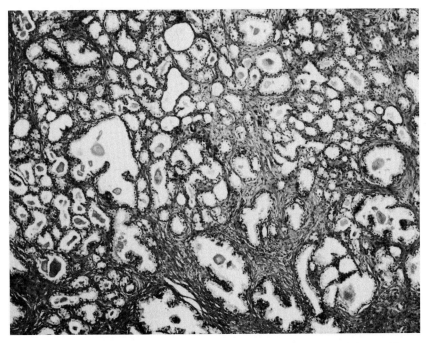

FIG. 7.4. Adenosis with numerous small glands with pale-to-clear cytoplasm. ×55.

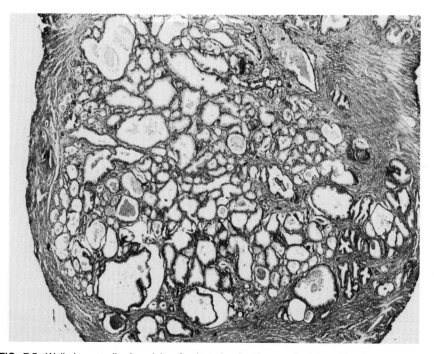

FIG. 7.5. Well-circumscribed nodule of adenosis showing gradual transition between small pale-staining glands suspicious for cancer to larger, more irregular-shaped benign-appearing glands. ×75.

cinoma has a haphazard, irregular, infiltrative growth pattern (see Figs. 6.16–6.21). Despite the overall lobular pattern seen in adenosis, 19% of cases reveal minimal infiltration of glands into the surrounding stroma (Figs. 7.1 and 7.6).

Probably the most important differentiating feature of adenosis seen on hemoxylin and eosin (H&E) stain is that within a nodule of adenosis there are elongated glands with papillary infolding and branching lumina typical of more benign glands, yet in their nuclear and cytoplasmic features they look similar to the adjacent small glands suspicious for carcinoma (Figs. 7.7 and 7.8). Another common feature seen is the budding off of glands of adenosis from obviously benign glands (Fig. 7.9). Glands of adenocarcinoma, even in the unusual case when the tumor is fairly lobular, shows a pure population of small crowded glands without benign architectural features that do not merge in with adjacent larger benign glands (Fig. 7.10).

At higher power, adenosis is typically composed of small glands with pale to clear cytoplasm, as opposed to some carcinomas, which have more amphophilic cytoplasm (Figs. 7.11–7.13). In order for this feature to be diag-

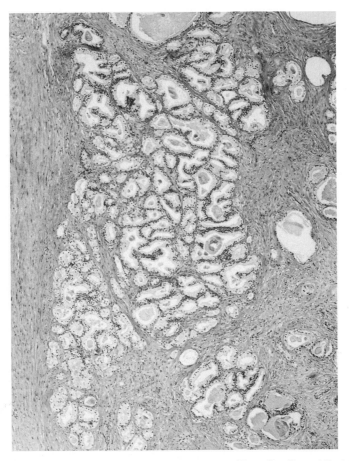

FIG. 7.6. Adenosis with minimal infiltration at its perimeter. (From Gaudin and Epstein, ref. 1, with permission.) Antibodies to high molecular weight cytokeratin demonstrated basal cells, verifying the diagnosis.

nostically useful, the cytoplasm of benign prostate glands should appear pale or clear on routinely stained slides. A diagnosis of carcinoma should not be rendered based on what appears to be either a few individual cells or poorly formed glands within a nodule that is otherwise typical of adenosis. Occasional single cells or poorly formed glands are not uncommon in a nodule of adenosis and probably represent tangential sections of small glands (Table 7.3).

Usually, adenosis has been described as having totally bland appearing nuclei without nucleoli. This is generally valid; most (60%) lesions contain no or at most rare prominent nucleoli. In the other 40%, fairly prominent (>1.6

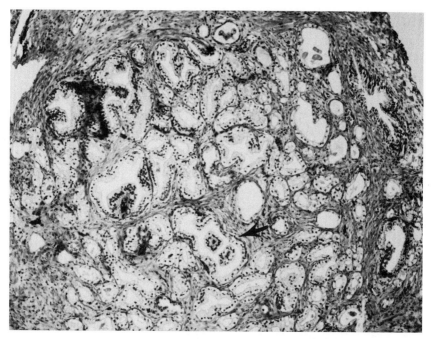

FIG. 7.7. Adenosis. Note gland with small papillary projections typical of a benign gland *(arrow)* with the same nuclear and cytoplasmic features of surrounding small glands. ×55.

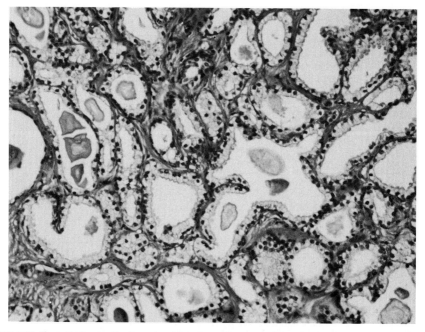

FIG. 7.8. Typical glands of adenosis with pale-to-clear cytoplasm containing scattered, irregularly shaped, more benign-appearing glands. ×160.

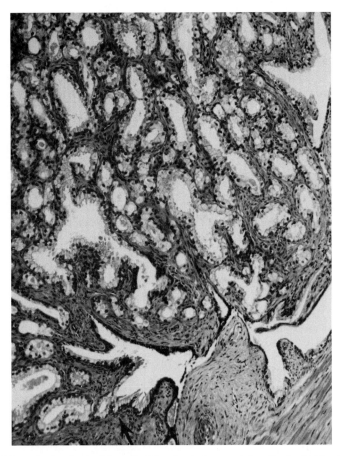

FIG. 7.9. Adenosis showing budding off of the glands from peripherally situated benign-appearing glands *(arrow).* ×145.

microns) nucleoli are present, which should not lead to the diagnosis of carcinoma (Fig. 7.14) (6). In another study, 18% contained nucleoli larger than 1 micron (3). Only huge nucleoli (>3 microns) are incompatible with a diagnosis of adenosis (Fig. 7.15). In contrast, the majority (70%) of foci of low-grade adenocarcinoma have occasional or frequent large nucleoli. The remaining low-grade carcinomas have either no prominent or at most rare prominent nucleoli (Fig. 7.16). These findings emphasize that, although nucleoli are generally helpful in differentiating adenosis from adenocarcinoma, there is overlap between the two entities.

The luminal contents also may be useful in this differential diagnosis. Corpora amylacea are commonly seen in adenosis, and are rare in carcinoma. Only 2% of cases of adenosis contain blue intraluminal secretions visible on H&E-stained

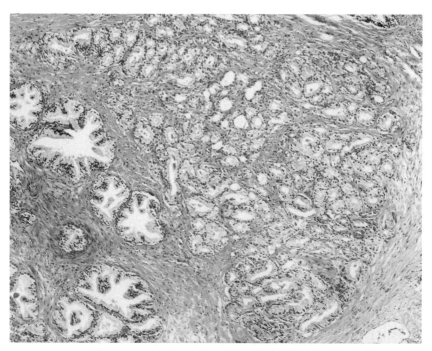

FIG. 7.10. Lobular pattern of adenocarcinoma. Note lack of merging in of small glands with adjacent larger benign glands *(left)*.

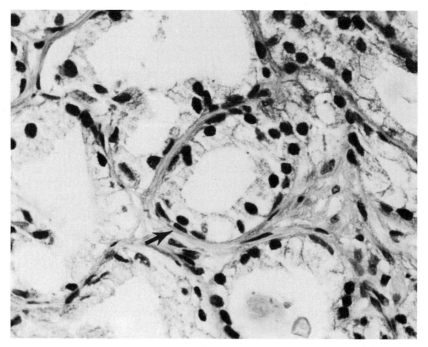

FIG. 7.11. High magnification of glands of adenosis showing focally identifiable basal cell layer *(arrow)*. ×575.

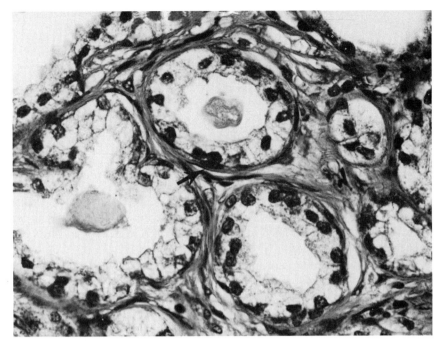

FIG. 7.12. High magnification of adenosis showing focal basal cell layer *(arrow)*. Compare to stromal fibroblasts with elongated nuclei having pointed edges. ×550.

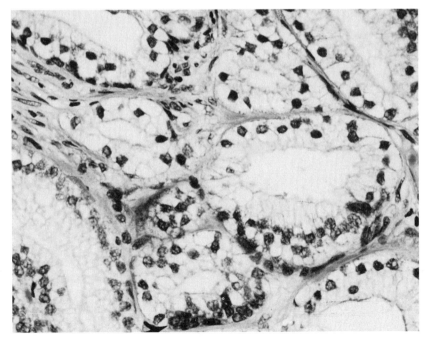

FIG. 7.13. Glands of adenosis with focal areas of piling up of the basal cell layer *(arrow)*. ×370.

TABLE 7.3. *Nondiagnostic features in adenosis and carcinoma*

Features shared in adenosis and cancer

Crowded (back-to-back glands)
Intraluminal crystalloids
Medium-sized (<3 microns) nucleoli
Scattered poorly formed glands and single cells
Minimal infiltration at periphery of nodule

sections, a feature common in low-grade carcinomas. It is not helpful to perform special stains for mucin. Despite earlier studies' claims that acid mucin was diagnostic of carcinoma, a later work found that 54% of foci of adenosis contained acid mucin secretions (7).

Crystalloids are intraluminal structures that have been touted as distinguishing adenosis from carcinoma. However, 18% to 39% of foci of adenosis contain crystalloids, sometimes in great number. Crystalloids should not be used to differentiate adenosis and carcinoma (Table 7.3).

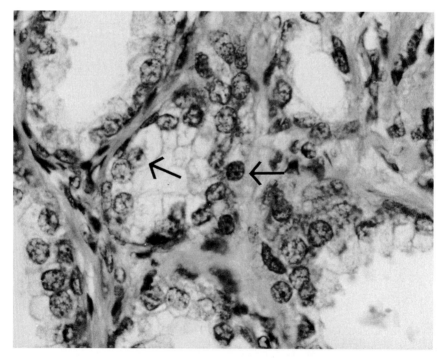

FIG. 7.14. Adenosis with prominent nucleoli *(arrows)*. (From Kramer and Epstein, ref. 6, with permission.)

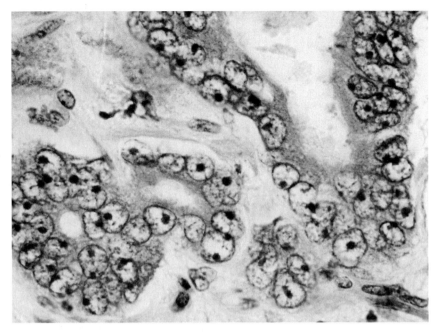

FIG. 7.15. Atypical glands with huge nucleoli, diagnostic of adenocarcinoma.

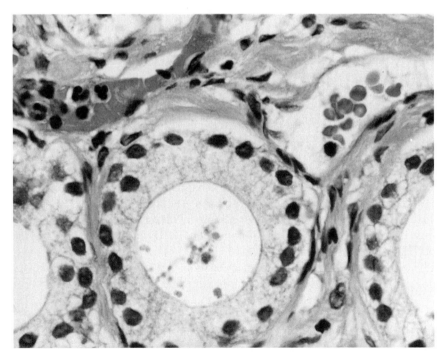

FIG. 7.16. Low-grade adenocarcinoma (high magnification of Fig. 6.17) with benign-appearing nuclei. (From Kramer and Epstein, ref. 6, with permission.)

The presence of basal cells is the one feature seen in adenosis that is typically not seen in carcinoma. Although basal cells may be difficult to identify within many of the glands, a flattened basal cell layer can be seen in at least some of the glands. As long as the glands with a basal cell layer are otherwise identical to the glands where a basal cell layer can not be identified, then the entire lesion is benign. It is important to distinguish basal cells from adjacent fibroblasts. While fibroblasts have elongated pointed hyperchromatic nuclei, basal cell nuclei that are recognizable in routine sections have a more cigar-shaped ovoid contour with chromatin similar to that of the overlying secretory cells (Figs. 7.14–7.16). Basal cells may sometimes be apparent as a cluster of cells with scant cytoplasm polarized at the edge of a gland. In foci of glandular crowding where all of the features are typical of adenosis and there is no cytologic atypia, adenosis can be diagnosed without immunohistochemical stains even if basal cells are not visible on routine sections.

In cases where the architectural pattern favors adenosis yet there are visible nucleoli, the diagnosis can be clarified using immunohistochemistry for basal cells. The use of a basal cell specific antibody to high molecular weight keratin is helpful since some glands will show a thin rim of keratin immunoreactivity beneath the cuboidal or columnar secretory cells (1,2,8). As few as 10% of the glands in a nodule of adenosis may be labeled with antibodies to high molecular keratin, although usually more than half of the glands will show some staining. The stain is also patchy within a given gland, with sometimes only one to two basal cells identified (Color Plate 23). If some glands suspicious for adenosis lack high molecular weight cytokeratin immunoreactivity, yet are otherwise indistinguishable from adjacent glands which demonstrate basal cell keratin immunoreactivity, the absence of a basal cell layer in some glands should not be used to diagnose the lesion as carcinoma. Some of the variability in basal cell immunoreactivity within adenosis and other lesions may be caused by tissue fixation since more uniform immunoreactivity has been observed in frozen tissue.

Adenosis often appears to be multifocal. In a few cases on TURP, foci are so numerous that, if misdiagnosed as carcinoma, they would be classified as stage T1b, leading to unwarranted radical therapy. The distinction between adenosis and low-grade adenocarcinoma in even a single focus may be critical, since diagnosis of even a single focus of carcinoma on TURP in a relatively young man may lead to aggressive surgery.

The diagnosis of adenosis on needle biopsy is more difficult, since it is more difficult to appreciate the architectural pattern on needle biopsy (efig 677-679;680-681;682-684;685-688;689-692;693-695;696-698;699-702;703-704;705-708;709-712;713-714;715-718;719-722;723-724;725-727). In a study of 77 foci of adenosis on needle biopsy, adenosis on needle biopsy appeared as a relatively well localized nodule of closely packed glands with pale to clear cytoplasm (Figs. 7.17–7.18)(2). In only 7% of foci was the entire

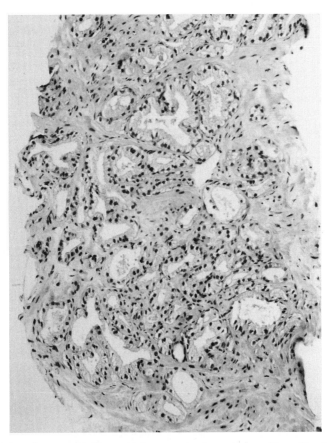

FIG. 7.17. Adenosis on needle biopsy. Note some glands are larger with papillary infolding, yet similar to surrounding smaller glands.

lobular lesion visualized on needle biopsy. In 45% of foci, one edge of the nodule could be appreciated and was circumscribed; yet the other side was not visible since the lesion was bisected by one edge of the needle biopsy (Fig. 7.19). The remaining 48% of foci were transected in the middle of the nodule of adenosis such that the lesion extended to both edges of the needle biopsy (Figs. 7.20–7.23). Although in these cases assessment of circumscription was difficult, in all but three cases the foci of adenosis occupied a small portion of the core length. In three cases, adenosis occupied >3 mm of the core length. Other than not having an entire nodule available for evaluation, the histologic features of adenosis on needle biopsy are the same as on TURP. On needle biopsy, due to the limited number of glands in question, basal cell specific antibodies must be interpreted with caution. Because basal cell staining

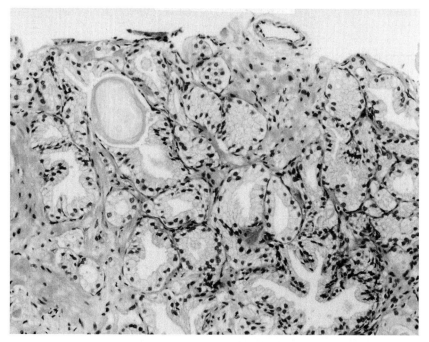

FIG. 7.18. Adenosis on needle biopsy. Note several benign glands with papillary infoldings and corpora amylacea merging in with smaller crowded glands sharing similar cytologic features.

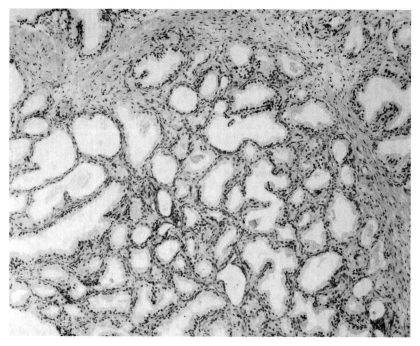

FIG. 7.19. Adenosis on needle biopsy. Note lobular organization with larger, more benign-appearing glands merging in with smaller crowded glands.

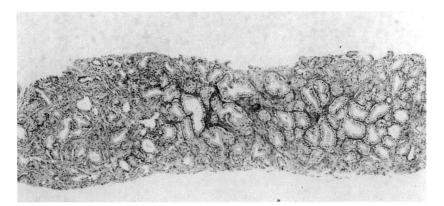

FIG. 7.20. One of the few cases of extensive adenosis on needle biopsy. Antibodies to high molecular weight cytokeratin demonstrated basal cells, verifying the diagnosis.

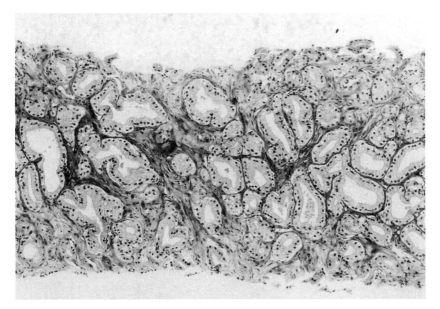

FIG. 7.21. Higher magnification of Fig. 7.20. Note more benign-appearing glands *(left)* merging in with glands suspicious for carcinoma *(right)*.

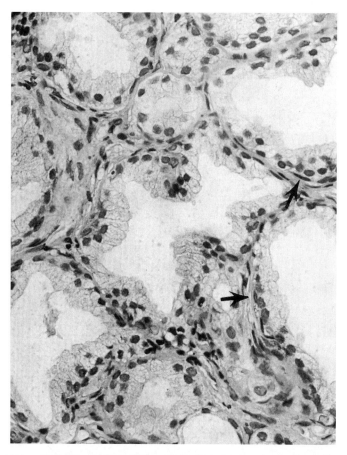

FIG. 7.22. High magnification of Figs. 7.20 and 7.21. Note benign gland with papillary infolding, sharing similar cytology and cytoplasm to surrounding smaller glands suspicious for cancer. Note the focal presence of basal cell layer *(arrows)*.

may be patchy in adenosis, negative staining in a small focus of glands is not necessarily indicative of malignancy. However, if some of the glands within a crowded glandular focus on needle biopsy demonstrate a basal cell layer, then adenosis can be diagnosed. Because of the difficulty in diagnosing adenosis on needle biopsy, it is useful to verify the diagnosis with high molecular weight cytokeratin antibodies. When the small crowded glands have identical nuclear and cytoplasmic features as surrounding more recognizable glands, then the focus may be adenosis. In the evaluation of a nodule of adenosis, it is difficult to determine where the atypical glands end and the benign glands begin, since the small glands of adenosis merge in with the surrounding more

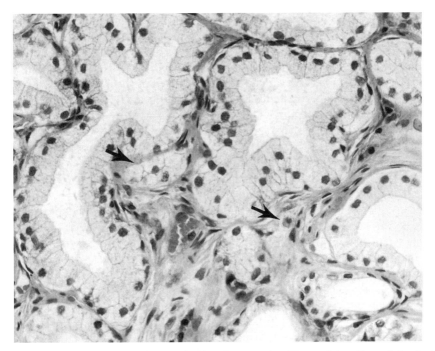

FIG. 7.23. High magnification of adenosis. Note that occasional tangential sections of glands of adenosis result in poorly formed glands and individual cells *(arrows)*. Antibodies to high molecular weight cytokeratin demonstrated basal cells, verifying the diagnosis.

recognizable benign glands. In contrast, with cancer one should be able to identify each gland as either benign or malignant based on cytologic differences (efig 728-730;731-732;733-734;735-736;737-739;740-741;742-744; 745-748).

Although adenosis mimics carcinoma, there is no conclusive evidence suggesting that patients with adenosis have an increased risk of harboring or developing adenocarcinoma of the prostate. In our series of adenosis, 14% of the transurethral resection (TUR) specimens examined also contained incidental foci of adenocarcinoma of the prostate (1). This is similar to the reported frequency of incidental adenocarcinomas found in TURs performed for clinically benign disease (9). Prior reports of transitions between adenosis and carcinoma were not verified with the use of basal cell specific antibodies, and may have been adenosis with foci of individual cells, minimal infiltration, or visible nucleoli. Another argument that has been raised to suggest that adenosis is a precursor to prostate cancer is that the two entities share certain morphologic features. Several studies have shown that adenosis may contain acid mucin, crystalloids, nucleoli, and have a patchy basal cell layer. Rather than proving a relation between adenosis and carcinoma, these findings demonstrate that any one of these features, by itself, is not specific for carcinoma. For example, acid mucin may be seen in atrophy (7), a patchy basal cell layer in clear cell cribriform hyperplasia, and nucleoli in basal cell hyperplasia (10). None of these lesions is a precursor to prostate cancer. The interpretation of these features must be made in the context of the totality of a lesion's architectural and cytologic features.

A study from M.D. Anderson Cancer Center supports the lack of association between adenosis and cancer (11). They studied 60 prostates from men who underwent cystoprostatectomy for bladder cancer. Forty-one prostates were found to have incidental prostate cancer and 12 were found to have adenosis, which they termed "atypical small glandular proliferations." They subcategorized cases of adenosis into cases with and without architectural and/or cytologic atypia. The overall prevalence of adenosis in prostates with and without carcinoma was not significantly different. The distribution of adenosis with and without atypical features also did not differ significantly between cases with and without carcinoma. There was no topographic association between either form of adenosis and carcinoma. Those studies suggesting a higher risk of carcinoma in men with adenosis have defined it differently, including many examples of what most authorities would call carcinoma (12,13).

Adenosis is closer to benign prostatic hyperplasia than carcinoma in terms of its proliferation (14,15). There have been a limited number of studies looking at the genetic findings in adenosis. Qian, using fluorescence in situ hybridization (FISH) analysis, demonstrated chromosomal anomalies in only 9% of cases of adenosis as compared to 55% of carcinomas (16). There was also no relationship between the chromosomal anomalies seen in adenosis and matched foci of carcinoma. In another study by the same group, Cheng noted allelic imbalances in 7/15 (47%) cases of adenosis (17). A subsequent study by Doll et al., however, found allelic imbalances in only 12% of cases of adenosis (18). One potential difference between the two studies was that the cases with foci of adenosis in the study by Doll et al. lacked associated carcinomas. Also, Doll et al. used the more stringent allelic imbalance criteria of a 50% reduction of allelic intensity in adenosis samples as compared to the patient matched normal samples, whereas Cheng et al. used a 30% reduction criterion. These results suggest that genetic alterations in adenosis may be infrequent.

The most critical issue in terms of patient management is whether patients with adenosis on histologic examination are at increased risk of subsequently being diagnosed with adenocarcinoma. In the only study to address this issue, Renedo studied 24 men with foci of adenosis compared to 61 men with benign prostatic hyperplasia (19). Men with adenosis were followed on average 6 1/2 years. There was no difference in the subsequent development of adenocarcinoma between the two groups. When diagnosing adenosis, we include the following statement, "Adenosis, although mimicking cancer, has not been shown to be associated with an increased risk of prostate cancer."

Atrophy

Typically considered to be a process affecting the elderly, atrophy has been demonstrated in at least 70% of 19 to 29 year old men (20). Atrophy may result in prostatic induration or give rise to a hypoechoic lesion on transrectal ultrasound, and may be biopsied as a lesion suspicious for cancer.

Atrophy is best diagnosed at medium to low magnification. Although the glands may appear infiltrative, they appear invasive as a patch not as individual glands infiltrating in between larger benign glands. At low power, atrophic glands have a very basophilic appearance. This basophilic appearance is due to their scant cytoplasm and crowded nuclei such that at low magnification one is merely seeing a nuclear outline of the gland (efig 749-751;752-753;754-756; 757-758;759-761;762;763-766;767-768;769-772;773-775). Longitudinal tangential sections of atrophic glands results in cords of cells that can further mimic cancer (efig 776-777;778-779). In some cases there may be associated fibrosis, which gives the atrophic glands a more infiltrative appearance that has been termed sclerotic atrophy (Figs. 7.24–7.26, efig 780-781;782-784, Color Plates 24-25). A characteristic finding in some cases is the presence of a centrally dilated atrophic gland surrounding by fibrosis and clustered smaller glands, which has been termed "postatrophic hyperplasia (PAH)" (efig 785-787;788-

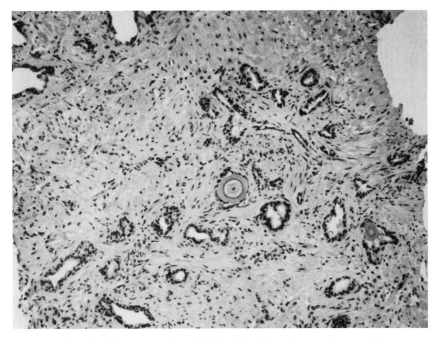

FIG. 7.24. Sclerotic atrophy mimicking infiltrating adenocarcinoma. ×110.

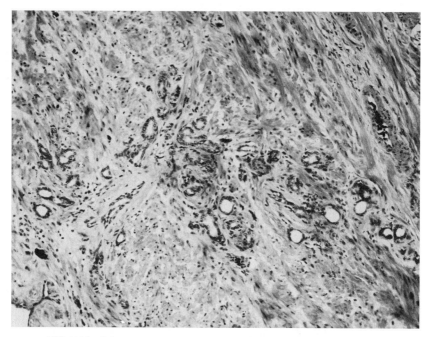

FIG. 7.25. Sclerotic atrophy mimicking infiltrating adenocarcinoma. ×100.

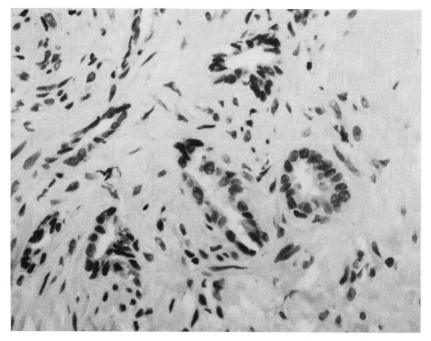

FIG. 7.26. Sclerotic atrophy showing well-formed glands with high nuclear-to-cytoplasmic ratio owing to atrophic cytoplasm with relatively benign-appearing nuclei. ×420.

790;791, Color Plate 26) (21). We do not use this term, but rather diagnose these cases as "benign prostate tissue with atrophy," although there is nothing wrong with using "PAH" in one's report. In contrast to what one might think, crowded atrophic glands have a much higher proliferation rate than nonatrophic benign glands (22). Compared to atrophy, gland-forming adenocarcinomas of the prostate typically have a greater amount of cytoplasm so that at low magnification the neoplastic glands are not as basophilic. Atrophy's very basophilic appearance is distinctive even when compared to adenocarcinoma with very amphophilic cytoplasm (Color Plate 27). Atrophy may show enlarged nuclei and prominent nucleoli, although not the huge eosinophilic nucleoli seen in some prostate cancers. Although prominent nucleoli are more common in atrophic glands associated with inflammation, we have also seen prominent nucleoli in atrophy without inflammation. Furthermore, the inflammation associated with atrophy may be trivial and chronic in nature but still give rise to significant nuclear atypia (Fig. 7.27). In deciding whether an atypical focus represents carcinoma, the presence of atrophic cytoplasm should, in general, dissuade one from diagnosing carcinoma. When there are concerns as to whether a focus represents atrophy or adenocarcinoma, immunohistochemistry with antibodies to high molecular weight cytokeratin can be performed to resolve the issue. Atro-

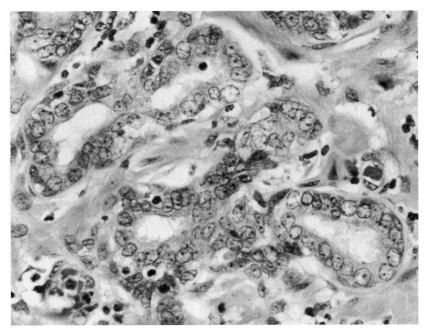

FIG. 7.27 Atrophic glands with enlarged vesicular nuclei and prominent nucleoli. Note trivial lymphocytic infiltrate.

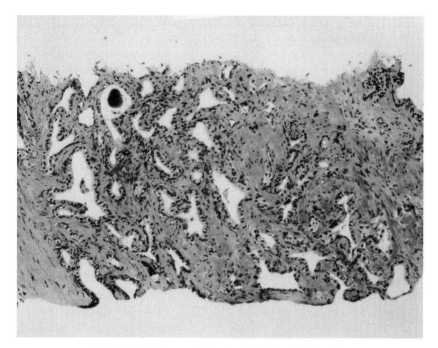

FIG. 7.28. Benign prostate glands with partial atrophy.

phy uniformly labels with high molecular weight keratin in contrast to negative staining in adenocarcinoma (Color Plate 28).

Rarely, carcinoma with an atrophic appearance may be present on needle biopsy. The diagnosis of carcinoma in these cases is made on (a) a truly infiltrative process with individual small atrophic glands situated between larger benign glands; (b) the concomitant presence of ordinary less atrophic carcinoma; and (c) greater cytologic atypia than is seen in benign atrophy (see Chapter 6).

A variant of atrophy that may cause confusion with carcinoma is "partial atrophy" (23) (efig 792-793;794-795;796-797;798-799;800-801;802-803;804-805; 806-807;808-812;813-815;816-818;819-820;821). Partial atrophy may still retain the lobular pattern of atrophy, or as seen in Figure 7.28, have more of a disorganized diffuse appearance. Partial atrophy lacks the basophilic appearance of fully developed atrophy as the nuclei are more spaced apart. The presence of crowded glands with pale cytoplasm may lead to an overdiagnosis of low-grade adenocarcinoma. At higher power, however, the glands have benign features characterized by undulating luminal surfaces with papillary infolding. Most carcinomas have more straight, even luminal borders. In addition, the glands are partially atrophic with nuclei in areas reaching the full height of the cytoplasm (Figs. 7.29 and 7.30). The nuclear features in partial atrophy tend to be relatively benign without prominent nucleoli. One should hesitate diagnosing cancer when

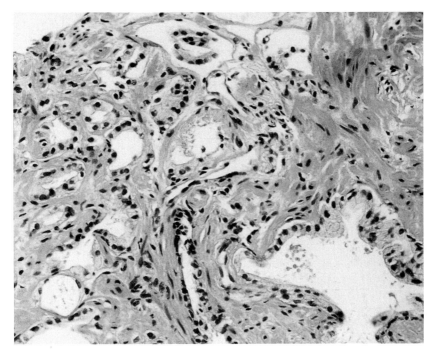

FIG. 7.29. Disorganized benign glands with partial atrophy.

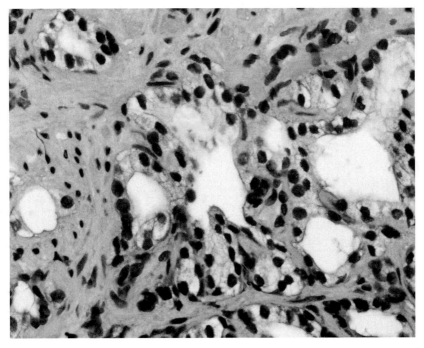

FIG. 7.30. High magnification of partial atrophy with bland nuclei and scant cytoplasm.

the nuclei occupy almost the full cell height and the cytoplasm has the same appearance as surrounding more obvious benign glands.

Basal Cell Hyperplasia

A spectrum of basaloid lesions ranging from hyperplasia to carcinoma exists in the prostate. Basal cell hyperplasia may resemble prostate acini seen in the fetus, accounting for the synonyms "fetalization" and "embryonal hyperplasia" of the prostate (24).

The most common form of basal cell hyperplasia consists of tubules or glands with piling up of the basal cell layer (24–26). Although they are often over-looked, small glands with basal cell hyperplasia are not uncommonly found focally within nodules of benign prostatic hyperplasia (Fig. 7.31). Glandular-stromal nodules in which a majority of glands show basal cell hyperplasia may also be identified (Figs. 7.32 and 7.33). In these cases, there is usually no con-fusion with carcinoma given the well-circumscribed nature of the lesion, the abundant stroma, as well as the intermingling of the glands of basal cell hyper-plasia with normal glands.

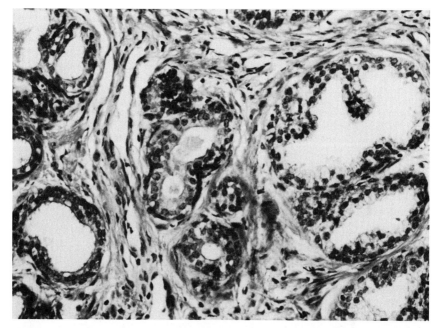

FIG. 7.31. Several glands showing piling up of the basal cell layer *(center)* within a nodule of hyperplasia. ×270.

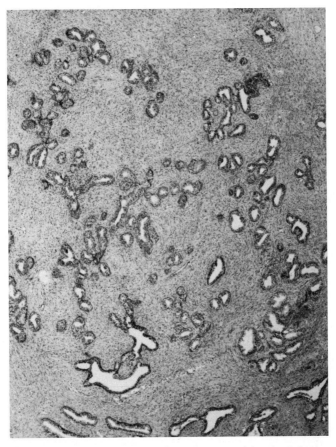

FIG. 7.32. Glandular-stromal nodule of hyperplasia with many of the glands having a basophilic appearance owing to piling up of the basal cell layer. ×40.

Basal cell hyperplasia may be more florid in some cases, whereby it may be confused with prostatic adenocarcinoma (efig 822-823;824-825;826-828;829-831;832-833;834;835-836;837-839;840-841;842-843;844-845). In some cases of florid basal cell hyperplasia the basal cell proliferation still retains a lobular configuration (Figs. 7.34 and 7.35). In other instances the lobular configuration may either be lost or not appreciated because of the fragmented nature of the transurethral resection specimen (Fig. 7.36). Even at low magnification, basal cell hyperplasia can be distinguished from carcinoma by its very basaloid appearance. The glands appear basophilic at low power due to multilayering of the basal cells which have scant cytoplasm. In contrast, gland-forming adeno-

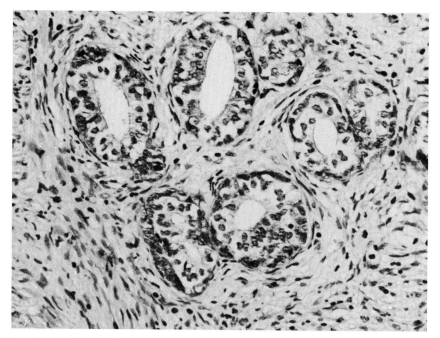

FIG. 7.33. Higher magnification of Fig. 7.32 showing glands with a multicell layer of basal cells. ×175.

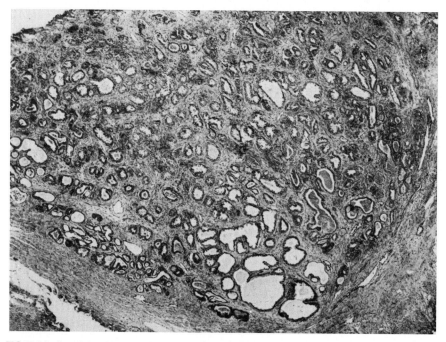

FIG. 7.34. A nodule of basal cell hyperplasia composed of open larger glands with minimal piling up of the basal cell layer. ×40.

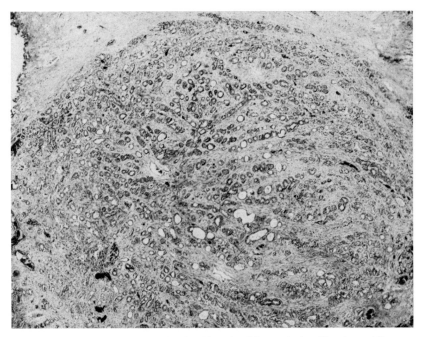

FIG. 7.35. Numerous small, closed glands of basal cell hyperplasia with a basophilic appearance growing in a lobular configuration. ×40.

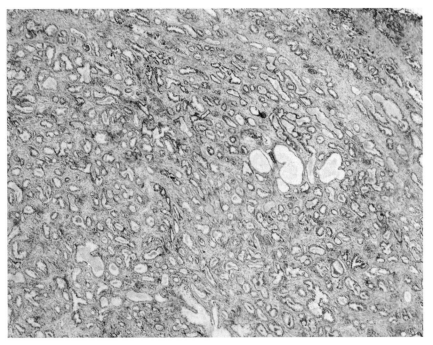

FIG. 7.36. Diffuse pattern of basal cell hyperplasia composed of open glands with minimal piling up of the basal cell layer.

carcinomas of the prostate almost always have more abundant cytoplasm result-ing in a more eosinophilic appearance to the glands at low magnification. Within basal cell hyperplasia, there is piling up of the nuclei within the lumen ranging from a single cell layer in a few glands, to three to four cells thick in other glands, to solid nests of epithelium (Figs. 7.31, 7.37, 7.38). Basal cell hyperpla-sia may reveal focal cribriform glands. Cribriform basal cell hyperplasia in most cases resembles back-to-back glands of basal cell hyperplasia rather than true cribriform glands (Fig. 7.39,efig 831;838-839;846-848;849-850;851-853;854-855;856-857). Adjacent to cribriform basal cell hyperplasia are usually more typical individual glands of basal cell hyperplasia. Basal cell hyperplasia is also one of the few prostatic entities that contain intraluminal calcifications (efig 858-859;860-862;863-864;865, Color Plate 29). These calcifications consist of well-formed lamellar calcifications. Carcinomas rarely contain calcifications, and when present usually consist of fine calcified grains usually within central necrosis in high-grade cancers (efig 866-867;868-869). Another unique feature seen within the cells of basal cell hyperplasia is the presence of intracytoplasmic eosinophilic globules (efig 870-872;873-875;876-878). Basal cell lesions are preferentially located in the transition zone and are seen on TURP, although

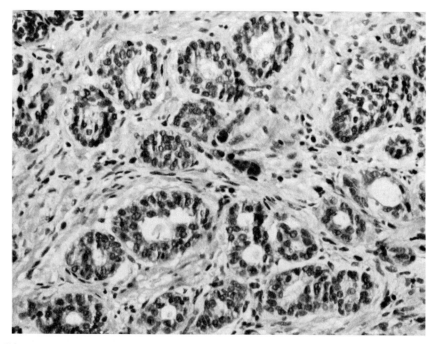

FIG. 7.37. Higher magnification of Fig 7.35 showing small glands with multilayering of the basal cells. ×300.

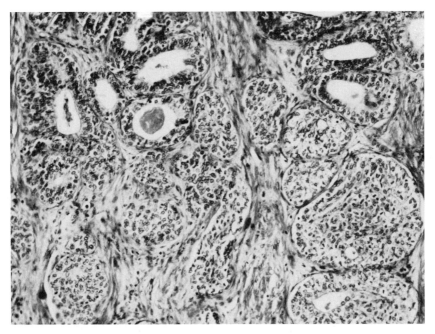

FIG. 7.38. Spectrum of basal cell hyperplasia from open glands with multilayering of the basal cells to solid nests of basal cells. ×165.

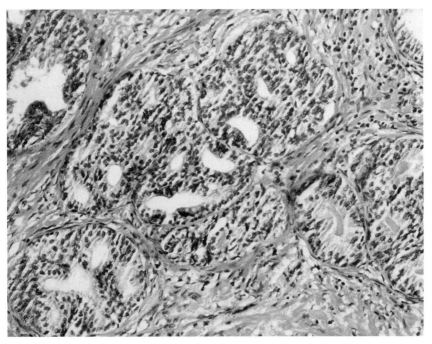

FIG. 7.39. Cribriform pattern of basal cell hyperplasia.

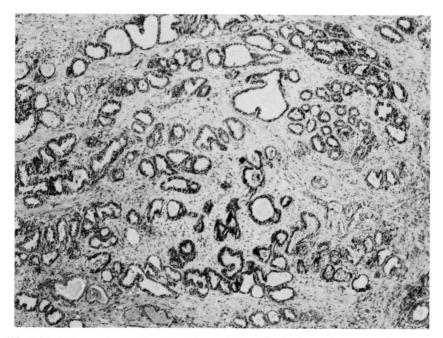

FIG. 7.40. Diffuse pattern of basal cell hyperplasia with glands set in a somewhat myxoid stroma. ×55.

occasionally, we have seen basal cell hyperplasia on needle biopsy (efig 879-881;882-883;884-885).

As shown in the preceding photomicrographs, glands of basal cell hyperplasia appear to be situated within the stroma without a desmoplastic response. In between the glands of basal cell hyperplasia is relatively unremarkable smooth muscle or on occasion a minimally myxoid stroma (Fig. 7.40).

If by light microscopy there is difficulty in distinguishing basal cell hyperplasia from prostatic adenocarcinoma, utilization of immunohistochemistry with a basal cell specific antibody such as high molecular weight cytokeratin can differentiate between the two lesions (efig 886-888;889-891;892-894). On the average, over 80% of the glands of basal cell hyperplasia are immunoreactive with antibodies to high molecular weight cytokeratin and often the staining is very intense (8,26–29). Adenocarcinomas of the prostate lack reactivity with high molecular weight cytokeratin, and normal glands reveal only a single basal layer of immunoreactivity, contrasted to the multilayered staining seen with basal cell hyperplasia.

Basal cell hyperplasia may have prominent nucleoli, but is otherwise identical to ordinary basal cell hyperplasia (30,31) (efig 887;895-897;898-899;900-901;902-905, Fig. 7.41, Color Plate 6). In the past, these cases were referred to as atypical basal cell hyperplasia. As these lesions are not associated with an adverse prognosis, we have dropped the word "atypical" so as not to cause undue concern for clinicians or patients. The enlarged nucleoli in general are seen diffusely throughout the lesion. In some cases of basal cell hyperplasia with prominent nucleoli, nuclei are seen undermining the overlying secretory cells that are cytologically normal (Fig. 5.14). Other features usually attributable to carcinoma that may be seen in basal cell hyperplasia with prominent nucleoli are nuclear hyperchromatism, rare mitotic figures, nuclear enlargement, individual cell necrosis, necrotic intraluminal secretions, and blue-tinged mucinous secretions. Basal cell hyperplasia with prominent nucleoli is distinguished from acinar adenocarcinoma by the multilayering of its nuclei, solid nests, and atrophic cytoplasm. There is no known association between basal cell hyperplasia showing prominent nucleoli and either acinar adenocarcinoma or basaloid carcinoma. Distinguishing basal cell hyperplasia with prominent nucleoli from PIN is more difficult (see Chapter 5).

Another form of basal cell hyperplasia is composed of basaloid nests with areas of luminal differentiation resembling basal cell adenomas or adenoid cystic carcinomas of the salivary gland (Fig. 7.42). We denote these lesions as the adenoid basal form of basal cell hyperplasia. When a well-formed distinct nodule of basaloid nests is formed, the term "basal cell adenoma" or "adenoid basal cell tumor" is sometimes employed, though others prefer to consider these lesions as more pro-

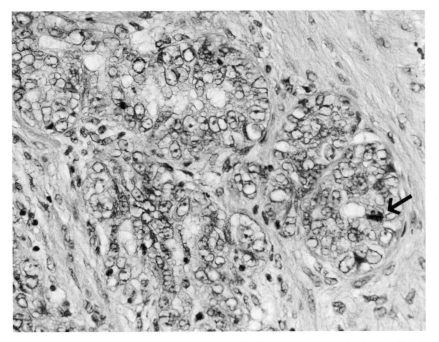

FIG. 7.41. Cytologically atypical basal cell hyperplasia. Note prominent nucleoli and mitotic figure *(arrow)*. (From Epstein and Armas, ref. 10, with permission.)

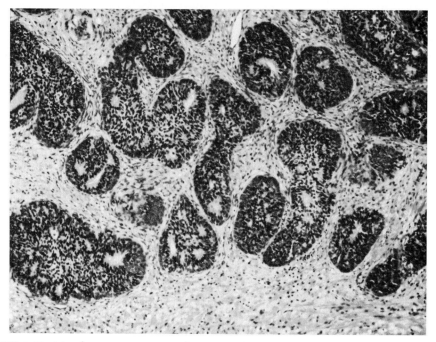

FIG. 7.42. Adenoid basal form of basal cell hyperplasia composed of nests of basal cells with focal lumen formation, resembling certain salivary gland lesions. Note the lack of desmoplastic response in the stroma between the basaloid nests. ×205.

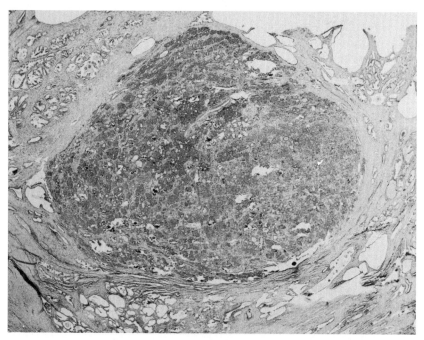

FIG. 7.43. Basal cell adenoma composed of well-circumscribed expansile nodule of basaloid nests. ×12.

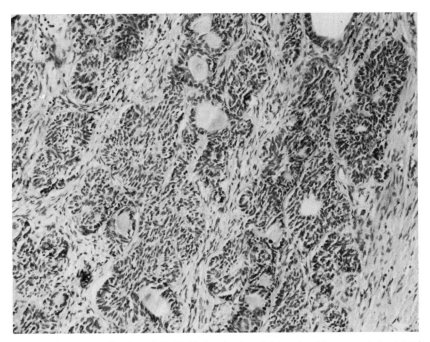

FIG. 7.44. Higher magnification of Fig 7.43 showing basaloid nests with areas of glandular formation. Note lack of desmoplastic response within basal cell adenoma. ×125.

nounced examples of basal cell hyperplasia (Figs. 7.43 and 7.44, efig 906-908) (26,32). The term "basal cell adenoma" is reasonable for these lesions given that the nodules grow in an expansile fashion compressing the adjacent normal prostatic stroma (33). In contrast to basal cell carcinomas, basal cell adenomas are well circumscribed, lack necrosis, and the stroma between the basaloid nests is similar to that of the surrounding normal prostatic stroma (see Chapter 17).

Colonic Mucosa

Rarely, distorted fragments of colonic mucosa on transrectal biopsies of the prostate can be confused with adenocarcinoma of the prostate (efig 909-910). Features that can mimic prostate cancer are the presence of luminal blue-tinged mucinous secretions and reactive/reparative atypia. The presence of goblet cells and other features of colonic tissue, such as a potentially thickened basement membrane, lamina propria, and muscularis should prevent a misdiagnosis. Immunohistochemistry with prostatic markers can verify the nonprostatic nature of the lesion. Assessing the colonic mucosa can also be helpful in diagnosing limited prostate cancer on biopsy. In some cases the H&E stain is so basophilic that the colonic mucosa has a blue hue, such that the significance of blue-tinged mucinous secretions in atypical prostatic glands is not as discriminatory as in cases where the H&E stain is not as basophilic (efig 911).

Cowper's Glands

Initially, Cowper's glands were identified on TUR as a potential pitfall in the diagnosis of prostate cancer. Subsequently, it was noted that they may be sampled on needle biopsy (34). Cowper's glands may resemble both low-grade adenocarcinoma and the more recently described foamy gland carcinoma, both of which may have bland cytology (35)(efig 912-913;914-915;916-917;918-919;920-926, Fig. 7.45). The presence of glands in skeletal muscle may further mimic cancer if the lesion is not recognized as Cowper's glands. The diagnosis of Cowper's glands rests on the recognition of a noninfiltrative lobular pattern of a dimorphic population of ducts and mucinous acini in Cowper's glands, with the caveat that the ducts may not be obvious in all foci. The presence of abundant mucin-filled cytoplasm also distinguishes this lesion from carcinoma (color plate 30). Although prostate cancer cytoplasm may contain neutral mucinous secretions, none of the studies describe abundant mucinous cytoplasm to the extent that the lumina are almost occluded. Foamy gland carcinomas have almost as abundant cytoplasm, yet the glands are larger and mucin stains are negative.

In difficult cases where ducts in Cowper's glands may not be obvious, immunohistochemistry with a panel of antibodies may be useful. In our study,

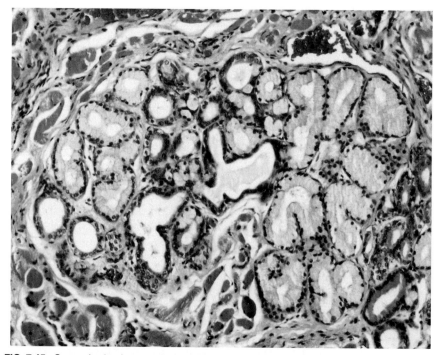

FIG. 7.45. Cowper's gland on needle biopsy. Note dimorphic population with ducts (*central*) surrounded by mucinous glands. These glands are situated in skeletal muscle.

prostate-specific acid phosphatase (PSAP) was negative in all cases, although the abundant cytoplasm of the acinar cells decorated focally with prostate-specific antigen (PSA) in a heterogeneous "clumped" fashion in four of ten cases. The ductal epithelium failed to react with either antibody. High molecular weight cytokeratin (34BE12) decorated the ductal epithelium, hybrid cells, and an attenuated basal layer at the periphery of acini. Muscle-specific actin was positive in a basal distribution about the acini in three of five cases. Saboorian reported conflicting results, demonstrating that Cowper's glands were negative for PSA in all cases, negative for high molecular weight cytokeratin in nine of ten cases, and positive for smooth muscle actin in all cases (36).

Mesonephric Hyperplasia

Identical to the lesion seen in the female genital tract, mesonephric hyperplasia has rarely been seen in the prostate on either TURP or in radical prostatectomy specimens (37,38)(Fig. 7.46, efig 927-928;929-930;931-936). It is distinguished from carcinoma by the atrophic appearance of the glands, occasional papillary tufting, lack of stromal reaction, dense colloid secretions, and negative immunoreactivity for PSA and PSAP.

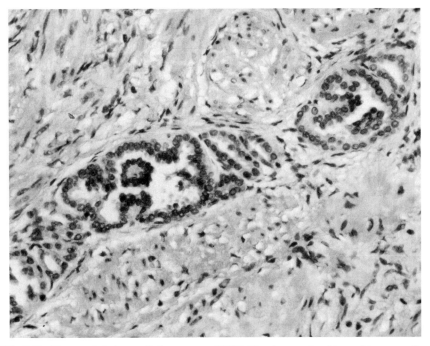

FIG. 7.46. Mesonephric hyperplasia seen on TURP. Glands are atrophic and have papillary infoldings and tufts in contrast to adenocarcinoma of the prostate.

Nephrogenic Adenoma

Nephrogenic adenoma, thought to be a benign metaplastic response of the urothelium to injury, can rarely affect the prostatic urethra. Extension of small tubules of nephrogenic adenoma into the underlying prostatic fibromuscular stroma can lead to the misdiagnosis of low-grade prostatic adenocarcinoma in TUR specimens and rarely on prostate biopsies. As this lesion is mainly associated with the prostatic urethra, it is discussed in Chapter 18.

Radiation Atypia

Radiation changes in benign prostate glands can mimic adenocarcinoma of the prostate. This subject is discussed in Chapter 14 along with other manifestations of therapy-related morphologic changes.

Seminal Vesicles

The incidence of transurethral resection material containing seminal vesicle epithelium in our institution is approximately 3%. There are differences in the literature as to the clinical significance of resecting seminal vesicle epithelium. In one study there was a high incidence of postoperative epididymitis, whereas there was no significant morbidity in another study (39,40). Although the overdiagnosis of seminal vesicles as carcinoma is less likely in TUR material given the greater amount of tissue to evaluate, there are some instances where seminal vesicle epithelium is composed of closely packed glands resembling adenocarcinoma (Fig. 7.47, efig 937-938;939-942). Occasionally seminal vesicles sampled on needle biopsy can also be a source of overdiagnosing prostatic adenocarcinoma (efig 943-944;945-946;947-948;949-952;953-954). The recognition of seminal vesicle rests on appreciating its architectural as well as cytologic features. Seminal vesicles are characterized by a central large dilated lumina with numerous small glands clustered around the periphery. Often the glands appear to bud off from the central lumen. Although on needle biopsy it may be difficult to recognize the architectural pattern of seminal vesicles due to the limited tissue, certain features may be present. A common finding on needle biopsy of the seminal vesicle is the dilated irregular lumen of the seminal vesicle seen at the edge of the tissue core, where the core has fragmented as it entered the seminal vesicle lumen. Surrounding this dilated structure are clusters of smaller glands (Fig. 7.48). Recognition that the small glands suspicious for carcinoma are all clustered around this dilated glandular structure, is the first step in not overdiagnosing seminal vesicle epithelium as carcinoma. A variation on this architectural pattern can be seen in Figure 7.49 where there is a dilated branching gland surrounded by similar appearing smaller acinar structures. Verification that one is dealing with seminal vesicle epithelium can readily be accomplished at higher magnification examination. Seminal vesicle epithelium characteristi-

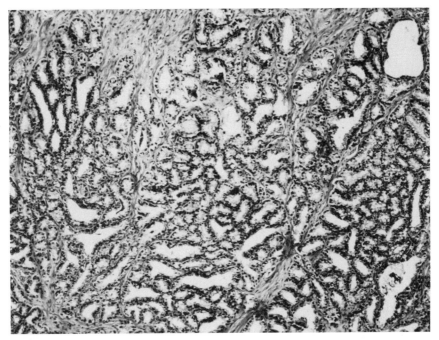

FIG. 7.47. Seminal vesicle epithelium composed of closely packed glands mimicking low-grade adenocarcinoma. ×75.

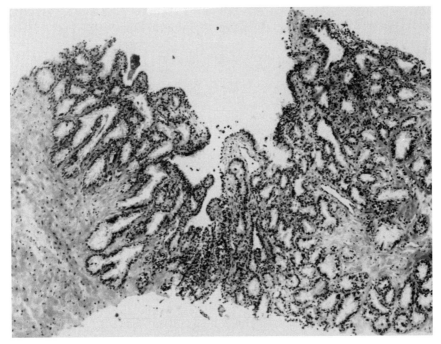

FIG. 7.48. Needle biopsy of seminal vesicle with central lumen of seminal vesicle toward the top. ×85.

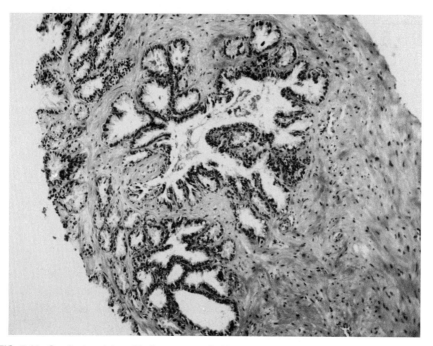

FIG. 7.49. Seminal vesicle epithelium on needle biopsy with dilated glands surrounded by out-pouchings of smaller glandular structures. ×100.

cally have scattered cells showing prominent nuclear atypia (41,42). These nuclei are markedly enlarged with bizarre shapes and have marked hyperchromasia that often obscures nuclear details (Color Plate 31). Despite these pleomorphic features, these nuclei lack mitotic activity. The atypia appears degenerative in nature, similar to that which is seen with radiation atypia. The common finding within seminal vesicles of markedly atypical nuclei present within well-formed glandular structures differs from prostate cancer in which gland-forming well- to moderately-differentiated carcinomas have only slight to moderate nuclear atypia. Even in poorly-differentiated prostatic carcinoma that lacks glandular differentiation, one rarely sees the severe atypia that is present within scattered seminal vesicle epithelial cells. Prominent globular golden brown lipofuscin granules are typical of seminal vesicle epithelium. Benign prostate tissue, high-grade PIN, and rarely carcinoma may contain lipofuscin pigment, but it differs in that the granules are smaller and more red-orange or blue (43) (efig 955-956;957;958;959;960). If there still exists questions as to whether the lesion is seminal vesicle epithelium or prostatic adenocarcinoma, immunohistochemistry for high molecular weight cytokeratin will label basal cells surrounding seminal vesicle epithelium, whereas basal cells are absent in prostate adenocarcinoma. Caution must be used with immunohistochemistry using polyclonal antibodies to PSA, as it will label seminal vesicle tissue; monoclonal antibodies to PSA do not exhibit this cross-reactivity (44).

Verumontanum Mucosal Gland Hyperplasia

Gagucas and colleagues reported the presence of a distinctive small acinar proliferation in radical prostatectomy specimens involving the verumontanum and adjacent posterior urethra (45). This lesion, termed "verumontanum mucosal gland hyperplasia" (VMGH), is a potential mimic of adenocarcinoma and should be included in the differential diagnosis of small acinar proliferations of the prostate (Fig. 7.50, efig 961-963;964-967). We have encountered similar lesions in prostatic needle biopsy specimens submitted for consultation (46). The verumontanum is situated along the posterior prostatic urethral wall and is the

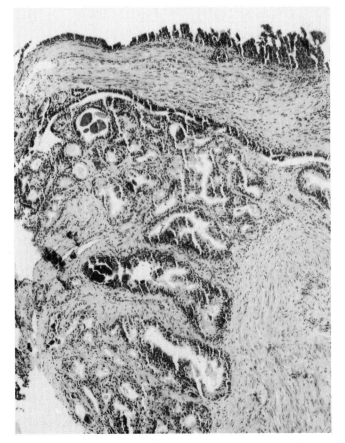

FIG. 7.50. Needle biopsy of crowded glands at the verumontanum beneath urothelium *(top)*.

point at which the utricle and ejaculatory ducts merge with the prostatic urethra. The mimicry of adenocarcinoma that is produced by VMGH is particularly evident at low magnification. Here, the small size and crowded nature of verumontanum mucosal glands may simulate low-grade prostatic adenocarcinoma. Further confusion with carcinoma may arise from the presence of VMGH in multiple cores or from extensive involvement (i.e., >50%) of a single biopsy core. The glands of VMGH lack the infiltrative and haphazard arrangement of the glands typically found in prostatic adenocarcinoma. Moreover, the glands of prostatic adenocarcinoma are often found infiltrating between benign prostatic glands, a feature that is absent in VMGH. In addition, VMGH is characteristically identified adjacent to and often contiguous with urothelium. Contents of these mucosal glands are sufficiently distinct to allow discrimination from prostatic adenocarcinoma. Unlike prostatic adenocarcinoma, corpora amylacea are a feature typical of VMGH. Also, in VMGH one characteristically finds distinctive brown-orange concretions. Verumontanum mucosal glands are immunophenotypically similar to prostatic acini; thus, the secretory cells of these mucosal glands stain positively with antibodies to PSA whereas the basal cells stain with antibodies to high molecular weight cytokeratin.

MIMICKERS OF GLEASON SCORE 7–10 ADENOCARCINOMA
Clear Cell Cribriform Hyperplasia

One of the mimickers of Gleason score 7–10 adenocarcinoma is clear cell cribriform hyperplasia, which occurs within the transition zone and is mostly seen in TURP specimens removed for urinary obstructive symptoms, and rarely seen on needle biopsy (Table 7.4). It is considered by some to be a cribriform variant of benign prostatic hypertrophy (BPH). While its classification within a conceptual framework is unresolved, it remains useful from the practical standpoint to consider it as a distinct entity, as it may be confused with either PIN or adenocarcinoma of the prostate (47).

In its most readily recognized form, clear cell cribriform hyperplasia is composed of numerous cribriform glands separated from one another by a modest amount of stroma in a pattern of nodular hyperplasia (Fig. 5.10) (47). In florid

TABLE 7.4. *Benign mimickers of gleason score 7–10 adenocarcinoma*

Entity	Predominant mode of sampling
Nonspecific granulomatous prostatitis	TURP = Needle
Paraganglia	TURP > Needle
Clear cell cribriform hyperplasia	TURP > Needle
Sclerosing adenosis	TURP >> Needle
Xanthoma	Needle > TURP
Signet ring cell lymphocytes	TURP

cases, the glands infiltrate the stroma more diffusely (Fig. 5.12, efig 968-971; 972-976;977-981;982-984;985-986). If it were to be misdiagnosed as adenocarcinoma, it would be classified as cribriform Gleason score 4+4=8. The epithelial cells have distinctive clear cytoplasm and small bland nuclei with inconspicuous or small nucleoli. Around many of the glands of clear cell cribriform hyperplasia is a strikingly prominent basal cell layer, consisting of a row of cuboidal darkly staining cells beneath the clear cells (Fig. 5.13). The basal cells may form small knots at the periphery of some of the glands (Fig. 5.11). Occasionally, the basal cells may have small nucleoli. The basal cell layer may be incomplete and in some glands may be invisible in routine sections. Tangential sections can also result in the appearance of occasional nests of clear cells without cribriform architecture or basal cells (Fig. 5.11). Although usually unnecessary, immunostains for high molecular weight cytokeratin can highlight the basal cell layer (48).

The distinction between clear cell cribriform hyperplasia and cribriform PIN may be difficult (see Chapter 5). The distinction between clear cell cribriform hyperplasia and infiltrating cribriform carcinoma is easier. The presence of basal cells around some of the glands in clear cell cribriform hyperplasia rules out carcinoma, even though some glands with identical nuclear and cytoplasmic features may not have an apparent basal cell layer. The glands in clear cell cribriform hyperplasia lack cytologic atypia, in contrast to infiltrating cribriform carcinoma. Also it is uncommon to see cribriform carcinoma unaccompanied by small infiltrating neoplastic glands.

Clear cell cribriform hyperplasia is uncommon, and its natural history is unknown. Although three of 25 reported cases were associated with adenocarcinoma of the prostate, there were no areas of transition from clear cell cribriform hyperplasia to carcinoma of the prostate (47,48). Taking into account prostate cancer's high incidence in elderly men, it is felt that clear cell cribriform hyperplasia is unrelated to adenocarcinoma of the prostate.

Nonspecific Granulomatous Prostatitis

One of the principle entities that can be confused with high-grade prostate cancer is nonspecific granulomatous prostatitis (49). Although discussed in general in Chapter 4, it is discussed here in the context of its differentiation from adenocarcinoma. Nonspecific granulomatous prostatitis (NSGP) can closely mimic cancer clinically. In a series of cases on needle biopsy, prostatic carcinoma was suspected or considered prior to biopsy in 55% of cases (50). Prostate-specific antigen levels greater than 4 ng/nL were seen in 84% of NSGP and digital rectal exam was frequently abnormal.

Although most cases of NSGP seen on needle biopsy do not histologically resemble prostate cancer, 4% of cases can closely resemble cancer. These cases of NSGP consists of sheets of epithelioid histiocytes, some with prominent nucleoli with abundant granular cytoplasm (efig 987-988;989-990;991-993; 994-997, Color Plate 32). Reactive cribriform nonneoplastic prostatic glands further mimicking cancer may be seen in 7% of NSGP cases on biopsy (efig 998-999). The key feature to avoid a misdiagnosis of cancer is to recognize the other inflammatory cells in NSGP, such as scattered neutrophils, lymphocytes, plasma cells, and eosinophils. The presence of scattered multinucleated giant cells may also aid in the diagnosis of NSGP. However, despite its name, approximately 50% of cases of NSGP lack multinucleated giant cells on needle biopsy (50). In contrast, most adenocarcinomas of the prostate lack an associated inflammatory component (51). Although it may be difficult to appreciate on needle biopsy specimens, NSGP initially is localized around ruptured ducts and acini. As seen in Fig. 7.51, the epithelioid cells are not present diffusely throughout the needle biopsy core but surround an acinus or duct with attenuated partially disrupted epithelium. If this were carcinoma, the epithelioid cells would show no relationship to acini and ducts but would infiltrate throughout the core.

If there are difficulties in distinguishing NSGP from poorly differentiated adenocarcinoma, immunohistochemistry can be utilized. These epithelioid cells will be negative for PSA, PSAP, and pancytokeratin (Color Plate 33), and positive for various histiocytic markers (52). Just as isolated architecturally atypical glands can be seen on H&E stains in a heavily inflamed prostate, there may be focal architectural abnormalities when evaluating sections labeled with PSA, PSAP, or pancytokeratin. Out of context, focal collections of individual immunoreactive

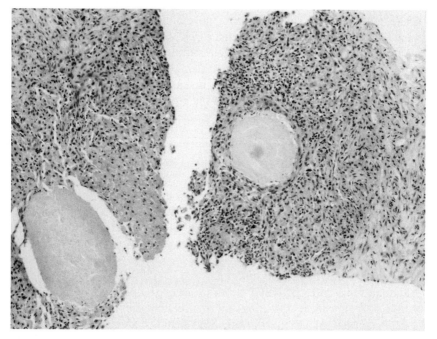

FIG. 7.51. Nonspecific granulomatous prostatitis surrounding ruptured ducts with corpora amylacea.

epithelial cells may be suspicious for cancer (Color Plate 34). However, these foci are localized and the vast majority of epithelioid cells are negative for epithelial markers indicating that these areas represent ruptured ducts and acini.

Paraganglia

Paraganglia have been identified in 8% of radical prostatectomies (53). They are usually present in the posterolateral soft tissue exterior to the prostate. Uncommonly, they may be found in the lateral prostatic stroma or in the bladder neck smooth muscle. Rarely, paraganglia may be seen on TURP or on needle biopsy where their distinction from carcinoma must be made (54). They consist of clusters of clear or amphophilic cells with fine cytoplasmic granules and a prominent vascular pattern, often intimately related to nerves (Fig. 7.52, efig 1000; 1001-1002;1003-1005;1006-1007). Nucleoli are not prominent, and if nuclear atypia is present, it is degenerative in appearance as seen in endocrine lesions. Paraganglia are situated in smooth muscle, not admixed with benign prostate glands. Although this lesion closely mimics high-grade adenocarcinoma of the prostate, the highly vascular setting along with the degenerative atypia are clues to prevent a misdiagnosis. Also before diagnosing a small focus of high-grade carcinoma on TURP or needle biopsy, where the atypical focus appears entirely extraprostatic, paraganglia

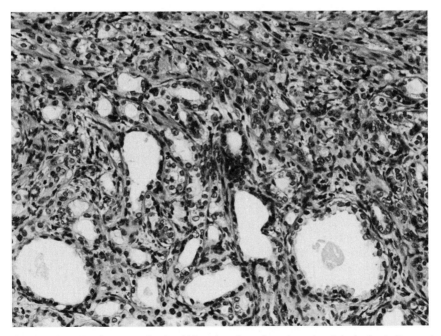

FIG. 7.52. Transition between glands within sclerosing adenosis and crytologically similar cords and infiltrating individual cells. ×300.

should be considered in the differential diagnosis. Verification of the diagnosis can be accomplished with positive immunostaining for neuroendocrine markers and S100, and negative reactivity for PSA and PSAP.

Sclerosing Adenosis

Lesions with the morphology of sclerosing adenosis were first reported in 1983 as an adenomatoid prostatic tumor (55). More recently, the designation sclerosing adenosis has been preferred (56–60). In one series, sclerosing adenosis was found in approximately 2% of prostatic specimens. In most reported cases and in those seen at our institution, the lesions were discovered incidentally in TURs performed for urinary obstructive symptoms. Usually, only one or two small foci are present, although in one report as many as ten prostatic chips contained the lesion. As with any lesion seen on TUR, true multifocality as opposed to multiple sections through a single lesion cannot be distinguished. Very rarely sclerosing adenosis may be seen on needle biopsy. The major differential diagnosis rests between sclerosing adenosis and adenocarcinoma. Sclerosing adenosis consists of a mixture of well-formed glands, single cells, and a cellular spindle cell component (Fig. 7.53, efig 1008-1012;1013-1016;1017-1018;1019-1020;1021-1025;1026-1027;1028-1032;1033-1036;1037-1038).

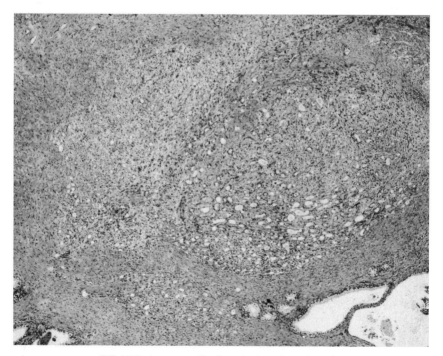

FIG. 7.53. Low magnification of sclerosing adenosis.

There are several features that should prevent a misdiagnosis of malignancy:

1. Adenocarcinomas of the prostate composed of an admixture of glands, poorly formed glandular structures, and single cells would be assigned a high Gleason score (7 or 8). Prostatic adenocarcinomas with these scores are only rarely seen as limited foci within a TURP. The finding of only one or several small foci of a cellular lesion suspicious for high-grade carcinoma should prompt a consideration of sclerosing adenosis or paraganglia (Fig. 7.54). Furthermore, although sclerosing adenosis may be minimally infiltrative at its perimeter, the lesion is still relatively circumscribed in contrast to high-grade prostate adenocarcinoma.

2. The glandular structures in sclerosing adenosis resemble those seen in ordinary adenosis. They are composed of cells with pale to clear cytoplasm and relatively benign-appearing nuclei. In many of the glandular structures, a basal cell layer can be identified on H&E-stained sections. This contrasts to carcinoma, where basal cells are absent.

3. Sclerosing adenosis contains a dense spindle cell component that is typically lacking in adenocarcinomas (Fig. 7.55). Usually, adenocarcinomas of the prostate show no apparent stromal response or at most a hypocellular fibrotic reaction.

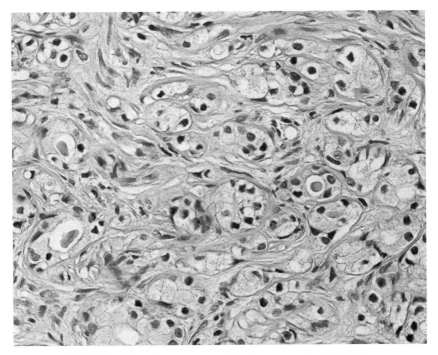

FIG. 7.54. Sclerosing adenosis with glands and cellular stroma.

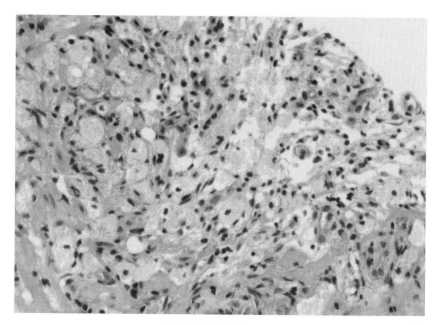

Fig. 7.55. Xanthoma.

4. A rather unique feature of sclerosing adenosis is the presence of a hyaline sheath-like structure around some of the glands (Color Plate 35). The glands in ordinary adenocarcinoma lack such a collarette and have a "naked" appearance as they infiltrate the stroma.
5. The relatively bland cytology may also help in distinguishing sclerosing adenosis from adenocarcinoma, although some nuclei within sclerosing adenosis may be moderately enlarged and contain prominent nucleoli.

These light microscopic features are classic for sclerosing adenosis, and it is usually not necessary to perform immunohistochemistry to clarify the diagnosis. However, immunohistochemistry is definitive in difficult cases. Ordinary adenocarcinomas of the prostate of all grades lack basal cells and thus high molecular weight cytokeratin immunoreactivity. Sclerosing adenosis contains a basal cell layer around most of the glandular structures as well as among the individual cells and cords of cells. The basal cells within sclerosing adenosis, however, are distinctive in their immunophenotypical staining and differ from ordinary basal cells. Ordinary basal cells of the prostate show no myoepithelial cell differentiation. They lack staining for muscle specific actin and ultrastructurally do not show contractile elements. Within sclerosing adenosis, the basal cells show muscle specific actin positivity consistent with myoepithelial cell differentiation (56,57). The dense spindle cell component in sclerosing adenosis also shows partial staining with keratin and muscle-specific actin consistent with myoepithelial cell differentiation. Ultrastructural examination of several of these cases has verified their myoepithelial differentiation (59). There is no known association between sclerosing adenosis and adenocarcinoma of the prostate.

Signet Ring Lymphocytes

TURP specimens may frequently show aggregates of degenerated lymphocytes with a signet ring cell appearance (61). This finding results from thermal injury and is not seen in needle biopsy or open prostatectomy specimens. Only rarely are these changes so prominent to be confused with signet ring cell carcinoma (efig 1039-1041;1042).

Xanthoma

Although rare, prostatic xanthoma can be a source of diagnostic confusion, particularly with small tissue fragments such as those obtained from needle biopsies (Fig. 7.55, efig 1043-1045;1046-1049;1050-1051;1052;1053-1055; 1056-1057;1058;1059)(62). Features that aid in the recognition of xanthoma include circumscription, clustering of uniform cells that lack gland formation, vacuolated cytoplasm, and benign-appearing nuclei without prominent nucleoli; immunohistochemical studies for histiocytic markers are confirmatory.

REFERENCES

1. Gaudin PB, Epstein JI. Adenosis of the prostate: histologic features in transurethral resection specimens. *Am J Surg Pathol* 1994;18:863–870.
2. Gaudin PB, Epstein JI. Adenosis of the prostate: histologic features in needle biopsy specimens. *Am J Surg Pathol* 1995;19:737–747.
3. Bostwick DG, Srigley J, Grignon D, et al. Atypical adenomatous hyperplasia of the prostate: morphologic criteria for its distinction from well-differentiated carcinoma. *Hum Pathol* 1993;24:819–832.
4. Mittal BV, Amin MD, Kinare SG. Spectrum of histological lesions in 185 consecutive prostatic specimen. *J Post Grad Med* 1989;35:157–161.
5. Srigley JR, Toth P, Hartwick RWJ. Atypical histologic patterns in cases of benign prostatic hyperplasia. *Lab Invest* 1989;60:69A.
6. Kramer CE, Epstein JI. Nucleoli in low-grade prostate adenocarcinoma and adenosis. *Hum Pathol* 1993;24:618–623.
7. Epstein JI, Fynheer J. Acidic mucin in the prostate: can it differentiate adenosis from adenocarcinoma? *Human Pathol* 1992;23:1321–1325.
8. Hedrick L, Epstein JI. Use of keratin 903 as an adjunct in the diagnosis of prostate carcinoma. *Am J Surg Pathol* 1989;13:389–396.
9. Eble JN, Epstein JI. Stage A carcinoma of the prostate. In: Bostwick DG consultant ed. *Pathology of the Prostate, Seminal Vesicles, and Male Urethra.* New York, NY: Churchill Livingstone; 1990:61–82. Roth LM, ed. *Contemporary Issues in Surgical Pathology.*
10. Epstein JI, Armas OA. Atypical basal cell hyperplasia of the prostate. *Am J Surg Pathol* 1992;16:1205–1214.
11. Troncoso P, Ayala AG. Atypical small gland proliferations of the transition zone in cystoprostatectomy specimens. *Mod Pathol* 1994;7:85A.
12. Brawn PN. Adenosis of the prostate: a dysplastic lesion that can be confused with prostate adenocarcinoma. *Cancer* 1982;49:826–833.
13. Brawn PN. *Interpretation of Prostate Biopsies.* New York, NY: Raven Press, 1983;48–81.

14. Helpap B. Cell kinetic studies in prostatic intraepithelial neoplasia and atypical adenomatous hyperplasia of the prostate. *Pathol Res Pract* 1995;171:904–907.

15. Häussler O, Epstein JI, Amin MB, et al. Cell proliferation, apoptosis, oncogene, and tumor suppressor gene status in adenosis with comparison to benign prostatic hyperplasia, prostatic intraepithelial neoplasia, and cancer. *Hum Pathol* 1999;30:1077–1086.

16. Qian J, Jenkins RB, Bostwick DG. Chromosomal anomalies in atypical adenomatous hyperplasia and carcinoma of the prostate using fluorescence in situ hybridization. *Urology* 1995;46:837–842.

17. Cheng L, Shan A, Cheville JC, et al. Atypical adenomatous hyperplasia of the prostate: a premalignant lesion? *Cancer Res* 1998;58:389–391.

18. Doll JA, Zhu X, Furman J, et al. Genetic analysis of prostatic atypical adenomatous hyperplasia (adenosis). *Am J Pathol* 1999;155:967–971.

19. Renedo D, Poy E, Wojno KJ. Clinical significance and distinction of adenosis from low-grade adenocarcinoma of the prostate on TURP. *Mod Pathol* 1995;8:82A.

20. Gardner WA, Jr, Culberson DE. Atrophy and proliferation in the young adult prostate. *J Urol* 1987; 137:53–56.

21. Amin MB, Tamboli P, Varma M, et al. Postatrophic hyperplasia of the prostate gland: a detailed analysis of its morphology in needle biopsy specimens. *Am J Surg Pathol* 1999;23:925–931.

22. Ruska KM, Sauvageot J, Epstein JI. Histology and cellular kinetics of prostatic atrophy. *Am J Surg Pathol* 1998; 22:1073–1077.

23. Oppenheimer JR, Epstein JI. Partial atrophy in prostate needle cores—another diagnostic pitfall for the surgical pathologist. *Am J Surg Pathol* 1998;22:440–445.

24. Bennett ED, Gardner WA Jr. Embryonal hyperplasia of the prostate. *Prostate* 1985;7:411–417.

25. Cleary KR, Choi HY, Ayala AG. Basal cell hyperplasia of the prostate. *Am J Clin* Pathol 1983;80: 850–854.

26. Grignon DJ, Ro JY, Ordonez NG, et al. Basal cell hyperplasia, adenoid basal cell tumor, and adenoid cystic carcinoma of the prostate: an immunohistochemical study. *Hum Pathol* 1988;19:1425–1433.

27. Shah IA, Schlageter M, Stinnett P, et al. Cytokeratin immunohistochemistry as a diagnostic tool for distinguishing malignant from benign epithelial lesions of the prostate. *Mod Pathol* 1991;4:220–224.

28. Brawer MK, Peehl DM, Stamey TA, et al. Keratin immunoreactivity in the benign and neoplastic human prostate. *Cancer Res* 1985;45:3663–3667.

29. O'Malley FP, Grignon DJ, Shum DT. Usefulness of immunoperoxidase staining with high-molecular-weight cytokeratin in the differential diagnosis of small-acinar lesions of the prostate gland. *Virchows Archiv A Pathol Anat* 1990;417:191–196.

30. Epstein JI, Armas OA. Atypical basal cell hyperplasia of the prostate. *Am J Surg Pathol* 1992;16: 1205–1214.

31. Devaraj LT, Bostwick DG. Atypical basal cell hyperplasia of the prostate: immunophenotypic profile and proposed classification of basal cell proliferations. *Am J Surg* Pathol 1993;17:645–659.

32. Ronnett BM, Epstein JI. A case showing sclerosing adenosis and an unusual form of basal cell hyperplasia of the prostate. *Am J Surg Pathol* 1989;13:866–872.

33. Lin JI, Cohen EL, Villacin AB, et al. Basal cell adenoma of prostate. *Urology* 1978;11:409–410.

34. Cina SJ, Silberman MA, Kahane H, et al. Diagnosis of Cowper's glands on prostate needle biopsy. *Am J Surg Pathol* 1997;21:550–555.

35. Nelson RS, Epstein JI. Prostatic carcinoma with abundant xanthomatous cytoplasm: foamy gland carcinoma. *Am J Surg Pathol* 1996;20:419–426.

36. Saboorian MH, Huffman H, Ashfaq R, et al. Distinguishing Cowper's glands from neoplastic and pseudoneoplastic lesions of prostate: immunohistochemical and ultrastructural studies. *Am J Surg Pathol* 1997;21:1069–1074.

37. Gikas PW, Del Buono EA, Epstein JI. Florid hyperplasia of mesonephric remnants involving prostate and periprostatic tissue: possible confusion with adenocarcinoma. *Am J Surg* Pathol 1993;17: 454–460.

38. Jiminez RE, Raval MFT, Spanta R, et al. Mesonephric remnants hyperplasia: pitfall in the diagnosis of prostatic adenocarcinoma. *J Urol Pathol* 1998;9:83–92.

39. Jensen KM, Sonneland P, Madsen PO. Seminal vesicle tissue in "resectate" of transurethral resection of prostate. *Urology* 1983;22:20–23.

40. Tsuang MT, Weiss NA, Evans AT. Transurethral resection of the prostate with partial resection of the seminal vesicle. *J Urol* 1981;126:615–617.

41. Arias-Stella J, Takano-Moron J. Atypical epithelial changes in the seminal vesicles. *Arch Pathol* 1958; 66:761–766.

42. Kuo T, Gomez LG. Monstrous epithelial cells in human epididymis and seminal vesicles: a pseudo-malignant change. *Am J Surg Pathol* 1981;5:483–490.

43. Brennick JB, O'Connell JX, Dickersin GR, et al. Lipofuscin pigmentation (so-called "melanosis") of the prostate. *Am J Surg Pathol* 1994;18:446–454.

44. Varma M, Morgan M, Amin MB. Immunohistochemical detection of PSA: comparison of monoclonal and polyclonal antibodies with implications for diagnostic pathology. *Mod Pathol* 2001;14:126A.

45. Gagucas RJ, Brown RW, Wheeler TM. Verumontanum mucosal gland hyperplasia. *Am J Surg Pathol* 1995;19:30–36.

46. Gaudin PB, Wheeler TM, Epstein JI. Verumontanum mucosal gland hyperplasia in prostatic needle biopsy specimens: a mimic of low grade prostatic adenocarcinoma. *Am J Clin* Pathol 1995;104: 620–626.

47. Ayala AG, Srigley JR, Ro JY, et al. Clear cell cribriform hyperplasia of prostate: report of ten cases. *Am J Surg Pathol* 1986;10:665–671.

48. Frauenhoffer EE, Ro JY, El-Naggar AK, et al. Clear cell cribriform hyperplasia of the prostate: immunohistochemical and flow cytometric study. *Am J Clin Pathol* 1991;95:446–453.

49. Stillwell TJ, Engen DE, Farrow GM. The clinical spectrum of granulomatous prostatitis: a report of 200 cases. *J Urol* 1987;138:320–323.

50. Oppenheimer JR, Kahane H, Epstein JI. Granulomatous prostatitis on needle biopsy. *Arch Pathol Lab Med* 1997;121:724–729.

51. Blumenfeld W, Tucci S, Narayan P. Incidental lymphocytic prostatitis: selective involvement with nonmalignant glands. *Am J Surg Pathol* 1992;16:975–981.

52. Presti B, Weidner N. Granulomatous prostatitis and poorly differentiated prostate carcinoma: their distinction with the use of immunohistochemical methods. *Am J Clin Pathol* 1991;95:330.

53. Ostrowski ML, Wheeler TM. Paraganglia of the prostate: location, frequency, and differentiation from prostatic adenocarcinoma. *Am J Surg Pathol* 1994;18:412–420.

54. Kawabata K. Paraganglion of the prostate in a needle biopsy specimen: a potential diagnostic pitfall. *Arch Pathol Lab Med* 1997; 121:515–516.

55. Chen KTK, Schiff JJ. Adenomatoid prostatic tumor. *Urology* 1983;21:88–89.

56. Sakamoto N, Tsuneyoshi M, Enjoji M. Sclerosing adenosis of the prostate: histopathologic and immunohistochemical analysis. *Am J Surg Pathol* 1991;15:660–667.

57. Jones EC, Clement PB, Young RH. Sclerosing adenosis of the prostate gland: a clinicopathological and immunohistochemical study of 11 cases. *Am J Surg Pathol* 1991;15:1171–1180.

58. Ronnett BM, Epstein JI. A case showing sclerosing adenosis and an unusual form of basal cell hyper-plasia of the prostate. *Am J Surg Pathol* 1989;13:866–872.

59. Grignon DJ, Ro JY, Srigley JR, et al. Sclerosing adenosis of the prostate gland: a lesion showing myoepithelial differentiation. *Am J Surg Pathol* 1992;16:383–391.

60. Young RH. Pseudoneoplastic lesions of the prostate gland. *Pathol Ann* 1988; 23(pt.1):105–128.

61. Alguacil-Garcia A. Artifactual changes mimicking signet ring cell carcinoma in transurethral prosta-tectomy specimens. *Am J Surg Pathol* 1986;10:795–800.

62. Sebo TJ, Bostwick DG, Farrow GM, et al. Prostatic xanthoma: a mimic of prostatic adenocarcinoma. *Hum Pathol* 1994;25:386–389.

8

Reporting Cancer

Influence on Prognosis and Treatment

NEEDLE BIOPSY

Use of Macros (Canned Text)

We have made extensive use of abbreviations in our pathology reports concerning prostate specimens. The advantages of these macros are multiple: (a) shorten transcription time with reduction in typographical errors; (b) create uniform terminology for clinicians; (c) prevent omission of important points relating to treatment and prognosis; (d) save pathologists' time by not having to "reinvent the wheel" each time he or she has to add a comment; and (e) allow one to search for prior diagnoses based on standard verbiage used. The macros that we use are listed in the appendix. The only potential disadvantage of using macros is if one relies on them too heavily. For the occasional case that does not fit a macro, it is necessary to abandon them for the use of free text or to add free text at the end of the macro.

Quantification of Amount of Cancer on Needle Biopsy

Multiple techniques of quantifying the amount of cancer found on needle biopsy have been developed and studied, including measurement of the (a) number of positive cores; (b) total millimeters of cancer amongst all cores; (c) percentage of each core occupied by cancer; and (d) total percent of cancer in the entire specimen. There are multiple studies claiming superiority of one technique over the other with no one method being clearly superior to the others.

Numerous studies show a correlation between the number of positive cores and various prognostic variables, including risk of extraprostatic extension of cancer found at radical prostatectomy (1–6) (Table 8.1). These studies have shown that the involvement of multiple biopsy cores on systematic prostate biopsy is a powerful predictor of adverse pathologic findings at radical prostate-

TABLE 8.1. *Correlation between number of prostate biopsy cores revealing cancer and pathologic stage at radical prostatectomy*

Number of positive cores	Percent of men with extraprostatic extension at RP					
	(Reference #)					
	(6)	(3)	(2)	(4)	(5)	(1)
1	7	10	—	—	38	40
2	—	33	—	—	38	47
<3	11	—	—	—	—	—
3	—	38	—	—	60	54
<4	21	—	—	44	—	—
4	—	77	—	—	—	69
≥4	47	—	—	70	75	—
5	—	100	—	—	—	63
5–6	48	—	83	—	—	—
6	71	83	—	—	—	100

RP, radical prostatectomy.

ctomy. The converse is not true. Prostate cancer limited to even one or two needle biopsy cores offers no guarantee of favorable findings at final surgical staging. The number of cores containing prostate cancer also correlates with the presence of seminal vesicle invasion (2,3,7), lymph node metastases (8), radical prostatectomy tumor volume (3,9), the presence of positive surgical margins (10,11), and postprostatectomy cancer progression (2,4,12).

The other widely used method of quantifying the amount of cancer on needle biopsy is measurement of the percentage of each biopsy core containing cancer, which is correlated with the likelihood of extraprostatic extension (1,7,13–17), seminal vesicle invasion (13), and positive surgical margins (7). Multiple studies have demonstrated that a limited extent (<3 mm.) of cancer on biopsy does not necessarily predict "insignificant" amounts of tumor in the entire prostate (9,14, 18–22). One feasible and rationale approach would be to have pathologists report the number of cores containing cancer, as well as one other system quantifying tumor extent. At our institution, the number of cores containing cancer is reported, along with the percentage of cancer present on each involved core. Calculating the percent of each core involved by cancer is based on a visual estimate of the length of the cancer involvement divided by the length of the core. An example of how we report our needle biopsy findings is as follows: "Adenocarcinoma of the prostate, Gleason score 3+3=6, involving 3 cores (10%, 15%, 30%)." In cases where the cores are fragmented and difficult to assess, we state that the specimen is fragmented and give an estimate as to the percentage of the entire slide involved by cancer. Occasionally, there will be scattered small foci of cancer occupying, for example, 80% of the length of the core, yet only 5% of the total core volume. Merely reporting such a case as showing 80% involvement by cancer may be misleading, as one would expect to see extensive cancer on the biopsy. On the other hand, such a case should be distinguished from one with only a single minute focus of cancer involving 5% of the core. An example of how we report such a case is as follows: "Scattered small foci of adenocarcinoma, Gleason score 3+3=6, discontinuously involving 80% of the length of one core." We would predict that such a tumor would not be "insignificant" and would need definitive therapy, in contrast to some cases with only a single minute focus of cancer.

Location of Positive Biopsy Cores

Some urologists hesitate to submit routine sextant needle biopsies as six separate cores in six separate containers, and instead submit them as left- and right-sided cores. Evidence to support lumping the cores together is provided by a study reporting that the positive predictive value of an individual positive core for the location of extraprostatic extension was not sufficient to guide the surgical decision to spare or excise a neurovascular bundle (23). However, biopsy core location is of potentially critical importance in the 5% to 10% of biopsies diagnosed as atypical and suspicious for cancer. We advocate the precise labeling of the initial biopsies to localize the sites of an initial atypical diagnosis and to direct the location of repeat biopsies, as increased sampling of the initial atypical site and adjacent ipsilateral and adjacent contralateral sites will increase the yield of cancer detection on repeat biopsy (24).

Several studies have demonstrated that the location of a positive biopsy core is predictive of adverse findings at radical prostatectomy. Badalament reported that the percentage of cancer in the biopsies from the base and apex correlated with extraprostatic extension and positive margins, respectively (1). In a study by Calvanese, the presence of Gleason score 7–9 cancer in the midprostate or prostatic base correlated with risk of seminal vesicle invasion and lymph node metastases (25). The presence of cancer in multiple sextant sites is predictive of the presence of multifocal rather than solitary cancer at radical prostatectomy; however, these differences do not correlate with pathologic stage or margin positivity (26).

The submission of needle biopsy specimens in separate containers may lead to much larger pathology charges, although the payments for the pathologists' services are less than the charges. If this is an issue, it is important for urologists and pathologists to come up with alternative strategies that result in agreeable charges while preserving the maximum possible predictive value for biopsy specimens. One option is to put the biopsies from the left gland and the biopsies from the right gland in separate containers. Biopsy cores from the mid and basal areas can be marked with different colors of dye, with the apex unstained, such that the specimens could be submitted together with their sextant origin preserved. A third option would be to dye only biopsies from one side of the gland (i.e., left), with three separate containers (apex, mid, base) submitted to the pathologist. With these options, the pathologist would still be able to identify the site of the atypical focus, and the patient would only be charged for either two or three parts to a case.

Needle Biopsy Perineural Invasion

Perineural invasion is defined as the presence of prostate cancer tracking along or around a nerve (efig 1060;1061). Although the finding of perineural invasion on pathologic analysis of a radical prostatectomy specimen has no significance, the role of prostate needle biopsy perineural invasion in treatment planning has been a source of considerable debate (27). Perineural invasion has been demonstrated to be one of the major mechanisms of extension of prostate cancer from the prostatic parenchyma to the periprostatic soft tissue. Perineural invasion extensive enough to be sampled on needle biopsy signals an increased risk of extraprostatic extension of cancer (28).

The reported positive predictive value of biopsy perineural invasion for extraprostatic cancer extension at radical prostatectomy is summarized in Table 8.2 (4,16,29–33). In many studies of perineural invasion, assessment of extraprostatic extension was performed on only partially submitted prostates such that it was most likely underrecognized. The absence of perineural invasion on biopsy does not indicate that organ-confined disease will be present at radical prostatectomy. No clear consensus exists on whether perineural invasion on needle biopsy provides independent prediction of extraprostatic extension beyond that provided by biopsy Gleason grade and preoperative prostate-specific antigen (PSA) level. Although one study reported that extraprostatic extension could be directly seen on biopsy in 45% of biopsies, we have found this to be a rare event (4). The discrepancy in perceived significance of biopsy perineural invasion may relate to different biopsy techniques or the presence of patient populations with different likelihood's of harboring advanced disease. The presence of perineural invasion on needle biopsy has also been shown to independently predict lymph node metastases and postoperative cancer progression (34,35). When perineural invasion is seen on biopsy, the urologists should consider excising the neurovascular bundle on that side (30).

Some clinicians may counsel men with biopsy perineural invasion against radical prostatectomy. This strategy may be excessively conservative, as men with biopsy perineural invasion may not have extraprostatic extension at radical prostatectomy and, even if extraprostatic extension is found at radical prostatectomy, these

TABLE 8.2. *Perineural invasion on needle biopsy: risk of extraprostatic extension*

Author (reference)	% EPE	Independent[a]
Vargas (33)	38%	Yes
Egan (32)	49%	No
Taille (31)	52%	Yes
Ukimura (16)	61%	Yes
Ravery (4)	74%	Not Assessed
Holmes (30)	78%	Not Assessed
Bastacky (29)	93%	Not Assessed

[a]Independently significant in multivariate analysis.
EPE, extraprostatic extension.

men still have between a 77% and 41% risk of being progression-free 10 years after surgery depending on prostatectomy Gleason score and margin status (36).

Perineural invasion has also been shown to be predictive of results following radiotherapy. The finding of perineural invasion on biopsy may alter treatment strategies, favoring the use of external beam radiotherapy over brachytherapy (interstitial seed therapy) in order to treat disease with a high risk of being exterior to the prostate (37).

Needle Biopsy and DNA Ploidy

We have demonstrated that in the presence of accurate grading of biopsy specimens, ploidy is not helpful in predicting prostatectomy findings (38). However, ploidy does correlate with prostatectomy stage and grade, and may be of value if accurate Gleason grading is of concern (39,40).

Emerging Adjuncts to Needle Biopsy Interpretation

A host of new and emerging techniques offer potential for increasing the prognostic power available from prostate needle biopsy. The mean number of microscopic blood vessels in tissue is higher in prostate cancer and prostatic intraepithelial neoplasia (PIN) than normal prostate tissue. One study has shown that microvessel density analysis on needle biopsy, when combined with Gleason score and preoperative PSA, provided improved ability to predict extraprostatic extension at radical prostatectomy (41). Although microvessel density was significant in the multivariate analysis, Gleason score and serum PSA were much more powerful predictors of extraprostatic disease. Although statistically significant, the clinical benefit of evaluating microvessel density may still be marginal in terms of the management of individual patients.

A single study has demonstrated that proliferation of cancer on biopsy as measured by ki67 and percentage of cells in S-phase and G_2M better correlated than biopsy grade with PSA failure after radical prostatectomy (42). In a separate work, needle biopsy P53 and Gleason score were independent predictors of biochemical relapse after radical prostatectomy (43). Neuroendocrine differentiation on needle biopsy has not been shown to be of prognostic significance (44). Nuclear morphometric measurements on needle biopsy have also been demonstrated in limited studies to correlate with prostate cancer prognosis (45). While offering promise that new methods applied to needle biopsy will be able to enhance our prognostication for prostate cancer, further studies are needed before these techniques can be considered part of routine clinical practice.

Use of Nomograms

Various nomograms have been developed to predict pathologic stage and postradical prostatectomy progression (46–49). These nomograms use preoperative variables such as Gleason score, clinical stage, serum PSA, and in a more recent study the extent of cancer on biopsy to predict the risk of extraprostatic disease, seminal vesicle invasion, and lymph node metastases. Nomograms using the same preoperative variables have also been formulated to predict the risk the outcome after radiotherapy (50). The most widely used of these are the Partin tables, which are used by urologists, radiotherapists, oncologists, and patients to predict pathologic stage. The validity of these tables in part rests on accurate Gleason scoring, which will be dealt with in the next chapter.

Direct Staging on Needle Biopsy

Skeletal muscle fibers admix within the normal prostate, especially distally (apically) and anteriorly. Recognition of this finding is important for two reasons. First, nonneoplastic prostate glands may be seen admixed with skeletal muscle fibers occasionally in both transurethral resection (TUR) material as well as on needle biopsy (Fig. 3.3), and should not be diagnosed as prostate carcinoma. Also, the finding of adenocarcinoma of the prostate admixed with skeletal muscle fibers is not diagnostic of extraprostatic extension by carcinoma (Fig. 8.1, efig 1062-1063).

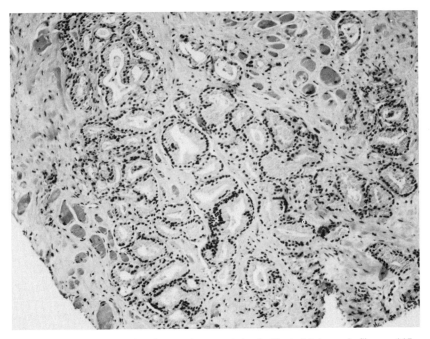

FIG. 8.1. Needle biopsy showing carcinoma admixed with skeletal muscle fibers. ×115.

In order to diagnose extraprostatic extension on needle biopsy, it is necessary to demonstrate adenocarcinoma infiltrating periprostatic adipose tissue, which is not a common finding (Fig. 8.2, efig 1064;1065;1066). Cancer can sometimes be identified infiltrating thick well-formed smooth muscle bundles, which is diagnostic of bladder neck muscle (efig 1067-1068;1069). As ganglion cells are sometimes located within the prostate, cancer invading ganglion cells are not diagnostic of extraprostatic extension. On occasion, the urologist may purposely biopsy the seminal vesicle to detect whether there is invasion. Those who recommend this procedure restrict this procedure to patients with abnormal seminal vesicles on ultrasound, markedly elevated PSA levels, or abnormal seminal vesicles on digital rectal examination (51,52). In some cases, carcinoma may be identified invading the seminal vesicle (Fig. 8.3, efig 1070-1071;1072;1073-1074;1075). If the urologist does not specify that he is biopsying the seminal vesicles, one has to be cautious in the interpretation of what appears to be seminal vesicle invasion by cancer. Cancer invading the ejaculatory ducts will appear identical on biopsy, yet does not indicate that the tumor is surgically incurable, as is the case with seminal vesicle invasion.

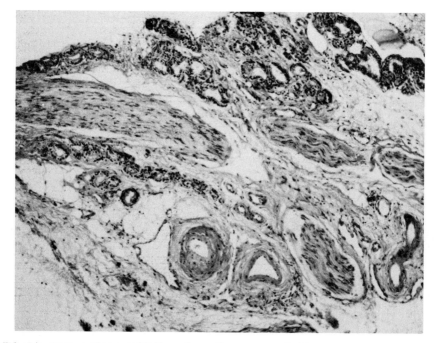

FIG. 8.2. Adenocarcinoma infiltrating adipose tissue on needle biopsy diagnostic of capsular penetration. ×115.

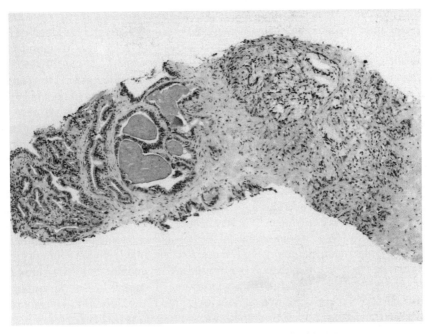

FIG. 8.3. Adenocarcinoma invading seminal vesicles *(left).*

Transurethral Resection

Currently, fewer cancers are incidentally detected on TUR as compared to a few years ago. This phenomenon results from a combination of factors. First, urologists are employing various medical therapies for the treatment of benign prostatic hyperplasia in an increasing number of men. Secondly, alternative surgical treatment options, such as lasers, cryosurgery, balloon dilatation, stents, and microwave therapy may not provide tissue for histological examination. Finally, in the workup of men with urinary obstructive symptoms, serum PSA tests and ultrasound studies may lead to a needle biopsy diagnosis of cancer. Nonetheless, TURs will continue to be performed either as an initial line of therapy in some men or in men who fail alternative treatment options.

Carcinoma that is unsuspected clinically and incidentally discovered in TUR specimens usually removed for benign prostatic hyperplasia is referred to as stage T1a and T1b disease. This situation occurs when either (a) the amount of carcinoma within the gland is very focal and not detectable by rectal exam, (b) when the tumor diffusely infiltrates the prostate without resulting in induration or a clinically detectable nodule, or (c) when the tumor is predominantly anteriorly or centrally located and not detectable on rectal examination even though there may be significant amount of tumor present. As one would expect, the behavior of the tumor in these various situations differs considerably. In fact, patients with a significant amount of clinically unsuspected tumor on transurethral resection of the prostate (TURP) tend to have higher pathologic stage in terms of extraprostatic extension, seminal vesicle involvement, and pelvic lymph node metastases than patients with unilateral palpable carcinoma (53). Because the tumor is not recognized clinically, the entire staging system used to evaluate these tumors is based on a histologic examination of the tumor. It is therefore the pathologists' responsibility to determine which system for classification of stage T1a and T1b disease is to be utilized and to advise the clinicians on the prognosis of incidental carcinomas of varying grades and quantities.

Subclassification

Approximately 16% (range 13% to 22%) of TURs performed for presumed benign prostatic hyperplasia reveal incidental adenocarcinoma of the prostate (54). Incidental adenocarcinoma of the prostate is divided into those tumors that are relatively low-volume and low-grade (stage T1a) and those that are high-volume or high-grade (stage T1b). The definition of stage T1a disease is tumor occupying ≤5% of the specimen *and* not high-grade (Gleason sum <7), and stage T1b is defined as higher volume *or* high-grade tumor (55). There have been several articles published on the long-term progression rate of untreated stage T1a disease (56). The progression rates in these studies ranged from 8% to 27% with the minimum follow-up ranging from 5 to 10 years. Data from these long-term studies shed some light on the question of whether low-volume intermediate grade tumor should be considered stage T1a or T1b. As long as the tumor occupies ≤5% of the specimen, there is no difference in the progression rate at 8 years following diagnosis whether the Gleason sum is ≤4 or 5 to 6 (54). Newer techniques, such as DNA ploidy and nuclear morphometry, have in some studies enhanced our ability to predict progression in stage T1a and T1b tumors, although these tests have not been adopted for clinical use (57,58).

It is important for the pathologist to accurately stage T1a or T1b disease when incidental adenocarcinoma is found on TURP. Depending on the age of the patient, stage T1b patients are treated definitively with surgery or radiotherapy, while most stage T1a patients are followed expectantly. There are two situations where subclassification is not as critical, since both T1a and T1b disease are treated definitively. Some young men with stage T1a disease may be offered radical prostatectomy as a treatment option because of their increased long-term risk of progression. The other situation where a man with stage T1a cancer might undergo radical prostatectomy is if his post-TURP serum PSA level is high, suggesting significant residual tumor (59).

Calculating the percent of the TUR involved by cancer is not always straightforward unless the amount of cancer is at the extremes (i.e., >30% or <1%). To assess the percentage of caner, first, only the cancer is circled on the glass slide, not the entire chip that contains the cancer. Second, choose the size of a chip that you are going to consider as a "typical chip." Then add on all the slides how many "typical chips" of cancer there are; two small areas of circled cancer on two chips may equal one "typical chip" of cancer. Next, calculate the total number of "typical chips" there are in the entire specimen by estimating the number of "typical chips" there are on one slide, and multiplying it by the total number of slides (assuming an approximately equal amount of tissue per slide). The percentage of the specimen involved by cancer is the number of "typical chips" with cancer divided by the total number of "typical chips".

REFERENCES

1. Badalament RA, Miller MC, Peller PA, et al. An algorithm for predicting nonorgan confined prostate cancer using the results obtained from sextant core biopsies with prostate specific antigen level. *J Urol* 1996;156:1375–1380.
2. Huland H, Hammerer P, Henke RP, et al. Preoperative prediction of tumor heterogeneity and recurrence after radical prostatectomy for localized prostatic carcinoma with digital rectal examination, prostate specific antigen and the results of 6 systematic biopsies. *J Urol* 1996;155:1344–1347.
3. Peller PA, Young DC, Marmaduke DP, et al. Sextant prostate biopsies: a histopathologic correlation with radical prostatectomy specimens. *Cancer* 1995; 75;530–538.
4. Ravery V, Boccon-Gibod LA, Dauge-Geffroy MC, et al. Systemic biopsies accurately predict extracapsular extension of prostate cancer and persistent/recurrent detectable PSA after radical prostatectomy. *Urology* 1994;44:371–376.
5. Wills ML, Sauvageot J, Partin AW, et al. Ability of sextant biopsies to predict radical prostatectomy stage. *Urology* 1998;51:759–764.
6. Sebo TJ, Bock BJ, Cheville JC, et al. The percent of cores positive for cancer in prostate needle biopsy specimens is strongly predictive of tumor stage and volume at radical prostatectomy. *J Urol* 2000; 163:174–178.
7. Terris MK, Haney DJ, Johnstone IM, et al. Prediction of prostate cancer volume using prostate-specific antigen levels, transrectal ultrasound, and systemic sextant biopsies. *Urology* 1995;45:75–80.
8. Conrad S, Graefen M, Pichlmeier U, et al. Systematic sextant biopsies improve preoperative prediction of pelvic lymph node metastases in patients with clinically localized prostatic carcinoma. *J Urol* 1998;159:2023–2029.
9. Humphrey PA, Baty J, Keetch D. Relationship between serum prostate specific antigen, needle biopsy findings, and histopathologic features of prostatic carcinoma in radical prostatectomy tissues. *Cancer* 1995;75:1842–1849.
10. Ackerman DA, Barry JM, Wicklund RA, et al. Analysis of risk factors associated with prostate cancer extension to the surgical margin and pelvic node metastasis at radical prostatectomy. *J Urol* 1993; 159:1845–1850.
11. Tigrani VS, Bhargava V, Shinohara K, et al. Number of positive systematic sextant biopsies predicts surgical margin status at radical prostatectomy. *Urology* 1999;54:689–693.
12. Presti JC Jr, Shinohara K, Bacchetti P, et al. Positive fraction of systematic biopsies predicts risk of relapse after radical prostatectomy. *Urology* 1998;52:1079–1084.
13. Bostwick DG, Qian J, Bergstralh E, et al. Prediction of capsular perforation and seminal vesicle invasion in prostate cancer. *J Urol* 1996;155:1361–1367.
14. Cupp MR, Bostwick DG, Myers RP, et al. The volume of prostate cancer in the biopsy specimen cannot reliably predict the quantity of cancer in the radical prostatectomy specimen on an individual basis. *J Urol* 1995;53:1543–1548.
15. Ravery V, Schmid HP, Toublanc M, et al. Is the percentage of cancer in biopsy cores predictive of extracapsular disease in T1-T2 prostate carcinoma? *Cancer* 1996;78:1079–1084.
16. Ukimura O, Troncoso P, Ramirez EI, et al. Prostate cancer staging: correlation between determined tumor contact length and pathologically confirmed extraprostatic extension. *J Urol* 1998;159: 1251–1259.
17. Rubin MA, Bassily N, Sanda M, et al. Relationship and significance of greatest percentage of tumor and perineural invasion on needle biopsy in prostatic adenocarcinoma. *Am J Surg Pathol* 2000;24: 183–189.

18. Bruce RG, Rankin WR, Cibull ML, et al. Single focus of adenocarcinoma in the prostate biopsy specimen is not predictive of the pathologic stage of disease. *Urology* 1996;48:75–79.
19. Dietrick DD, McNeal JE, Stamey TA. Core cancer length in ultrasound-guided systematic sextant biopsies: a preoperative evaluation of prostate cancer volume. *Urology* 1995;45:987–992.
20. Epstein JI, Walsh PC, CarMichael M, et al. Pathological and clinical findings to predict tumor extent of non-palpable (stage T1c) prostate cancer. *JAMA* 1994;271:368–374.
21. Wang X, Brannigan RE, Rademaker AW, et al. One core positive prostate biopsy is a poor predictor of cancer volume in the radical prostatectomy specimen. *J Urol* 1997;158:1431–1435.
22. Weldon W, Tavel FR, Neuwirth H, et al. Failure of focal prostate cancer on biopsy to predict focal prostate cancer: the importance of prevalence. *J Urol* 1995;154:1074–1077.
23. Taneja SS, Penson DF, Epelbaum A, et al. Does site specific labeling of sextant biopsy cores predict the site of extraprostatic extension in radical prostatectomy surgical specimen? *J Urol* 1999;162: 1352–1358.
24. Allen EA, Kahane H, Epstein JI. Repeat biopsy strategies for men with atypical diagnoses on initial prostate needle biopsy. *Urology* 1998;52:803–807.
25. Calvanese CB, Kahane H, Carlson GD, et al. Presurgical staging of prostate cancer. *Infect Urol* 1999; 12:22–28.
26. Epstein JI, Lecksell K, Carter HB. Prostate cancer sampled on sextant needle biopsy: significance of cancer on multiple cores from different areas of the prostate. *Urology* 1999;54:291–294.
27. Byar DP, Mostofi FK, Veterans Administration Cooperative Urological Research Group. Carcinoma of the prostate: prognostic evaluation of certain pathologic features in 208 radical prostatectomies. *Cancer* 1972;30:5–13.
28. Villers A, McNeal JE, Redwine EA, et al. The role of perineural invasion in the local spread of prostatic adenocarcinoma. *J Urol* 1989;142:763–768.
29. Bastacky SI, Walsh PC, Epstein JI. Relationship between perineural tumor invasion on needle biopsy and radical prostatectomy capsular penetration in clinical stage B adenocarcinoma of the prostate. *Am J Surg Pathol* 1993;17:336–341.
30. Holmes GF, Walsh PC, Pound CR, et al. Excision of the neurovascular bundle at radical prostatectomy in cases with perineural invasion on needle biopsy. *Urology* 1999;53:752–756.
31. De la Taille A, Katz A, Bagiella E, et al. Perineural invasion on prostate needle biopsy: an independent predictor of final pathologic stage. *Urology* 1999;54:1039–1043.
32. Egan AJM, Bostwick DG. Prediction of extraprostatic extension of prostate cancer based on needle biopsy findings: perineural invasion lacks significance on multivariate analysis. *Am J Surg Pathol* 1997;21:1496–1500.
33. Vargas SO, Jiroutek M, Welch WR, et al. Perineural invasion in prostate needle biopsy specimens. Correlation with extraprostatic extension at resection. *Am J Clin.Pathol* 1999;111:223–228.
34. Stone NN, Stock RG, Parikh D., et al. Perineural invasion and seminal vesicle involvement predict lymph node metastasis in men with localized carcinoma of the prostate. *J Urol* 1998;160:1722–1726.
35. De la Taille A, Rubin MA, Bagiella E, et al. Can perineural invasion on prostate needle biopsy predict prostate specific antigen recurrence after radical prostatectomy? *J Urol* 1999;162:103–106.
36. Epstein .JI, Partin AW, Sauvageot J, et al. Prediction of progression following radical prostatectomy: a multivariate analysis of 721 men with long-term follow-up. *Am J Surg Pathol* 1996;20:286–292.
37. Anderson PR, Hanlon AL, Patchefsky A, et al. Perineural invasion and Gleason 7–10 tumors predict increased failure in prostate cancer patients with pretreatment PSA <10 ng/ml treated with conformal external beam radiation therapy. *Int J Radiat Oncol Biol Phys* 1998;41:1087–1092.
38. Brinker DA, Ross JS, Tran TA, et al. Can ploidy of prostate carcinoma diagnosed on needle biopsy predict radical prostatectomy stage and grade? *J Urol* 1999;162:2036–2039.
39. Ross JS, Figge H, Bui HX, et al. Prediction of pathologic stage and postprostatectomy disease recurrence by DNA ploidy analysis of initial needle biopsy specimens of prostate cancer. *Cancer* 1994;74: 2811–2818.
40. Ross JS, Sheehan CE, Ambros RA, et al. Needle biopsy DNA ploidy status predicts grade shifting in prostate cancer. *Am J Surg Pathol* 1999;23:296–301.
41. Bostwick DG, Wheeler TM, Blute M, et al. Optimized microvessel density analysis improves prediction of cancer stage from prostate needle biopsies. *Urology* 1996;48:47–57.
42. Diaz JI, Mora LB, Austin PF, et al. Predictability of PSA failure in prostate cancer by computerized cytometric assessment of tumor cell proliferation. *Urology* 1999;53:931–938.
43. Brewster SF, Oxley JD, Trivella M, et al. Preoperative p53, bcl-2, CD44 and e-cadherin immunohistochemistry as predictors of biochemical relapse after radical prostatectomy. *J Urol* 1999;161:1238–1243.

44. Casella R, Bubendorf L, Sauter G, et al. Focal neuroendocrine differentiation lacks prognostic significance in prostate core needle biopsies. *J Urol* 1998;160:406–410.
45. Zhang YH, Kanamaru H, Oyama N, et al. Prognostic value of nuclear morphometry on needle biopsy from patients with prostate cancer: is volume-weighted mean nuclear volume superior to other morphometric parameters? *Urology* 2000;55:377–381.
46. Ross PL, Scardino PT, Kattan MW. A catalog of prostate cancer nomograms. *J Urol* 2001;165: 1562–1568.
47. Partin AW, Kattan MW, Subong EN, et al. Combination of prostate-specific antigen, clinical stage, and Gleason score to predict pathological stage of localized prostate cancer. A multi-institutional update. *JAMA* 1997;277:1445–1451.
48. Kattan MW, Eastham JA, Stapleton AMF, et al. A preoperative nomogram for disease recurrence following radical prostatectomy for prostate cancer. *J Natl Cancer Inst* 1998;90:766–771.
49. D'Amico AY, Whittington R, Malcowicz SB, et al. Combination of preoperative PSA level, biopsy Gleason score, percentage of positive biopsies, and MRI T-stage to predict early PSA failure in men with clinically localized prostate cancer. *Urology* 2000;55:572–577.
50. Kattan MW, Zelefsky MJ, Kupelian PA, et al. Pretreatment nomogram for predicting the outcome of three-dimensional conformal radiotherapy in prostate cancer. *J Clin Oncol* 2000;18:3352–3359.
51. Terris MK, McNeal JE, Freiha FS, et al. Efficacy of transrectal ultrasound-guided seminal vesicle biopsies in the detection of seminal vesicle invasion by prostate cancer. *J Urol* 1993;149:1035–1039.
52. Vallancien G, Bochereau G, Wetzel O, et al. Influence of preoperative positive seminal vesicle biopsy on the staging of prostatic cancer. *J Urol* 1994;152:1152–1156.
53. Christenson WN, Partin AW, Walsh PC, et al. Pathologic findings in stage A2 prostate cancer: relation of tumor volume, grade and location to pathologic stage. *Cancer* 1990;65:1021–1027.
54. Eble JN, Epstein JI. Stage A carcinoma of the prostate. In: Bostwick DG (consultant ed). *Pathology of the Prostate, Seminal Vesicles, and Male Urethra.* Roth LM, ed. *Contemporary Issues in Surgical Pathology.* New York, NY: Churchill Livingstone; 1990:61–82.
55. Cantrell BB, Deklerk DP, Eggleston JC, et al. Pathological factors that influence prognosis in stage A prostatic cancer: the influence of extent versus grade. *J Urol* 1981;125:516–520.
56. Matzkin H, Patel JP, Altwein JE, et al. Stage T1A carcinoma of prostate. *Urology* 1994;43:11–21.
57. McIntire TL, Murphy WM, Coon JS, et al. The prognostic value of DNA ploidy combined with histologic substaging for incidental carcinoma of the prostate gland. *Am J Clin Pathol* 1988;89:370–373.
58. Epstein JI, Berry SJ, Eggleston JC. Nuclear roundness factor: a predictor of progression in untreated state A2 prostate cancer. *Cancer* 1984;54:1666–1671.
59. Carter HB, Partin AW, Epstein JI, et al. The relationship of prostate-specific antigen levels and residual tumor volume in stage A prostate cancer. *J Urol* 1990;144:1222–1226.

9

Grading of Prostatic Adenocarcinomas

The Gleason System

OVERVIEW OF THE GLEASON SYSTEM
AS APPLIED TO NEEDLE BIOPSIES
AND TRANSURETHRAL RESECTIONS

An important role of the pathologist in evaluating adenocarcinoma of the prostate on biopsy and transurethral resection of the prostate (TURP) is to grade the tumor accurately. The grade is often critical for urologists, radiotherapists, and oncologists in planning treatment and predicting prognosis.

The Gleason grading system is the most commonly used grading system for prostate cancer in the United States and is gaining worldwide acceptance (Fig. 9.1). There are several unique aspects of the Gleason grading system. First, the Gleason grading system is solely based on the architectural pattern (1–3). Cytologic features are not factored in. Correspondingly, there is a schematic diagram showing the architectural patterns of the Gleason system. The second unique feature of the Gleason grading system is that the overall grade is not based on the highest grade within the tumor. Gleason and the Veteran's Administration Cooperative Study found that the prognosis of prostate cancer was intermediate between that of the most predominant pattern of cancer and that of the second most predominant pattern. Both the primary (predominant) and the secondary (second most prevalent) architectural patterns are identified and assigned a grade from 1 to 5, with 1 the most differentiated and 5 the least differentiated.

If a tumor had only one histologic pattern, then for uniformity the primary and secondary scores are given the same grade. The combined Gleason grades range from 2 (1+1=2), which represents tumors uniformly composed of Gleason pattern 1 tumor, to 10 (5+5=10), which represents totally undifferentiated

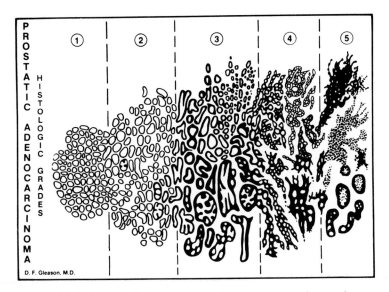

FIG. 9.1. Schematic diagram of Gleason's grading system (see text).

tumors. Synonyms for "combined Gleason grade" are "Gleason sum" and "Gleason score." A tumor that is predominantly Gleason pattern 3 with a lesser amount of Gleason pattern 5 has a combined Gleason grade of 8 (3+5=8), as does a tumor that is predominantly Gleason pattern 5 with a lesser amount of Gleason pattern 3 tumor (5+3=8) (Fig. 9.2, efig 1076;1077-1079;1080-1081). Most cases with divergent patterns, especially on needle biopsy, do not differ by more than one pattern.

Gleason Pattern 1

Gleason pattern 1 tumor is composed of circumscribed nodules of uniform, single, separate, closely packed glands (Fig. 9.3). Gleason pattern 1 is an extremely uncommon finding on transurethral resection and is even rarer as a pure pattern (i.e., Gleason grade 1+1=2) (efig 1082;1083-1085). We do not diagnose Gleason score 2–4 on needle biopsy (see below).

Gleason Pattern 2

In Gleason pattern 2, though the tumor is still fairly circumscribed, at the edge of the tumor nodule there can be minimal extension by neoplastic glands into the surrounding nonneoplastic prostate (efig 1086-1088;1089-1091). The glands are more loosely arranged and not quite as uniform as Gleason pattern 1 (Figs. 9.4

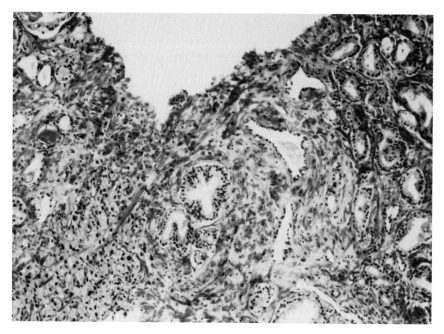

FIG. 9.2. Needle biopsy showing Gleason pattern 3 tumor *(right)* and focus of undifferentiated Gleason pattern 5 tumor *(lower left corner).* ×110.

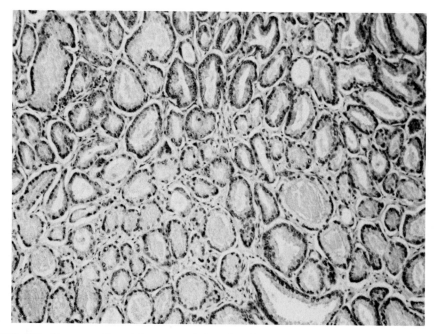

FIG. 9.3. Gleason pattern 1 tumor consisting of uniform, single, separate, closely packed glands. ×125.

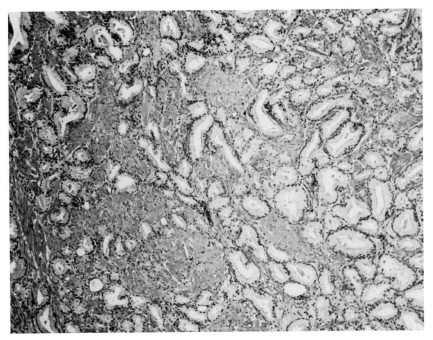

FIG. 9.4. Gleason pattern 2 carcinoma showing a less uniform and more loose arrangement of the neoplastic glands, as compared with Gleason pattern 1. ×50.

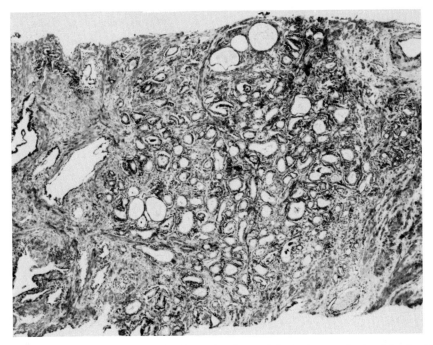

FIG. 9.5. Gleason pattern 2 on needle biopsy showing a relatively circumscribed nodule of open glands that show a somewhat greater variation in size and shape, as compared with Gleason pattern 1 tumor. ×45.

and 9.5, 6.16,6.18,6.19). The glands in Gleason pattern 1 and Gleason pattern 2 tumor tend to be larger than intermediate-grade carcinomas. Typically, both Gleason pattern 1 and Gleason pattern 2 carcinomas have abundant pale eosinophilic cytoplasm. It has been proposed that transition zone cancers be termed "clear cell carcinomas" (4). We do not feel that these tumors represent a unique histology, but rather reflect the finding that transition zone cancers are frequently low-grade. Carcinomas with pale cytoplasm may also be found in the peripheral zone.

Gleason Pattern 3

Gleason pattern 3 tumor infiltrates in and among nonneoplastic prostate acini as seen in Figures 9.6 and 9.7. The neoplastic glands show marked variation in size and shape. Gleason pattern 3 reveals smaller glands than seen in Gleason pattern 1 or 2 (Figs. 9.8 and 9.9, efig 1092-1093;1094-1095;1096-1098;1099-1100;1101-1102;1103-1104;1105, Color Plates 11, 12, 13, 14, 15, 16, 20). In contrast to Gleason pattern 4, the glands in Gleason pattern 3 are discrete units. If one can mentally draw a circle around well-formed individual glands, then it is Gleason pattern 3. One should assign a Gleason grade at rel-

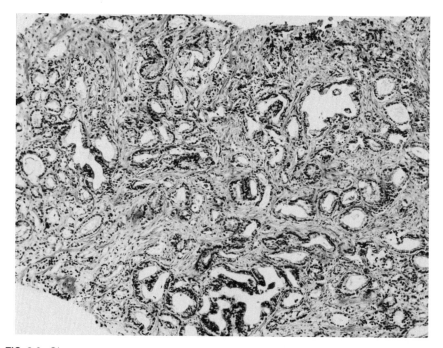

FIG. 9.6. Gleason pattern 3 tumor on needle biopsy showing large variation in size and shape of the neoplastic glands as well as an infiltrative pattern. ×60.

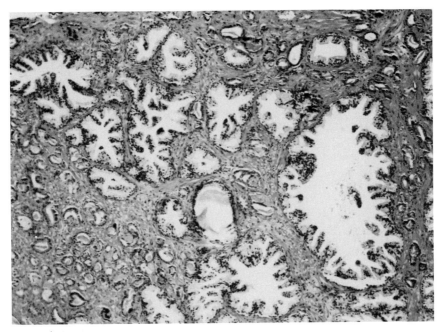

FIG. 9.7. Gleason pattern 3 tumor infiltrating among normal glands as opposed to more circumscribed Gleason patterns 1 and 2 tumor. ×145.

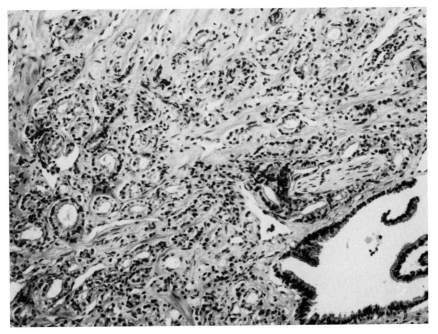

FIG. 9.8. Gleason pattern 3 tumor on needle biopsy showing discrete gland formation, yet smaller glands than seen in Gleason patterns 1 and 2. ×55.

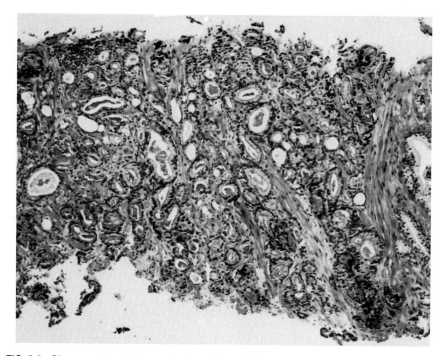

FIG. 9.9. Gleason pattern 3 tumor showing wide variation in size and shape in glands, ranging from very small glands to larger open glands. ×95.

atively low power (i.e., 2.5× or 4×); the presence of a few poorly formed glands at high power is still consistent with Gleason pattern 3 tumor (efig 1106-1107;1108-1109;1110-1111). Smoothly circumscribed small cribriform nodules of tumor are also classified as pattern 3 (Fig. 9.10, efig 1112;1113;1114; 1115;1116-1119;1120;1121-1122;1123). Small infiltrating glands of Gleason pattern 3 almost always accompany the cribriform glands. Although there is also subjectivity as to whether a tumor is Gleason sum 6 or 5, we have not found this distinction to be critical, since the prognosis and treatment of these tumors are similar (5).

Gleason Pattern 4

Gleason pattern 4 glands are no longer single and separate as seen in patterns 1 to 3 (Fig. 9.11). The glands appear fused and ill-defined, even at low magnification (Fig. 9.12, efig 1224;1125-1126;1127;1128-1129;1130;1131-1132;1133-1134;1135;1136-1137;1138-1139;1140;1141-1142;1143). Most cases on needle biopsy with mixed Gleason patterns, such as Gleason 3+4=7, consist of tumors such as those that we have illustrated where there are not discrete foci with different patterns, but rather tumors that tend to bridge between two patterns (Fig.

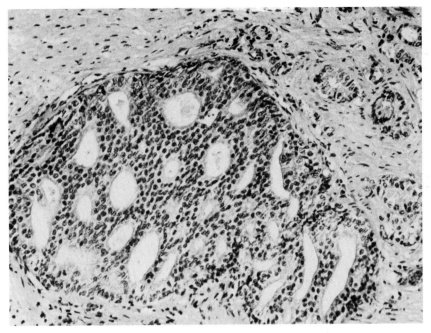

FIG. 9.10. Well-circumscribed cribriform nest of Gleason pattern 3 associated with surrounding small infiltrating glands of Gleason pattern 3. ×110.

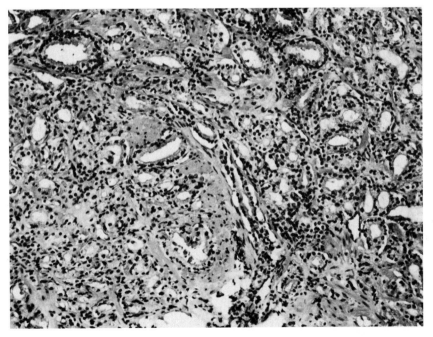

FIG. 9.11. Gleason 3+4=7 tumor with upper right corner showing individual small and larger glands (Gleason pattern 3) and lower left corner tumor showing loss of individual gland formation with only focal luminal differentiation (Gleason pattern 4). ×100.

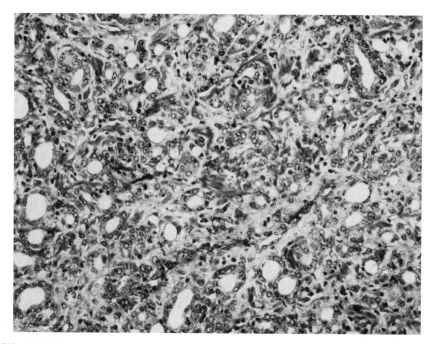

FIG. 9.12. Gleason pattern 4 tumor showing loss of glandular differentiation with only minimal lumen formation. ×195.

9.11, efig 1144;1145;1146;1147;1148;1149;1150;1151;1152;1153;1154). The potential for having discrete areas of different grades more frequently comes about when grading tumor on transurethral resection material given the greater amount of tumor sampled.

In Gleason pattern 4, one may also see large cribriform glands or cribriform glands with an irregular border (Figs. 9.13 and 9.14) as opposed to the smoothly circumscribed smaller nodules of cribriform Gleason pattern 3 (efig 1155;1156-1157;1158-1159;1160-1161;1162-1163;1164;1165-1166;1167-1169). On needle biopsy, cribriform Gleason pattern 4 tumor often manifests as fragments of cribriform tumor, as there is little supporting stroma. Another form of Gleason pattern 4 tumor resembles renal cell carcinoma and is referred to as a hypernephromatoid pattern (Fig. 9.15). It is important to recognize Gleason pattern 4 tumor, since tumors with this pattern have a significantly worse prognosis than those with pure Gleason pattern 3 (5–7).

Most examples of Gleason pattern 4 (3+4=7, 4+3=7, 4+4=8) seen on needle biopsy are fairly extensive. With increased screening for prostate cancer using serum prostatic-specific antigen (PSA) tests, we have seen an increased number of small foci of cancer on needle biopsy with Gleason pattern 4.

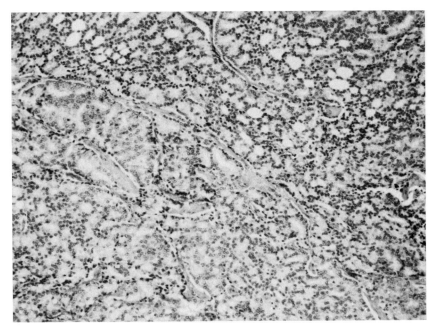

FIG. 9.13. Irregular nests and sheet-like cribriform formation of Gleason pattern 4 tumor. ×65.

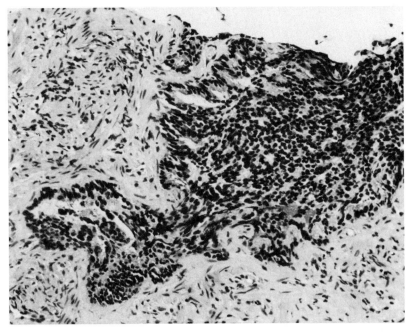

FIG. 9.14. Irregular nests of tumor with ragged boundaries and only minimal luminal differentiation typical of Gleason pattern 4 tumor. ×110.

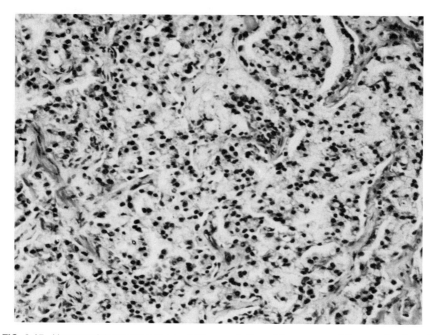

FIG. 9.15. Hypernephromatoid pattern of Gleason pattern 4 tumor resembling renal-cell carcinoma. ×195.

Gleason Pattern 5

Gleason pattern 5 tumor shows no glandular differentiation, composed of solid sheets, cords, or single cells (Figs. 9.16, 9.17, 9.18, efig 1170-1171;1172;1173-1175; 1176;1177; 1178;1179-1180;1181;1182;1183-1184;1185-1186;1187-1188). Solid nests of tumor with central comedonecrosis are also classified under Gleason pattern 5 (Fig. 9.19, efig 1189-1190;1191-1192). High-grade prostatic carcinomas often are not as pleomorphic or as mitotically active as poorly differentiated tumors in other organs such as the bladder (Fig. 9.20).

GLEASON SCORE 2–4 ADENOCARCINOMA OF THE PROSTATE ON NEEDLE BIOPSY

The vast majority of tumors graded as Gleason score 2–4 on needle biopsy, when reviewed by experts in urological pathology, are graded as Gleason scores 5–6 or higher (efig 1193-1194;1195-1196;1197-1198;1199-1200, Color Plate 36). In a study of men coming to The Johns Hopkins Hospital for radical prostatectomy, we concurred with the outside needle biopsy grade of Gleason score 2–4 in only four of 87 cases; 68 tumors were graded at our institution as Gleason score 5–6, 13 as Gleason score 7, and two as Gleason score 8–10 (8). Even the few cases diagnosed on biopsy as Gleason score 2–4 at our institution showed higher grade tumor at radical prostatectomy.

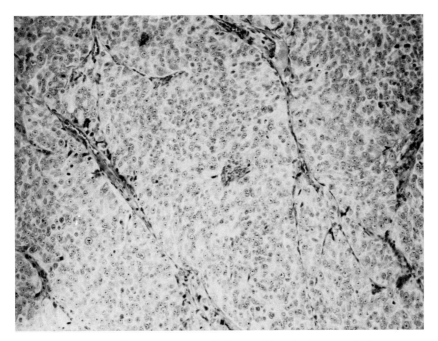

FIG. 9.16. Gleason pattern 5 with large solid nests of tumor. ×100.

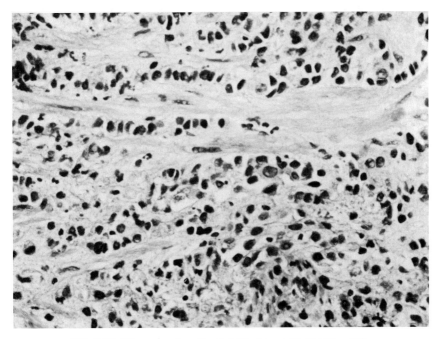

FIG. 9.17. Gleason pattern 5 with infiltrating cords of cells. ×310.

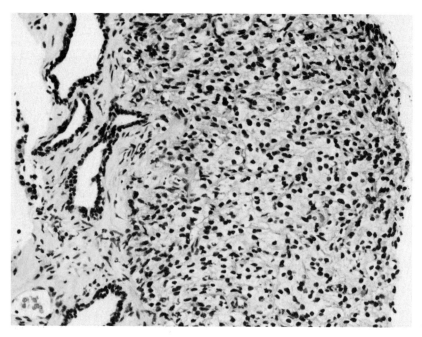

FIG. 9.18. Gleason pattern 5 tumor on needle biopsy consisting of infiltrating individual cells without luminal differentiation. ×125.

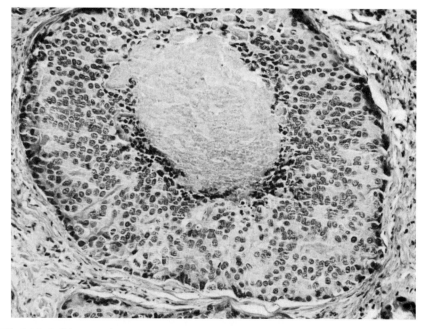

FIG. 9.19. Solid nests of tumor with central comedonecrosis, a variant of Gleason pattern 5 tumor. ×180.

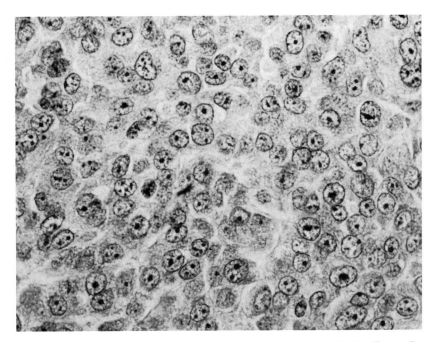

FIG. 9.20. Higher magnification of Gleason pattern 5 tumor showing relatively uniform cells, as opposed to poorly differentiated transitional-cell carcinoma of the bladder. ×420.

The second reason why Gleason score 2–4 should not be assigned as a grade on needle biopsy is poor reproducibility in its diagnosis even among urological pathology experts. In one study we sought to determine the interobserver reproducibility of the Gleason grading system among ten prostate pathology experts (9). There were four cases considered to represent Gleason score 2–4 cancer by the two authors who designed this study. However, in only one of the four cases was there a consensus by at least eight of the ten experts that it was low-grade. In the other three cases, the percentage of experts assigning a Gleason score 2–4 was 40%, 40%, and 70%. If the specialists cannot agree what is Gleason score 2–4 adenocarcinoma on needle biopsy, how can we expect general practicing pathologists to do so.

Most importantly, assigning a Gleason score 2–4 to adenocarcinoma on needle biopsies can adversely impact patient care, as clinicians may assume that low-grade cancers on needle biopsy do not need definitive therapy. In part, this treatment strategy is based on misinterpretation of medical articles that have received significant lay press. In one such article, the authors correlated Gleason score with prognosis in men managed conservatively for clinically localized prostate cancer (10). The authors concluded "Men whose prostate biopsy specimens show Gleason score 2–4 disease face a minimal risk of death from prostate cancer within 15 years of diagnosis." However, in this study almost all of the tumors assigned a Gleason score 2–4 were not diagnosed on needle biopsy, but rather on TURP. In contrast to the situation with needle biopsies, low volume Gleason score 2–4 adenocarcinoma of the prostate on TURP has a relatively indolent course. Some clinicians have generalized from this and other articles to consider all tumors with a Gleason score of 2–4, whether on biopsy or TURP, as having a low risk of progression. Consequently, some men with tumors diagnosed on needle biopsy, where the assigned grade is Gleason score 2–4, will potentially be undertreated or at the least improperly counseled as to their risk of tumor progression if expectant therapy is selected. The assurance that one is dealing with an indolent tumor based on a low Gleason score on needle biopsy is not well founded. Of 87 needle biopsies with cancers graded as Gleason score 2–4 by outside institutions, 48 (55%) showed extraprostatic extension at radical prostatectomy, including four cases with invasion of either seminal vesicles or lymph nodes (8).

By not assigning a Gleason score 2–4 to adenocarcinoma on needle biopsy, we are not denying the existence of low-grade prostate cancer. Gleason score 2–4 adenocarcinomas are typically seen on TURP. Low-grade cancers are rarely seen on needle biopsy because they are predominantly located anteriorly in the prostate within the transition zone and they tend to be small.

For the rare truly low-grade cancer sampled on needle biopsy, little harm will be done by assigning it a Gleason score 5 (Gleason score 2+3=5) as proposed, as compared to the current practice where many more cases of higher grade cancer are undergraded. For those who feel uncomfortable assigning a Gleason score 5–6 on biopsy, for the rare case that morphologically more resembles Gleason score 2–4 tumor, there are two alternatives. One option is to call the tumor Gleason score 2–4 and add a note stating "Tumors with a low-grade appearance on needle biopsy almost always show higher grade tumor in the prostate and in 50% of cases are associated with extraprostatic extension." Alternatively, these cases could be signed out as well-moderately differentiated adenocarcinoma (Gleason score 2–6). By adopting such a system, one would not have to feel that there is a conflict between one's observation and the classification system used. At the same time, the needle biopsy grade would more closely correlate with that found at radical prostatectomy and provide prognostically distinct groups to guide therapy.

PERCENTAGE PATTERN 4/5

The group from Stanford has been a strong proponent of using the proportion of high-grade tumor (Gleason pattern 4 and 5) as the preferred method for grading prostate cancer (11). However, percent pattern 4/5 is only very predictive for progression at the extremes (>70% or <20% pattern 4/5). In a more recent study, the same group did not demonstrate a good correlation between the percent Gleason pattern 4/5 on needle as compared to the corresponding radical prostatectomy specimen (12). For example, if there was no grade 4/5 in the biopsy, 27% of men had >10% grade 4/5 in the radical prostatectomy specimen. From the practical standpoint, often patterns 4 and 3 are intimately admixed such that their relative percentages are not readily calculatable. Assessing the percentage of Gleason pattern 4 is often difficult and not likely to be performed routinely.

PROGNOSIS

The Gleason grading system is one of the more powerful prognostic indicators in prostate cancer. Gleason score correlates with all of the important pathologic parameters seen in the radical prostatectomy specimen, with prognosis after radical prostatectomy, and with outcome following radiotherapy (Table 9.1)(5,7,13). The major shift in terms of the likelihood of having adverse findings in the prostatectomy, or with failure following prostatectomy or radiotherapy is between a Gleason score of 6 and 7. Gleason score 7 tumors behave significantly worse than Gleason score 5–6 tumors and should not be combined together as "intermediate-grade carcinoma." Gleason score 7 tumors do fare better than Gleason score 8–10 tumors. The following combination of Gleason scores results in groups of similar prognosis: Gleason score 2–4 (well-differentiated); Gleason score 5–6 (moderately differentiated); Gleason score 7 (moderately-poorly differentiated); and Gleason 8–10 (poorly differentiated).

The importance of grade is evidenced by the use of various nomograms to predict pathologic stage, postradical prostatectomy progression, and postradiotherapy failure (14–18). These nomograms use preoperative variables such as Gleason score, clinical stage, serum PSA and in a more recent study the extent of cancer on biopsy to predict the risk of extraprostatic disease, seminal vesicle invasion, and lymph node metastases. The validity of these tables in part rests on accurate Gleason scoring.

TABLE 9.1. *Correlation of Gleason score with pathology at radical prostatectomy*

Pathology	Gleason score			
	5	6	7	8–10
Nonfocal extraprostatic extension	16%	24%	62%	85%
Positive margins	20%	29%	48%	59%
Mean tumor volume	2.2	2.7	5.1	4.0
Seminal vesicle invasion	1%	4%	17%	48%
Lymph node metastases	1%	2%	12%	24%

IMPACT ON TREATMENT

Grade is one of the most influential factors used to determine treatment for prostate cancer. Whereas some younger men with limited amounts of Gleason score 5–6 on needle biopsy and low PSA values may be followed expectantly, almost all men with Gleason score 7 tumor will be treated more definitively (19,20).

Clinicians also use the grade as part of the nomograms to predict the likelihood of tumor extension out of the prostate. Based on these nomograms factoring in clinical stage and serum PSA values, a man with a Gleason score 6 tumor may be a candidate for interstitial radiotherapy (brachytherapy) as a monotherapy. However, if this man had a Gleason score 7 tumor, with a greater likelihood of extraprostatic extension by tumor, he would most likely be treated with external beam radiotherapy either as the sole therapy or as an adjunct to brachytherapy, as seed therapy cannot effectively treat extraprostatic disease. A surgeon may also be influenced by the grade of the tumor along with its extent on biopsy in deciding whether to resect the neurovascular bundle(s), which will impact on postoperative potency. An accurate diagnosis of Gleason scores 8 and above is also critical for patient management. A man with a Gleason score 8 or above cancer on biopsy might not be treated with surgery, depending on the extent of tumor and other clinical factors; the same man with a Gleason score 7 tumor would be offered radical prostatectomy as a treatment option.

Another use of the nomograms, which factor in the needle biopsy grade, is to predict the likelihood of a patient having lymph node metastases. In a man with a biopsy Gleason score of 6, a normal digital rectal examination, and a serum PSA value of <10 ng/mL, the likelihood of having lymph node metastases is so low that some urologists might forego lymphadenectomy at the time of radical prostatectomy. If the biopsy grade is Gleason score 7 or higher, lymph nodes would be sampled. At The Johns Hopkins Hospital, the biopsy grade dictates whether we do frozen sections on the pelvic lymphadenectomy specimens. We have found that the best predictor of which patients will not benefit from a radical prostatectomy who have positive nodes is the presence of high-grade cancer (Gleason 8–10) on needle biopsy. If these men with high-grade cancer on biopsy undergo radical prostatectomy with positive nodes, they proceed to distant metastases within a short period of time such that one cannot justify a radical prostatectomy for local control. Consequently, in men with a Gleason 8–10 cancer on needle biopsy, we recommend freezing multiple nodes or possibly having these patients undergo laparoscopic lymph node dissection prior to radical prostatectomy. If the nodes are positive in these cases then these men do not go on to radical prostatectomy. In men with Gleason 7 or less on needle biopsy we do not freeze the lymph nodes, since even if these men's lymph nodes are positive, they have a reasonably long life expectancy and our urologists proceed ahead with the radical prostatectomy for local control (21).

Grade on biopsy can therefore influence whether definitive treatment is given (watchful waiting or surgery/radiation), what type of treatment (surgery or radiation), and even decisions within a specific therapy (brachytherapy or external beam therapy; whether to resect the neurovascular bundle(s) or lymph nodes at surgery).

CORRELATION WITH SERUM PSA LEVELS

In general, serum PSA levels correlate with larger tumor volume, advanced pathologic stage, and higher grade. Although higher grade cancer produces less PSA per cell as compared to lower grade tumor, overall, poorly differentiated tumors are associated with higher PSA levels, as these tumors tend to be larger and of more advanced stage (22). There are exceptions where very high-grade prostate cancers are so poorly differentiated that associated serum PSA levels are disproportionably low. Certain subtypes of prostate cancer are also often associated with lower serum PSA levels as compared to the typical acinar prostate cancer; these include small cell carcinoma and ductal adenocarcinoma of the prostate.

APPLICATION WHEN MORE THAN TWO PATTERNS ARE PRESENT

In radical prostatectomy specimens, we have demonstrated that when there are three patterns present the prognosis is determined by the most common pattern combined with the highest grade (23). For example, if the tumor was Gleason score 3+4=7 with a tertiary pattern 5, the prognosis is that of Gleason score 8. Although comparable data does not exist for needle biopsy material, in the setting of three grades on biopsy where the highest grade is the least common, we incorporate the highest grade as the secondary pattern. The assumption is that a small focus of high-grade cancer on biopsy will correlate with a significant amount of high-grade cancer in the prostate, and that sampling artifact accounts for its limited nature on biopsy.

CORRELATION BETWEEN BIOPSY AND RADICAL PROSTATECTOMY SPECIMEN

There have been several studies correlating core biopsy and radical prostatectomy grade (8,24,25). As discussed above, when biopsies are assigned a Gleason score of 2–4, the tumor at radical prostatectomy is almost always higher. In a large study performed at Johns Hopkins Hospital, a Gleason score 5–6 on biopsy corresponded to the same grade in the radical prostatectomy in 64% of the cases (8). When the Gleason score was ≥7 on biopsy, the radical prostatectomy grade was the same in 87.5% of the cases. In general, adverse findings on needle biopsy accurately predict adverse findings in the radical prostatectomy specimen whereas favorable findings on the needle biopsy do not necessarily predict favorable findings in the radical prostatectomy specimens in large part due to sampling error.

GLEASON SCORE 5–6 TUMOR ON BIOPSY AND HIGHER GRADE IN THE RADICAL PROSTATECTOMY SPECIMEN: CAN THESE CASES BE IDENTIFIED PREOPERATIVELY?

One might assume that cases with Gleason score 5–6 on biopsy and extensive amounts of cancer on biopsy would be more likely to have higher grade tumor in the radical prostatectomy specimen. However, in the one study to analyze this issue it was found that regardless of how much cancer was on the biopsy there was no better correlation in predicting which of the biopsies were more likely to have higher grade on the radical prostatectomy specimen (8).

CORRELATION BETWEEN BIOPSY AND RADICAL PROSTATECTOMY GRADE WITH LIMITED CANCER ON BIOPSY

In a Johns Hopkins study, we analyzed a subset of 53 cases where there was less than 1 mm of cancer on one core (8). The grade assigned to these cases was just as accurate as compared to cases with more extensive cancer on biopsy. We, therefore, assign both a primary and secondary Gleason pattern to even minute foci of cancer on needle biopsy. The sampling error between cases with a limited amount of cancer on needle biopsy compared to those with a greater amount of cancer on needle biopsy is not as great as cases with greater amounts of cancer on needle biopsy compared to the entire tumor in the radical prostatectomy specimen. One core of prostatic tissue samples approximately 1/10,000 of the prostate gland. Even cases with fairly extensive cancer on needle biopsy are sampling only a small fraction of the tumor. There is also a practical reason to assign both a primary and secondary pattern to limited cancer on needle biopsy. We have seen some cases signed out as "Gleason grade 4" where the pathologist meant to convey that the tumor was high-grade (i.e., Gleason pattern 4). However, the urologist interpreted it to mean a Gleason score of 4 (i.e., Gleason grade 2+2=4). By assigning both a primary and secondary pattern even in cases with a limited amount of cancer, the urologist is clear as to the grade of the tumor.

SOURCES OF DISCREPANCIES BETWEEN RADICAL PROSTATECTOMY AND BIOPSY GRADE

In the study performed at our institution, we identified the three most common sources of discrepancy between biopsy and radical prostatectomy grade (8). Pathology error is most frequently seen when pathologists assigned a Gleason score of ≤4 on a needle biopsy which in fact was Gleason score 5–6. Many pathologists undergrade needle biopsies by confusing quantitative changes with qualitative changes. When there is a limited focus of small glands of cancer on needle biopsy, by definition this is a Gleason pattern 3. Gleason pattern 3 consists of small glands with an infiltrative pattern. Biopsying truly low-grade adenocarcinoma of the prostate could not result in just a few neoplastic glands but rather would be more extensive, as low-grade adenocarcinoma grows as nodules of closely packed glands rather than infiltrating in and amongst normal glands.

The other source of discrepancy between biopsy and radical prostatectomy grade is borderline cases. In the description of the Gleason grading system, there are some cases that are right at the interface between two different patterns where there will be interobserver variability and possibly even intraobserver variability.

The other common source of discrepancy is sampling error. The most common type of sampling error is when there is a higher grade component present within the radical prostatectomy specimen which is not sampled on needle biopsy. This typically occurs when a needle biopsy tumor is graded as Gleason grade 3+3=6. In the radical prostatectomy, there exists Gleason pattern 4 which was not sampled on the biopsy, resulting in a prostatectomy grade of Gleason grade 3+4=7.

CHANGE OF GRADE OVER TIME

There is limited data as to whether the grade of prostate cancer changes over time. In two studies addressing this issue, men who had two TURPs over time, each containing cancer, were compared. The second TURP tended to have higher grade cancer, with the conclusion that grade worsened over time (26,27). However, the reason why a second TURP was performed in these men was that the tumor progressed. The majority of men with cancer on the initial TURP who did not progress and whose grade may have not changed did not get a second TURP and were not factored in. Additional evidence of grade progression comes from the demonstration that there is a progressive worsening of grade from primary tumor to pelvic lymph node metastases to distant metastases (28,29). We looked at this issue in a series of men undergoing watchful waiting for cancer detected on needle biopsy. All men underwent repeat biopsy as part of the surveillance protocol. Over a 2- to 3-year period of time, the grade of cancer on needle biopsy did not tend to change (30). The implication of this study is that over the short term, men need not fear a dedifferentiation of their cancer if they defer treatment. Whether the grade will change with longer follow-up remains to be seen.

INTEROBSERVER REPRODUCIBILITY

In a major study to address this issue, 46 needle biopsies with adenocarcinoma of the prostate of varying grades were sent to 10 different urological pathologists (9). Gleason scores were grouped according to the following: 2–4; 5–6; 7; and 8–10. In 82.6% of the cases, at least seven of the ten pathologists agreed on the group. Of the 15 cases of Gleason score 5–6, in only 12 was there agreement of ≥70% of the urological pathologists and in only three cases did all urological pathologists agree on the grade. Of the 13 cases of Gleason score 7, nine cases had agreement of ≥70% of the pathologists, with only one case with 100% agreement. With Gleason score 8–10, there was agreement by seven or more of the urological pathologists in all of the 16 cases, although in only five cases was there 100% agreement in this grouping category.

Thirty-eight needle biopsies where there was ≥70% consensus among urological pathologists were then sent to 41 different general pathologists in the state of Georgia (31). Of the cases where there was a consensus score by the urological pathologists of 5–6, in only approximately half of the time was the score 5–6 by the general pathologists. In the remaining half of the cases, the tumors were undergraded as Gleason score 2–4. Of the nine cases with a consensus score of Gleason score 7, only approximately half of the cases were correctly assigned a Gleason score of 7 by the general pathologists. Again, there was undergrading with 43% of the cases being called a Gleason score 5–6 and 5% of the cases being called a Gleason score 2–4. Even with the 16 cases of having a consensus Gleason score 8–10 there was undergrading, with 17% called a Gleason score of 7 and 6% called a Gleason score of 5–6.

In an attempt to improve Gleason grading by pathologists, we have set up a web site (*www.pathology.jhu.edu/prostate*). We have demonstrated that both residents in pathology and practicing pathologists show significant improvements in Gleason grading following this relatively brief educational program (32,33).

SUMMARY

Whereas the Gleason grading system is a powerful tool to prognosticate and aid in the treatment of men with prostate cancer, there exists significant deficiencies in the practice of this grading system. Not only does there exist problems among practicing pathologists but also a relative lack of interobserver reproducibility among experts. Nonetheless, our studies have demonstrated that the Gleason system can be learned. Further educational endeavors are needed to arrive at a greater consensus and accuracy in the use of the Gleason grading system.

REFERENCES

1. Gleason DF, Mellinger GT, Veterans Administration Cooperative Urological Research Group. Prediction of prognosis for prostatic adenocarcinoma by combined histologic grading and clinical staging. *J Urol* 1974;111;58–64.
2. Gleason DF, Veterans Administration Cooperative Urological Research Group. Histologic grading and clinical staging of prostatic carcinoma. In: Tannenbaum M, ed. *Urologic Pathology: The Prostate.* Philadelphia, PA: Lea and Febiger; 1977:171–197.
3. Mellinger GT, Gleason D, Bailar J. The histology and prognosis of prostatic cancer. *J Urol* 1967; 97: 331–337.

4. McNeal JE, Redwine EA, Freiha FS, et al. Zonal distribution of prostatic adenocarcinoma: correlation with histologic pattern and direction of spread. *Am J Surg Pathol* 1988;12:897–906.
5. Epstein JI, Pizov G, Walsh PC. Correlation of pathologic findings with progression following radical retropubic prostatectomy. *Cancer* 1993;71:3582–3593.
6. McNeal JE, Villers AA, Redwine EA, et al. Histologic differentiation, cancer volume, and pelvic lymph node metastasis in adenocarcinoma of the prostate. *Cancer* 1990;66:1225–1233.
7. Epstein JI, Partin AW, Sauvageot J, et al. Prediction of progression following radical prostatectomy: a multivariate analysis of 721 men with long-term follow-up. *Am J Surg Pathol* 1996;20:286–292.
8. Steinberg DM, Sauvageot J, Piantadosi S, et al. Correlation of prostate needle biopsy and radical prostatectomy Gleason grade in academic and community settings. *Am J Surg Pathol* 1997; 21:566–576.
9. Allsbrook W, Lane R, Lance C, et.al. Interobserver reproducibility of Gleason's grading system. Urologic pathologists. *Hum Pathol* 2001:32;74–80.
10. Albertsen PC, Hanley JA, Gleason DF, et al. Competing risk analysis of men aged 55 to 74 years at diagnosis managed conservatively for clinically localized prostate cancer. *JAMA* 1998;280:975–980.
11. Stamey TA, McNeal JE, Yemoto CM, et al. Biological determinants of cancer progression in men with prostate cancer. *JAMA* 1999;281:1395–1400.
12. Noguchi M, Stamey TA, McNeal JE, et al. Relationship between systematic biopsies and histological features of 222 radical prostatectomy specimens: lack of prediction of tumor significance for men with nonpalpable prostate cancer. *J Urol* 2001;16:104–110.
13. Green GA, Hanlon AL, Al-Saleem T, et al. A Gleason score of 7 predicts a worse outcome for prostate carcinoma patients treated with radiotherapy. *Cancer* 1998;83:971–976.
14. Narayan P, Gajendran V, Taylor SP, et al. The role of transrectal ultrasound-guided biopsy-based staging, preoperative serum prostate-specific antigen, and biopsy Gleason score in prediction of final pathologic diagnosis in prostate cancer. *Urology* 1995;46:205–212.
15. Partin AW, Kattan MW, Subong EN, et al. Combination of prostate-specific antigen, clinical stage, and Gleason score to predict pathological stage of localized prostate cancer. A multi-institutional update. *JAMA* 1997; 277:1445–1451.
16. Kattan MW, Eastham JA, Stapleton AMF, et al. A preoperative nomogram for disease recurrence following radical prostatectomy for prostate cancer. *J Natl Cancer Inst* 1998;90:766–771.
17. D'Amico AY, Whittington R, Malcowicz SB, et al. Combination of preoperative PSA level, biopsy Gleason score, percentage of positive biopsies, and MRI T-stage to predict early PSA failure in men with clinically localized prostate cancer. *Urology* 2000;55:572–577.
18. Kattan MW, Zalefsky MJ, Kuppelian PA, et al. Pretreatment nomogram for predicting the outcome of 3-dimensional conformal radiotherapy in prostate cancer. *J Clin Oncol* 2000;18:3352–3359.
19. Epstein JI, Walsh PC, CarMichael M, et Al. Pathological and clinical findings to predict tumor extent of non-palpable (stage T1c) prostate cancer *JAMA* 1994;271:368–374.
20. Carter HB, Sauvageot J, Walsh PC, et al. Prospective evaluation of men with stage T1C adenocarcinoma of the prostate. *J Urol* 1997;157:2206–2209.
21. Sgrignoli AR, Walsh PC, Steinberg GD, et al. Prognostic factors in men with stage D1 prostate cancer: identification of patients less likely to benefit from radical surgery. *J Urol* 1994;152:1077–1081.
22. Partin AW, Carter HB, Chan DW, et al. Prostate-specific antigen in the staging of localized prostate cancer: influence of tumor differentiation, tumor volume, and benign hyperplasia. *J Urol* 1990;143: 747–752.
23. Pan CC, Potter SR, Partin AW, et al. The prognostic significance of tertiary Gleason patterns of higher grade in radical prostatectomy specimens: a proposal to modify the Gleason grading system. *Am J Surg Pathol* 2000;24:563–569.
24. Spires SE, Cibull ML, Wood DP Jr, et al. Gleason histologic grading in prostatic carcinoma: correlation of 18-guage core biopsy with prostatectomy. *Arch Pathol Lab Med* 1994;118:705–708.
25. Bostwick DG. Gleason grading of prostatic needle biopsies. Correlation with grade in 316 matched prostatectomies. *Am J Surg Pathol* 1994;18:796–803.
26. Brawn PN. The dedifferentiation of prostate carcinoma. *Cancer* 1983;52:246–251.
27. Cumming JA, Ritchies AW, Goodman CM, et al. De-differentiation with time in prostate cancer and the influence of treatment on the course of the disease. *Br J Urol* 1990;65:271–274.
28. Cheng L, Slezak J, Bergstralh EJ, et al. Dedifferentiation in the metastatic progression of prostate carcinoma. *Cancer* 1999;86:657–663.
29. Brawn PN, Speights VO. The dedifferentiation of metastatic prostate carcinoma. *Br J Cancer* 1989; 59:85–88.

30. Epstein JI, Carter HB. Is there dedifferentiation of prostate cancer grade change over time in men followed expectantly for stage T1C disease. *J Urol* (in press).
31. Allsbrook WC Jr, Mangold KA, Johnson MH, et al. Interobserver reproducibility of Gleason grading of prostatic carcinoma. II. General pathologists. *Hum Pathol* 2001;32:81–88.
32. Kronz JD, Silberman MA, Allsbrook WC Jr, et al. Pathology residents' use of a web-based tutorial to improve Gleason grading of prostate carcinoma on needle biopsies. *Hum Pathol* 2000;31:1044–1050.
33. Kronz JD, Silberman MA, Allsbrook WC Jr, et al. A web-based tutorial improves practicing pathologists' Gleason grading of prostate cancer on needle biopsies: validation of a new medical education paradigm. *Cancer* 2000;89:1818–1823.

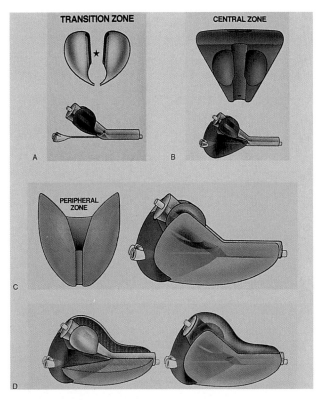

PLATE 1. McNeal's model of zonal anatomy of the prostate. (From Epstein JI, Wojno KJ. The prostate and seminal vesicles. In: Sternberg SS, ed. Diagnostic Surgical Pathology, 3rd ed. Philadelphia, Pa: Lippincott Williams & Wilkins, 1999, with permission.)

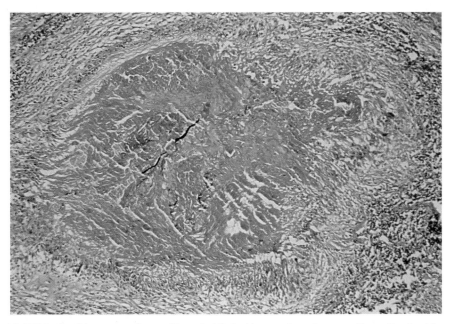

PLATE 2. Postbiopsy granuloma with central fibrinoid necrosis and surrounding palisading histiocytes.

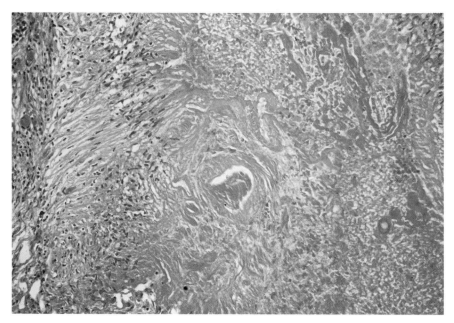

PLATE 3. Postbiopsy granuloma with coagulative necrosis showing residual outlines of vessels and connective tissue with peripheral palisading of histiocytes.

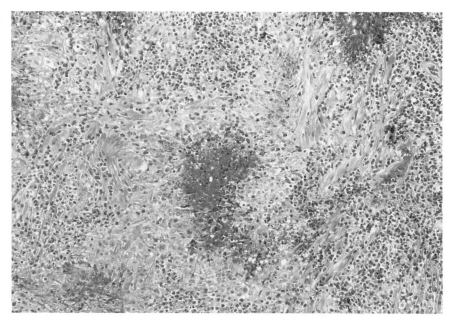

PLATE 4. Allergic granulomatous prostatitis with multiple eosinophilic foci of necrosis surrounded by granulomatous inflammation and abundant stromal eosinophils. (Courtesy of Dr. B. Bhagavan, Baltimore, MD.)

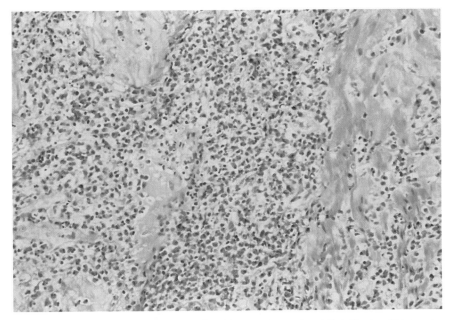

PLATE 5. Allergic granulomatous prostatitis with extensive eosinophilic infiltrate within prostatic stroma, both adjacent to and away from granulomas.

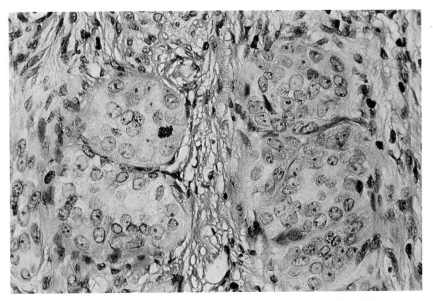

PLATE 6. Cytologically atypical basal cell hyperplasia with small, round basaloid nests. Note prominent nucleoli and mitotic figure.

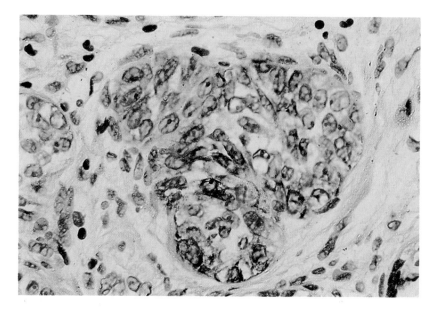

PLATE 7. High molecular weight cytokeratin staining of cytologic atypical basal cell hyperplasia. The cytologically atypical cells are demonstrated to be basal cells based on their positive immunoreactivity.

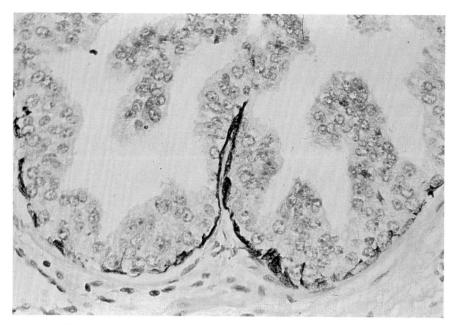

PLATE 8. High-grade prostatic intraepithelial neoplasia labeled with antibodies to high molecular weight cytokeratin.

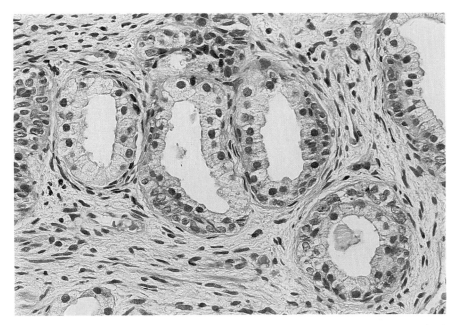

PLATE 9. Benign prostatic acini with basal cells showing enlargement and prominent nucleoli. In some hematoxylin and eosin preparations, the basal cells are violet with a halo in contrast to the secretory cells, which are more red-violet.

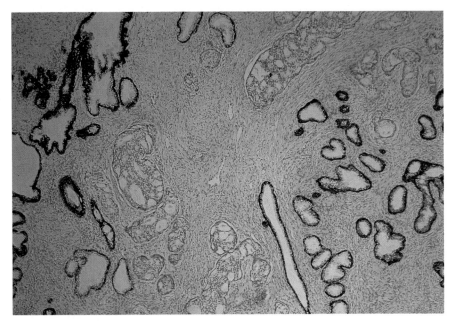

PLATE 10. Infiltrating cribriform carcinoma on transurethral resection of the prostate. Although on hematoxylin and eosin stain, glands could represent high-grade prostatic intraepithelial neoplasia, lack of staining for high molecular weight cytokeratin in numerous cribriform glands is diagnostic of infiltrating carcinoma.

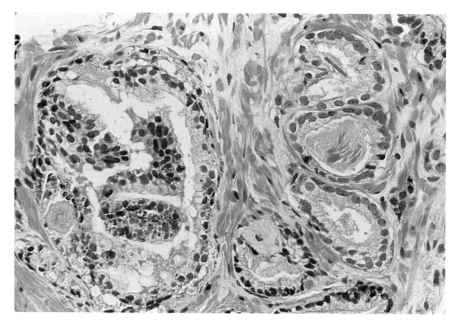

PLATE 11. Adenocarcinoma with crystalloids and mitotic figures.

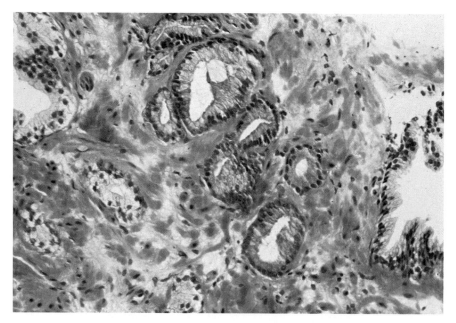

PLATE 12. Adenocarcinoma with amphophilic cytoplasm.

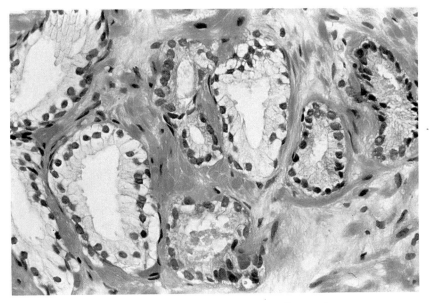

PLATE 13. Adenocarcinoma with amphophilic cytoplasm.

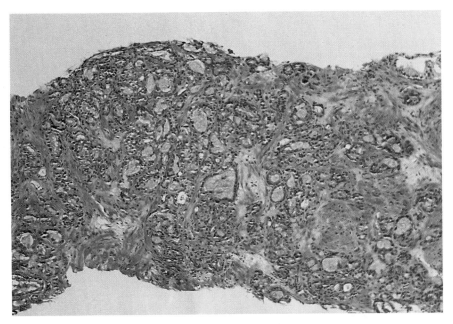

PLATE 14. Adenocarcinoma with blue-tinged mucinous secretions.

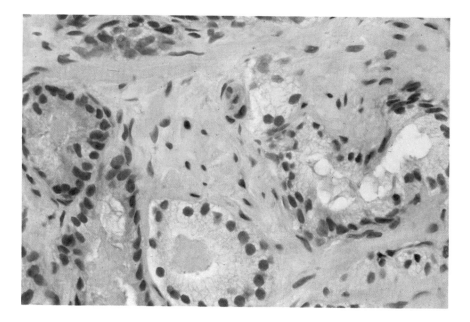

PLATE 15. Adenocarcinoma with blue-tinged and pink acellular intraluminal secretions.

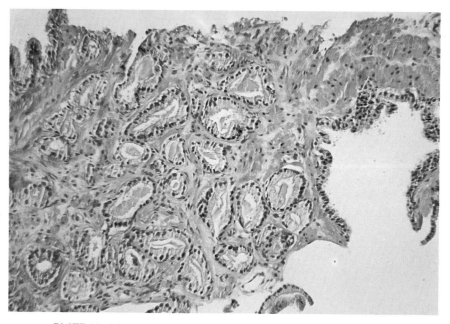

PLATE 16. Adenocarcinoma with pink amorphous intraluminal secretions.

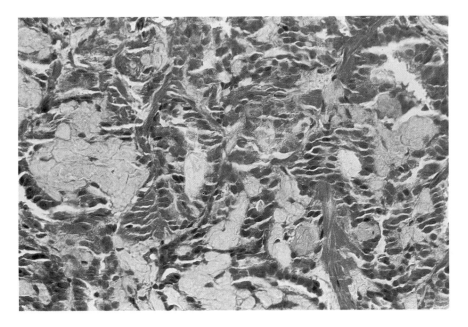

PLATE 17. Adenocarcinoma with mucinous fibroplasia.

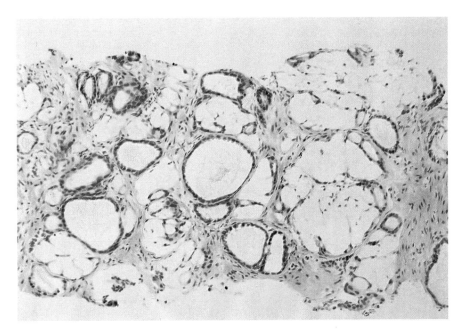

PLATE 18. Adenocarcinoma with abundant intraluminal and focal extracellular mucin.

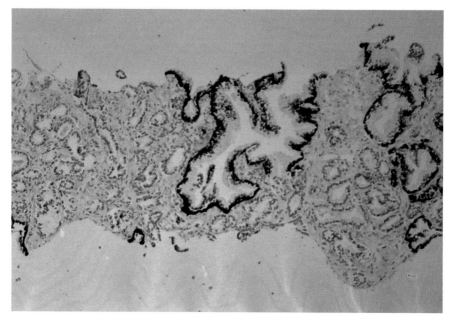

PLATE 19. Atypical glands seen in Figure 6.9 lack expression of high molecular weight cytokeratin consistent with lack of basal cells and consistent with a diagnosis of carcinoma.

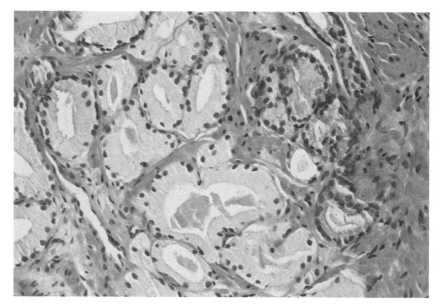

PLATE 20. Foamy gland carcinoma with glands containing abundant xanthomatous cytoplasm and dense intraluminal pink secretions. Contrast cytoplasm of more ordinary carcinoma *(right)* with foamy gland carcinoma.

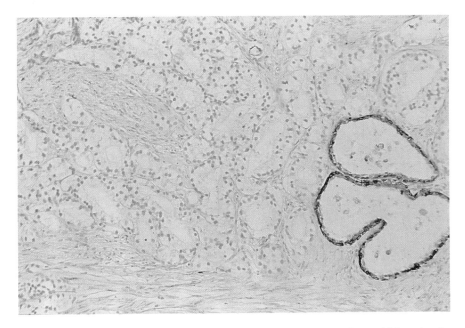

PLATE 21. Same case as shown in Figure 6.22 labeled with antibodies to high molecular weight cytokeratin. Neoplastic glands are negative in contrast to larger benign atrophic glands.

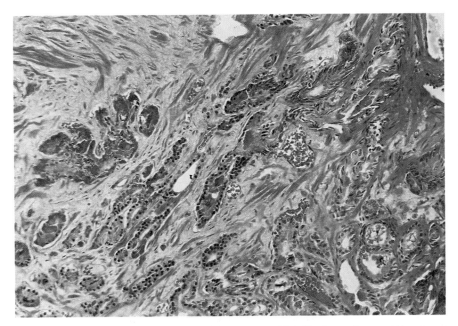

PLATE 22. Cauterized adenocarcinoma of the prostate with infiltrative pattern and blue-tinged mucinous secretions.

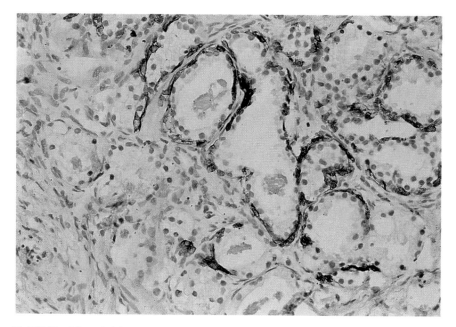

PLATE 23. Adenosis labeled with antibodies to high molecular weight cytokeratin. Note thin rim of immunoreactivity corresponding to flattened basal cells. Not all glands within a nodule are labeled.

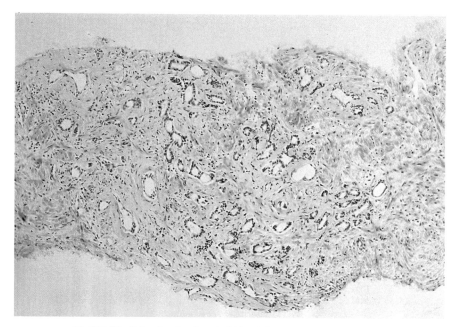

PLATE 24. Sclerotic atrophy mimicking infiltrating adenocarcinoma.

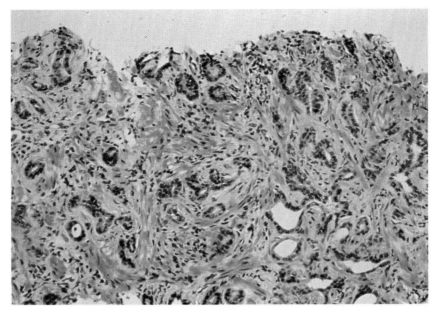

PLATE 25. Sclerotic atrophy resembling adenocarcinoma.

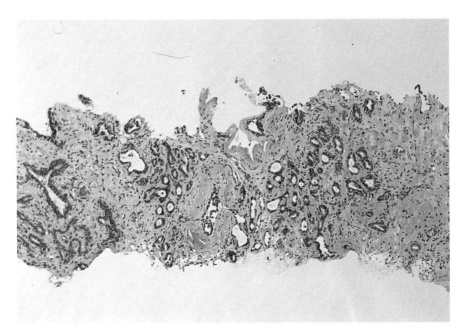

PLATE 26. Benign prostate glands with atrophy.

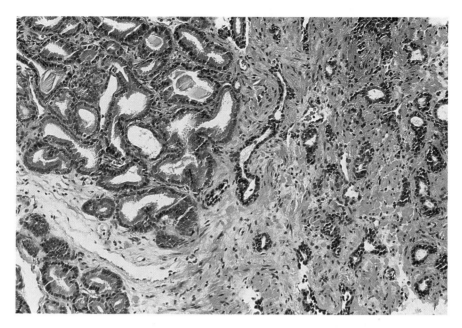

PLATE 27. Atrophy *(right)* contrasted with amphophilic carcinoma *(left).*

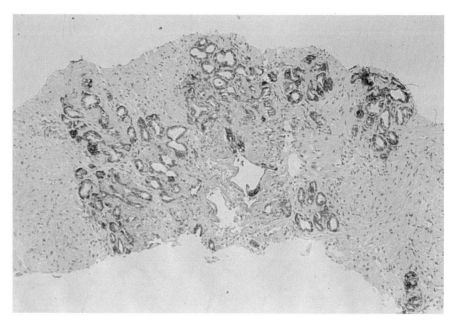

PLATE 28. High molecular weight cytokeratin staining of atrophy demonstrating presence of basal cell layer.

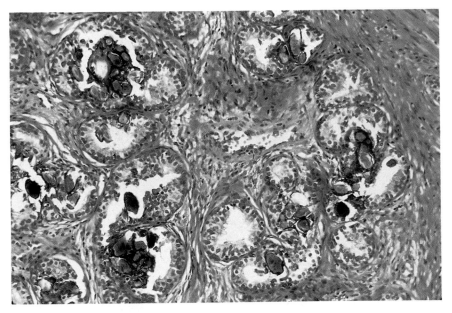

PLATE 29. Basal cell hyperplasia with calcifications.

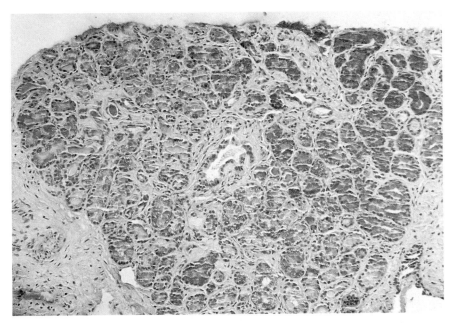

PLATE 30. Mucicarmine stain showing extensive positivity in Cowper's glands.

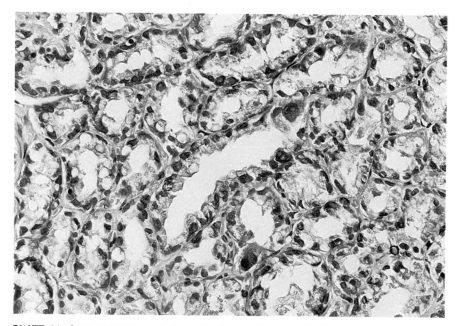

PLATE 31. Seminal vesicle epithelium showing scattered, markedly atypical hyperchromatic degenerative-appearing nuclei within well-formed glandular structures. Note more benign-appearing nuclei within the same glandular structures. Note abundant lipofuscin pigment.

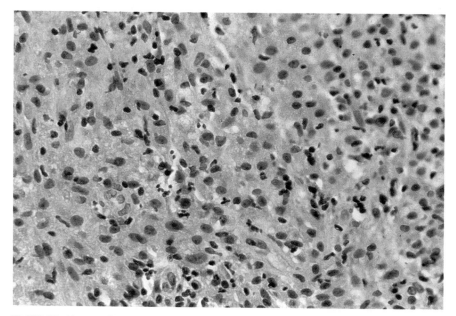

PLATE 32. Nonspecific granulomatous prostatitis with abundant epithelioid histiocytes resembling adenocarcinoma.

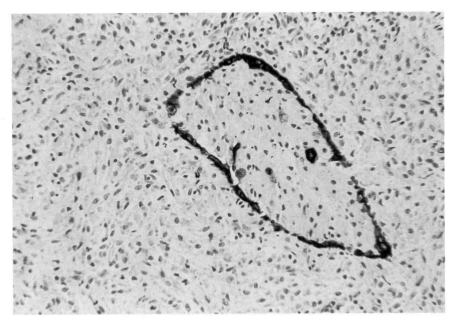

PLATE 33. Nonspecific granulomatous prostatitis stained with pancytokeratin.

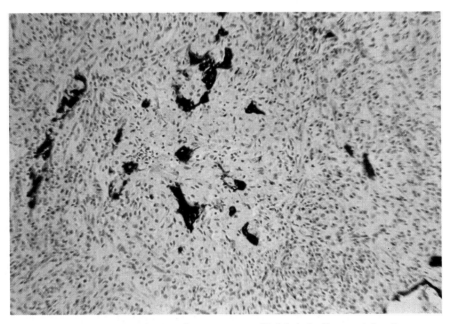

PLATE 34. Nonspecific granulomatous prostatitis labeled with pancytokeratin.

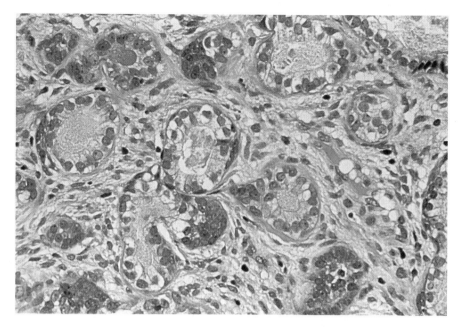

PLATE 35. Some glands within sclerosing adenosis are ensheathed by hyaline connective tissue. Note single basal cell layer in some glands and piled up basal cell layers in others.

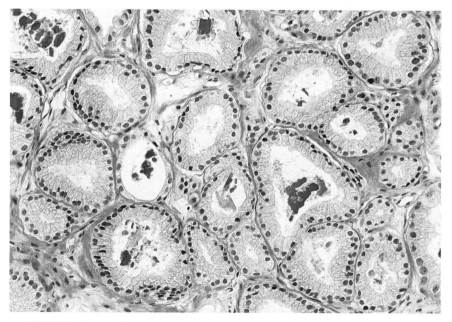

PLATE 36. Low-grade adenocarcinoma on needle biopsy with numerous crystalloids.

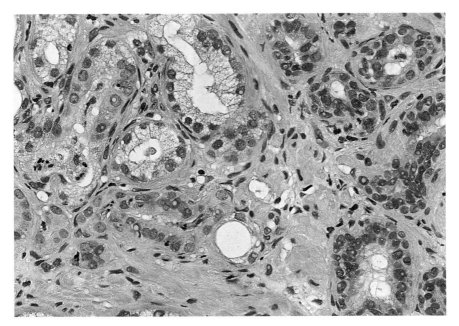

PLATE 37. Glands with intraluminal acute inflammation, suspicious but not diagnostic of adenocarcinoma. In areas, there is a suggestion of a basal cell layer surrounding some of the inflamed glands.

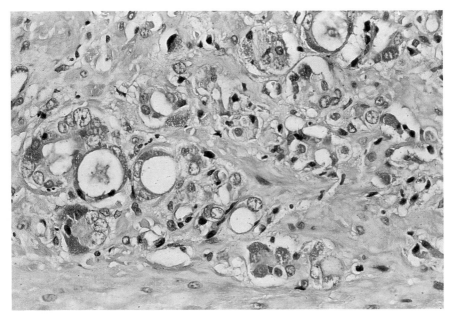

PLATE 38. Adenocarcinoma of the prostate with prominent neuroendocrine granules.

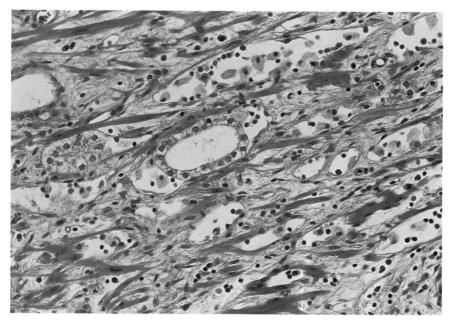

PLATE 39. Adenocarcinoma following Lupron therapy.

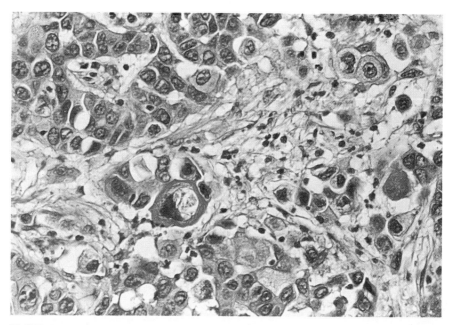

PLATE 40. Infiltrating, poorly differentiated transitional-cell carcinoma within the prostate, showing a cell with densely eosinophilic, hard cytoplasm typical of transitional-cell carcinoma.

10

Findings of Atypical Glands Suspicious for Cancer

TERMINOLOGY

The term "atypical hyperplasia" is nonspecific and has been used to denote such diverse entities as prostatic intraepithelial neoplasia (PIN), adenosis (a benign mimicker of cancer), and foci suspicious for infiltrating carcinoma. As the term "atypical hyperplasia" is nonspecific, it should not be used.

The term "atypical small acinar proliferation" (ASAP) has been proposed (1). Needle biopsies signed out as ASAP encompass such lesions as high-grade PIN, benign mimickers of cancer, reactive atypia, as well as many cases that in retrospect demonstrate focal carcinoma but contain insufficient cytological or architectural atypia to establish a definitive diagnosis of cancer. Urologists frequently equate ASAP with high-grade PIN. However, ASAP in contrast to high-grade PIN is not a specific entity, but rather a broad group of lesions of varying clinical significance. It is important not to equate ASAP with high-grade PIN, as the likelihood of finding cancer on repeat biopsy is higher with a diagnosis of ASAP than with a finding of high-grade PIN (2). The likely location of occult cancer and the optimum repeat biopsy strategy given an initial diagnosis of high-grade PIN is different than in ASAP. The potential risk with using the diagnostic term "ASAP" is that, although many of these lesions are in fact infiltrating carcinomas, the term does not fully convey this risk and patients with this diagnosis may thus not receive repeat biopsy.

We favor the use of descriptive terminology in pathology reports. At our institution, atypical biopsies are conveyed as "prostate tissue with small focus of atypical glands." We routinely note in needle biopsy reports that "while these findings are atypical and suspicious for adenocarcinoma, there is insufficient cytological and/or architectural atypia to establish a definitive diagnosis" (see appendix for macros). Pathologists may add further information detailing why a diagnosis is atypical but not diagnostic of cancer, such that PIN or atrophy or adenosis cannot be excluded with certainty. A recommendation for repeat biopsy is made in the pathology report if the patient is less than 70 years of age. In older men, we leave it up to the judgment of the urologist as to whether a repeat biopsy is justified.

INCIDENCE OF ATYPICAL DIAGNOSIS ON NEEDLE BIOPSY

Approximately 0.4% to 23.4% of all prostate needle biopsies obtained will be returned with a diagnosis of "atypical, suspicious for cancer" (3–12). The median incidence among these studies is 4.5% with a 4.1% incidence found at our institution.

PROSTATE CANCER RISK FOLLOWING A DIAGNOSIS OF ATYPIA

The likelihood of finding prostate cancer on subsequent biopsy in men with a diagnosis of atypia on initial biopsy varies from 21% to 49% (1,2,8,13,14). The largest studies document rates of subsequent carcinoma of 42%, 49%, and 57.1% (1,2,14). We have recently demonstrated that in a patient who has an initial diagnosis of "atypical, suspicious for cancer," a subsequent benign biopsy should not provide false optimism that the patient does not have cancer. Their risk of eventually being found with cancer is still high (52.8%) (14). Surprisingly, in men with an initial atypical biopsy, serum PSA levels and results of digital rectal examination do not correlate with the risk of finding cancer on subsequent biopsy. Consequently, regardless of PSA level, men with an atypical diagnosis should undergo repeat biopsy. There is no definitive data regarding when to obtain a repeat biopsy. We recommend performing a repeat biopsy within 3 months of the initial atypical diagnosis, as the purpose of the repeat biopsy is to rule out carcinoma in an individual at high-risk of harboring malignancy and no specific rationale exists for delaying repeat biopsy.

If repeat biopsy is negative this does not exclude the presence of carcinoma, since prostatic needle biopsies are associated with fairly high false-negative rates of up to 25% (15). We have seen numerous cases where the first biopsy was called atypical and a repeat biopsy was entirely benign, whereupon review of the initial biopsy it was diagnostic of cancer. It is incumbent upon the pathologist in these cases to have the initial biopsy sent off for consultation or try to resolve the initial biopsy with ancillary techniques such as immunoperoxidase with antibodies to high molecular weight keratin. If the pathologist is sufficiently worried with the initial biopsy to subject the patient to a surgical procedure (i.e., second needle biopsy), then there is an obligation to try to resolve that initial biopsy.

REBIOPSY TECHNIQUES FOLLOWING A DIAGNOSIS OF ATYPIA

Allen and associates studied men with initial atypical sextant biopsies and follow-up sextant biopsies in which cancer was detected. Cancer was found on rebiopsy in the same sextant site as the initial atypical biopsy in 48% of men (16). When the same sextant as the atypical biopsy core, the adjacent ipsilateral, and adjacent contralateral sextants were examined as a group, 85% of all cancers discovered on rebiopsy were included. These investigators concluded that sextant biopsy cores should be submitted separately to preserve the location of each biopsy and therefore allow localization of atypical biopsy cores. Based on these data, a rational approach for the rebiopsy of men with an initial atypical diagnosis includes collection of three cores from the site of the initial atypical biopsy, two cores from adjacent sites, and one core elsewhere. For example, if the patient had an atypical biopsy from the left apex, rebiopsy would include three cores from the left apex, two cores from the right apex, two cores from the left mid, and one core from every other sextant region, totaling ten cores.

HISTOLOGY–ATYPICAL SMALL GLANDS

A diagnosis of "atypical, suspicious for cancer" results when there are some features of cancer, yet the features are limited quantitatively or qualitatively. In some cases, cancer cannot be definitively diagnosed either due to atrophic features, where it is difficult to distinguish between benign atrophy and atrophic cancer (Fig. 10.1, efig 1201-1202;1203;1204;1205;1206;1207-1208;1209-1210; 1211). In other examples, adenosis (efig 1212-1213) or high-grade PIN (efig 1214-1215;1216-1217;1218-1219;1220-1222) cannot be ruled out. Cases where the atypical glands are at the edge of the core, where one cannot appreciate the infiltrative nature of the atypical glands among benign glands, are more likely to

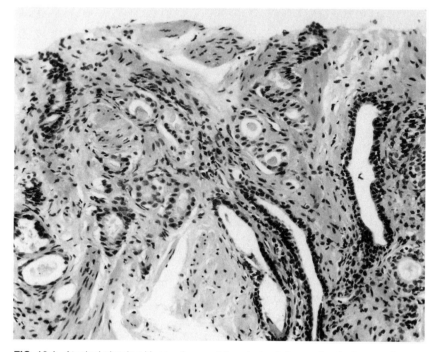

FIG. 10.1. Atypical glands with atrophy suspicious but not diagnostic of adenocarcinoma.

result in an atypical diagnosis. Another situation where an atypical diagnosis may result is in the presence of crush artifact as a result of mechanical distortion from the needle biopsy (efig 1223;1224), although a diagnosis of crushed cancer can sometimes be made (efig 1225-1227;1228-1229;1230). When certain features more typical of cancer, such as blue-tinged or dense pink mucinous secretions, are present yet the atypical findings are minimal, a diagnosis of atypical glands suspicious for cancer is rendered (efig 1231-1232;1233-1234;1235-1236;1237-1238;1239;1240;1241;1242).

In the presence of inflammation, one must be cautious in diagnosing cancer (Color Plate 37, efig 29-30;1243;1244-1246;1247-1248;1249-1253;1254-1255; 1256-1258). Rarely, one can establish a diagnosis of cancer associated with inflammation (efig 1259-1260;1261;1262-1263). Figure 10.2 demonstrates a focus of crowded small glands infiltrating in between larger benign glands associated with extensive inflammation. This focus is diagnostic of cancer because the pattern of numerous small glands in between larger benign glands cannot be attributed to inflammation. Furthermore, the degree of cytologic atypia present in the small atypical glands is significantly greater than the adjacent benign glands even though both are exposed to the same inflammatory milieu. Finally, there may be some cases where the pattern is suspicious for cancer yet the nuclei

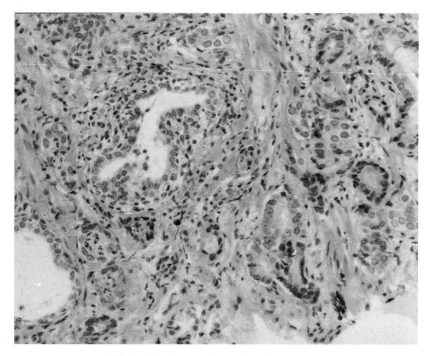

FIG. 10.2. Adenocarcinoma with inflammation.

are totally benign (Fig. 6.9, Color Plate 19). In these cases, stains for high molecular weight keratin may be helpful. If there are a sufficient number of atypical glands that are all negative with antibodies to high molecular weight keratin, and the surrounding benign glands are immunoreactive as an internal positive control, then the immunohistochemical results can lead to a definitive malignant diagnosis. However, there are other cases where the number of atypical glands are so few or the glands have no other atypical features other than that they are crowded that even in light of a negative high molecular weight cytokeratin stain, a definitive diagnosis of cancer cannot always be made (efig 1264-1265), as not every benign gland will react with antibodies to high molecular weight cytokeratin (efig 1266-1267;1268).

In the setting of an inflamed prostate, one should also be cautious in the evaluation of isolated glands with abnormal architecture. Although rarely carcinomas may be inflamed, inflammation tends to preferentially localize away from malignant glands. In areas of intense chronic inflammation, prostatic acini appear atrophic with a high nuclear to cytoplasmic ratio. These basophilic glands may show some architectural abnormalities such as pseudocribriform formation with budding off of little glands (Fig. 10.3, efig 1269-1270;1271-1272;1273). Streaming of basophilic epithelium in areas of

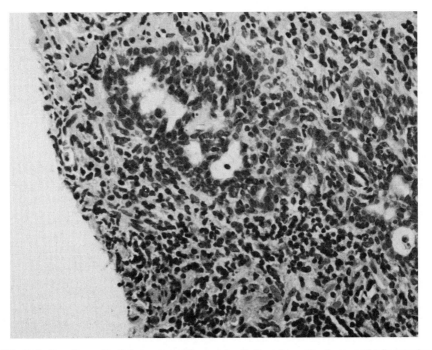

FIG. 10.3. Reactive epithelial changes with pseudocribriform formation in area of inflammation within nonspecific granulomatous prostatitis. ×320.

intense chronic inflammation resembles transitional cell metaplasia. The finding of occasional large nucleoli is not uncommon in areas of intense chronic or acute prostatitis. The distinction of these inflammatory atypias from carcinoma first relies on the recognition that the atypical glands are located in an area of intense inflammation. In addition, the glands have a very basophilic appearance in contrast to the usual gland-forming prostatic adenocarcinomas that have abundant often pale-staining cytoplasm. The high nuclear to cytoplasmic ratio seen in inflamed glands is predominantly seen in only the more poorly differentiated prostatic carcinomas that lack good gland formation. Careful examination of these basophilic glands will also demonstrate the finding of a basal cell layer in most instances.

Many mimickers of prostate cancer, illustrated in Chapter 7 are diagnosed as atypical. In addition, there are some other benign prostatic lesions that lack a specific name (i.e., crowded benign pale glands) which are often diagnosed as atypical (Fig. 10.4, efig 1274;1275-1276;1277;1278). Another situation where benign glands are diagnosed as atypical is when their basal cells contain prominent nucleoli (efig 1279). We have also seen some men whose "normal" prostate looks abnormal throughout, containing small clusters of crowded glands with at most mild cytological atypia (efig 1280-1282;1283-1285). Although the signif-

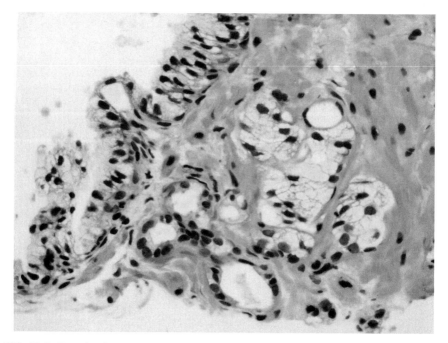

FIG. 10.4. Occasional tangential sections of benign glands give rise to artifactual small solid nests of epithelium.

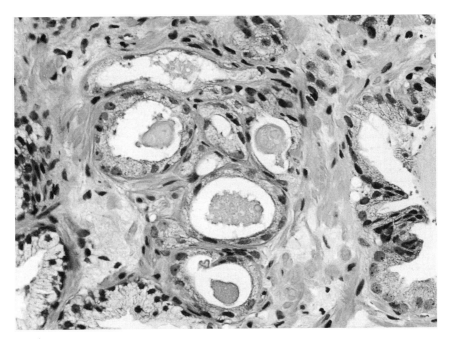

FIG. 10.5. Minute focus of adenocarcinoma with adjacent high-grade PIN *(right)*.

icance of these findings is unknown, one should hesitate diagnosing cancer in this setting unless there are overt malignant features. Small atypical glands of cancer adjacent to high-grade PIN can also be underdiagnosed as PINATYP (Fig. 10.5) (see Chapter 5).

HISTOLOGY–ATYPICAL CRIBRIFORM GLANDS

In some cases, there are atypical cribriform glands in which the differential is between cribriform PIN and cribriform Gleason pattern 3 cancer, where small glands of acinar adenocarcinoma are absent (efig 161-163;164-165;166-167). Glands diagnostic of cribriform PIN usually occur in the setting of more ordinary high-grade PIN. The cribriform glands tend to be few in number, may only focally involve a gland, and their glandular size, contour, and relationship to other glands are consistent with preexisting benign glands whose cells have been replaced by neoplastic cells. Also by convention, when basal cells are identified, these cribriform lesions have been designated cribriform high-grade PIN (see Chapter 5 for discussion of intraductal carcinoma). The diagnosis of cribriform Gleason pattern 3 cancer and its distinction from cribriform PIN in some cases is virtually impossible without the use of special stains for basal cells or the identification of the neoplastic glands exterior to the prostate.

REFERENCES

1. Iczkowski KA, MacLennan GT, Bostwick DG. Atypical small acinar proliferation suspicious for malignancy in prostate needle biopsies: clinical significance in 33 cases. *Am J Surg Pathol* 1997;21:1489–1495.
2. Chan TY, Epstein JI. Follow-up of atypical prostate needle biopsies suspicious for cancer. *Urology* 1999;53:351–355.
3. Bostwick DG, Qian J, Frankel K. The incidence of high grade prostatic intraepithelial neoplasia in needle biopsies. *J Urol* 1995;154:1791–1794.
4. Cheville JC, Reznicek MJ, Bostwick DG. The focus of "atypical glands, suspicious for malignancy" in prostatic needle biopsy specimens. Incidence, histologic features, and clinical follow-up of cases diagnosed in a community practice. *Am J Clin Path* 1997;108:633–640.
5. Hoedemaeker RF, Kranse R, Rietbergen JBW, et al. Evaluation of prostate needle biopsies in a population-based screening study. *Cancer* 1999;85:145–152.
6. Novis DA, Zarbo RJ, Valenstein PA. Diagnostic uncertainty expressed in prostate needle biopsies. A college of American pathologists Q-probes study of 15753 prostate needle biopsies in 332 institutions. *Arch Pathol Lab Med* 1999;123:687–692.
7. Orozco R, O'Dowd G, Kunnel B, et al. Observations on pathology trends in 62,537 prostate biopsies obtained from urology private practices in the United States. *Urology* 1997;51:186–195.
8. Renshaw AA, Santis WF, Richie JP. Clinicopathological characteristics of prostatic adenocarcinoma in men with atypical prostate needle biopsies. *J Urol* 1998;159:2018–2022.
9. Reyes AO, Humphrey PA. Diagnostic effect of complete histologic sampling of prostate needle biopsy specimens. *Am J Clin Pathol* 1998;109:416–422.
10. Kahane H, Sharp JW, Shuman GB, et al. Utilization of high molecular weight cytokeratin on prostate biopsies in an independent laboratory. *Urology* 1995;45:981–986.
11. Weinstein MH, Greenspan DL, Bhagavan B, et al. Diagnoses rendered on prostate needle biopsies in community hospitals. *Prostate* 1998;35:50–55.
12. Wills ML, Hamper UM, Partin AW, et al. Incidence of high-grade prostatic intraepithelial neoplasia in sextant needle biopsy specimens. *Urology* 1997;49:367–373.
13. Roehrborn CG, Pickens GJ, Sanders JS. Diagnostic yield of repeated transrectal ultrasound-guided biopsies stratified by specific histopathologic diagnoses and prostate-specific antigen levels. *Urology* 1996;47:347–352.
14. Allen EA, Kahane H, Epstein JI. Long-term follow–up of men with an initial atypical prostate needle biopsy. *Mod Pathol* 2001;14:100A.
15. Keetch DW, Catalona WJ, Smith DS. Serial prostatic biopsies in men with persistently elevated serum prostate specific antigen values. *J Urol* 1994;151:1571–1574.
16. Allen EA, Kahane H, Epstein JI. Repeat biopsy strategies for men with atypical diagnoses on initial prostate needle biopsy. *Urology* 1998;52:803–807.

11

Prostatic Duct
Adenocarcinoma

While most adenocarcinomas of the prostate are composed of cuboidal cells arranged in acini, 0.4% to 0.8% of prostate cancers show distinctive tall columnar cells in papillary or cribriform structures and are classified as prostatic duct adenocarcinomas (1–3). The initial impression in the pathology literature was that this was a truly "endometrial" tumor arising in a vestigial müllerian structure (4,5). However, subsequent reports on favorable response to orchiectomy (6), ultrastructure of tumor cells (7), histochemistry (8), and immunohistochemistry (2,7) have proven that this is a neoplasm of prostatic origin. Consequently, the terms "endometrioid" and "endometrial" adenocarcinoma of the prostate are no longer justified.

Prostatic duct adenocarcinomas may be the sole component, yet more frequently are seen in about 5% of prostatic adenocarcinomas admixed with tumor showing acinar differentiation. The term "prostatic duct carcinoma" should not be used, as it also refers to prostatic duct transitional cell carcinomas.

When prostatic duct adenocarcinomas arise in large primary periurethral prostatic ducts, they may grow as exophytic lesions into the urethra, most commonly in and around the verumontanum (Fig. 11.1, efig 1286-1288). These lesions cystoscopically closely resemble papillary transitional cell carcinomas. Often in these cases there are no abnormalities on rectal examination. Patients may present with either obstructive symptoms, or gross or microscopic hematuria. Tumors arising in the more peripheral prostatic ducts may or may not have a urethral component and may be palpable on rectal examination. Although ductal adenocarcinomas strongly express prostate-specific antigen (PSA) immunohistochemically, they are associated with variable expression in the serum (9).

Prostatic duct adenocarcinomas show a variety of architectural patterns. Tumors that grow into the urethra as exophytic lesions are often papillary (Fig. 11.2, efig 1289-1291;1292-1294;1295-1297). They are characterized by tall pseudostratified epithelial cells with abundant, usually amphophilic cytoplasm, in contrast to the cuboidal to columnar single cell layer of epithelium

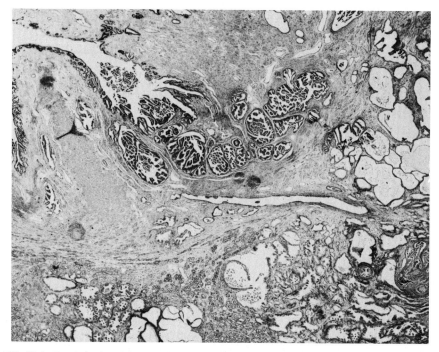

FIG. 11.1. Prostatic duct adenocarcinoma growing within large central prostatic ducts and into prostatic urethra *(top)*. Posterior peripheral portion of the prostate *(bottom)* shows separate typical acinar adenocarcinoma of the prostate. ×11.

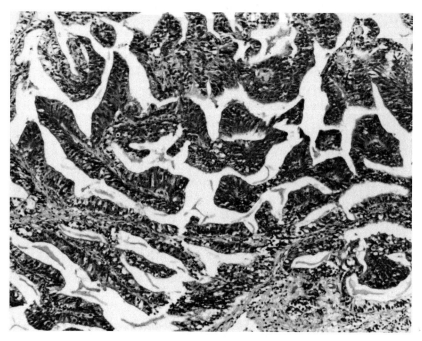

FIG. 11.2. Papillary prostatic duct adenocarcinoma. ×75.

seen with acinar prostatic carcinomas (efig 1298-1300). Occasionally the papillary fronds within prostatic duct adenocarcinoma may be composed of clear cells, yet have pseudostratification of the nuclei typical of prostatic duct adenocarcinomas (Fig. 11.3, efig 1301-1303). Although the papillary pattern of prostatic duct adenocarcinoma is most commonly seen on transurethral resection material, occasionally this papillary pattern may also be seen on needle biopsy material (Fig. 11.4).

The cribriform pattern of prostatic duct adenocarcinomas is more commonly seen deeper within the tissue, although it may also be noted in the exophytic urethral component of the lesion (Figs. 11.5 and 11.6). The cribriform pattern is formed by back-to-back large glands with intraglandular epithelial bridging resulting in the formation of slit-like lumens (efig 1304-1306). The epithelial lining is composed of pseudostratified tall columnar epithelium often with amphophilic cytoplasm. The pattern is somewhat reminiscent of endometrial adenocarcinoma within the female. This pattern of prostatic adenocarcinoma differs from the cribriform pattern of prostatic acinar adenocarcinoma which is composed of cuboidal epithelium and punched-out round lumina. It is not uncommon to find areas of papillary formation admixed with cribriform patterns (Fig. 11.7, efig 1307-1309).

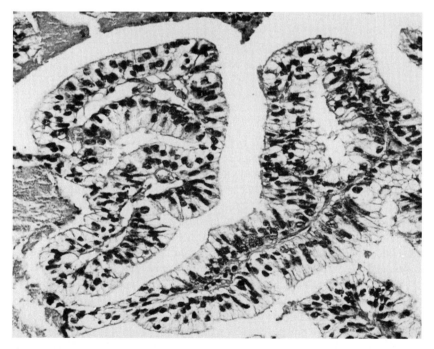

FIG. 11.3. Occasionally, prostatic duct carcinomas have abundant pale-staining cytoplasm, yet still have a pseudostratified columnar appearance in contrast to routine prostatic adenocarcinoma. ×280.

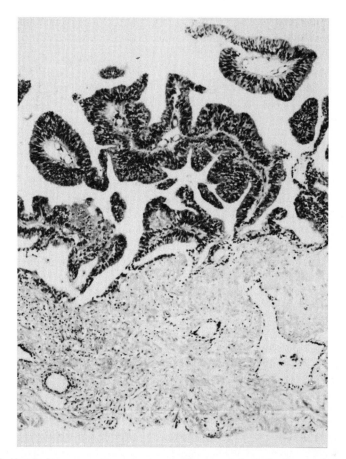

FIG. 11.4. Needle biopsy specimen showing papillary prostatic duct adenocarcinoma. ×115.

Other patterns of prostatic duct adenocarcinoma, which by themselves may be difficult to identify as being of prostatic duct origin, may be seen in association with either the papillary or cribriform pattern. Occasionally, solid tumor masses with numerous thin-walled vessels distend prostatic ducts (Fig. 11.8, efig 1310-1311). This pattern is a compact papillary form of prostatic duct adenocarcinoma, since areas can be seen where the solid pattern containing these thin fibrovascular cores open up into more recognizable papillary structures (Fig. 11.9). Prostatic duct adenocarcinomas may also grow as solid nests of tumors with central necrosis (Fig. 11.10). Without seeing this solid pattern in association with more recognizable prostatic duct adenocarcinoma, this pattern cannot be distinguished from poorly differentiated prostatic acinar adenocarcinoma. Prostatic duct adenocarcinomas may also invade as single glands lined by tall columnar epithelial cells unlike the cuboidal cells that characterize typical aci-

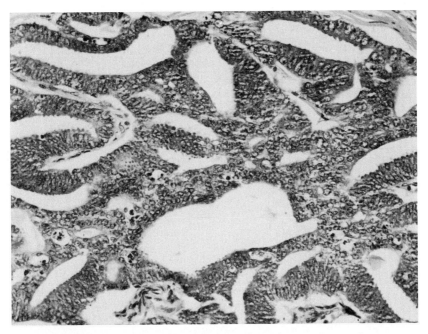

FIG. 11.5. Cribriform pattern of prostatic duct adenocarcinoma with irregular slit-like lumen formation and tall pseudostratified columnar cells with amphophilic cytoplasm.

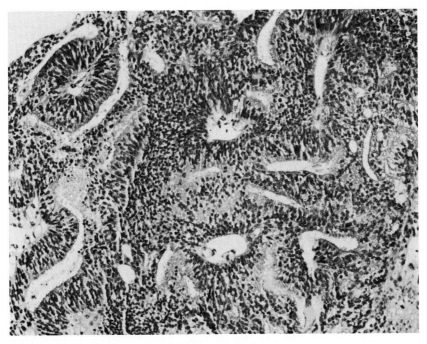

FIG. 11.6. Cribriform pattern of prostatic duct adenocarcinoma with focal papillary formation *(upper left).*

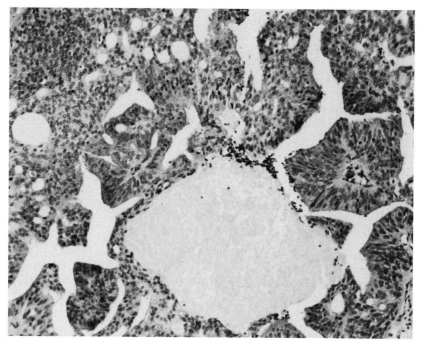

FIG. 11.7. Cribriform pattern of prostatic duct adenocarcinoma with focal necrosis and focal papillary formation *(right).*

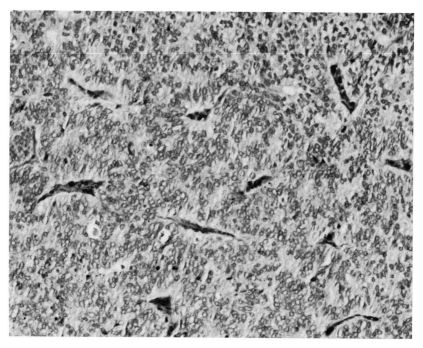

FIG. 11.8. Solid variant of prostatic duct adenocarcinoma with numerous, regularly distributed thin fibrovascular cores. ×110.

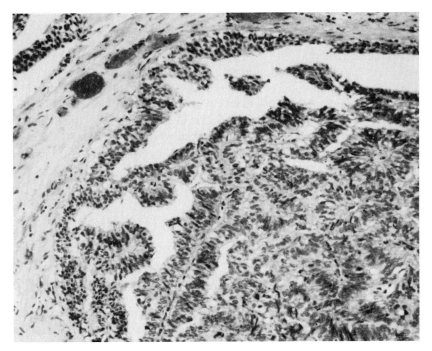

FIG. 11.9. Transition between solid pattern of prostatic duct adenocarcinoma *(lower right)* to more open typical papillary prostatic duct adenocarcinoma. ×170

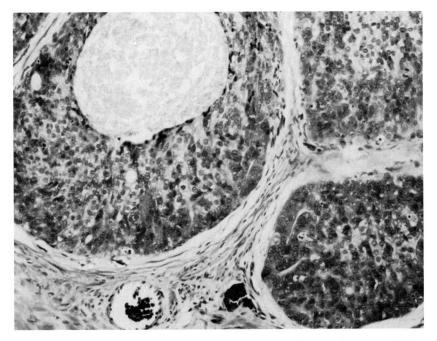

FIG. 11.10. Solid nests of prostatic duct adenocarcinoma with central necrosis. ×150.

nar prostatic carcinoma (Fig. 11.11, efig 1312-1314). The single infiltrating glands of prostatic duct adenocarcinoma resemble infiltrating colonic adenocarcinoma. The differentiation between prostatic duct adenocarcinoma and secondary involvement of the prostate by colonic adenocarcinoma can be made by finding more typical prostatic duct adenocarcinoma elsewhere within the biopsy, as well as by immunohistochemical demonstration of PSA and prostate-specific acid phosphatase (PSAP) in ductal adenocarcinoma (efig 1315-1316).

In most cases with mixed acinar and ductal features, the two components are intimately comingled (Fig. 11.12, efig 1317-1319;1320-1325). Other relationships seen between the two types include the co-existence of a centrally located duct carcinoma with a peripherally located acinar tumor (Fig. 11.1). A prostatic duct adenocarcinoma can also express acinar differentiation in either prior or subsequent biopsies. Similarly, metastases from a ductal carcinoma may be purely ductal, acinar, or mixed (2). As with other unusual subtypes of prostate cancer, we do not assign a Gleason score to ductal adenocarcinoma, but only to the conventional adenocarcinoma component if present.

Ductal adenocarcinoma on needle biopsy may be particularly difficult to diagnose in that there may be mild cytologic atypia without prominent nucleoli (9) (Figs. 11.13–11.15, efig 1326-1327;1328;1329-1330;1331-1332;1333-1334;

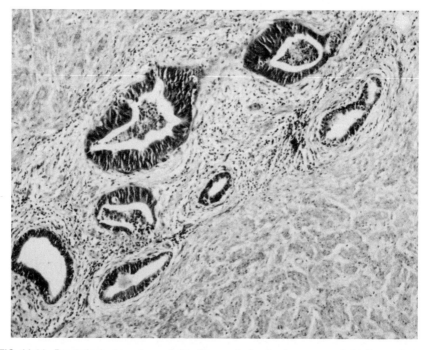

FIG. 11.11. Prostatic duct carcinoma infiltrating as single glands composed of tall pseudostratified columnar epithelium with amphophilic cytoplasm. ×115.

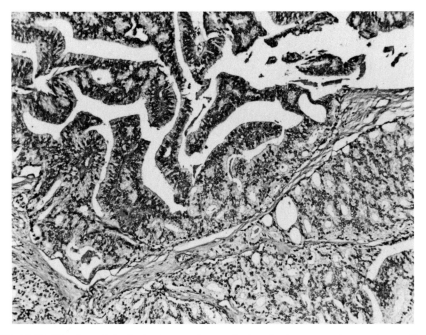

FIG. 11.12. Mixed prostatic duct adenocarcinoma *(top)* and acinar-appearing carcinoma *(bottom).* ×85.

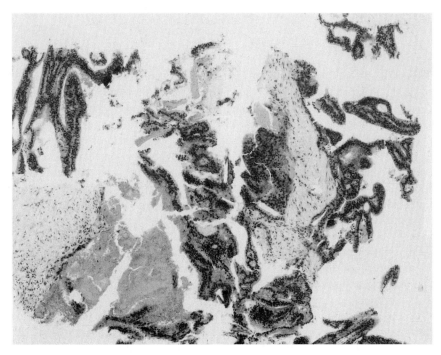

FIG. 11.13. Fragments of prostatic duct adenocarcinoma on needle biopsy.

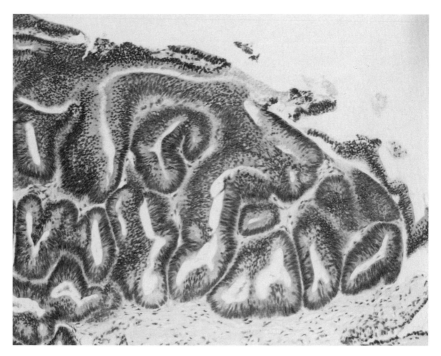

FIG. 11.14. Prostatic duct adenocarcinoma on needle biopsy.

1335-1336;1337-1339). The other feature that can result in underdiagnosis of prostatic duct adenocarcinoma on needle biopsy is tumor fragmentation, resulting in small detached foci of carcinoma. One of the lesions most frequently confused with cytologically bland ductal adenocarcinoma is prostatic urethral polyp. Whereas ductal adenocarcinomas are composed of tall pseudostratified columnar cells, prostatic urethral polyps are polypoid nodules made up of entirely benign-appearing prostate acini lined by prostatic glandular epithelium and urothelium (see Chapter 18). A more difficult distinction is between cribriform high-grade prostatic intraepithelial neoplasia (PIN) and ductal adenocarcinoma of the prostate (see Chapter 5).

We have found that the number of positive needle cores correlate with positive margins at radical prostatectomy, and with decreased time to progression. The proportion of ductal as opposed to acinar cancer on needle biopsy does not have predictive power, such that any ductal features on needle biopsy is an adverse prognostic feature.

Although one study has suggested a favorable prognosis (10), most consider ductal morphology to connote a more aggressive course than acinar prostate cancer (2,3,7,11). Data from our needle biopsy study support the assertion that this type of prostate carcinoma has a more aggressive course, as the men in our study

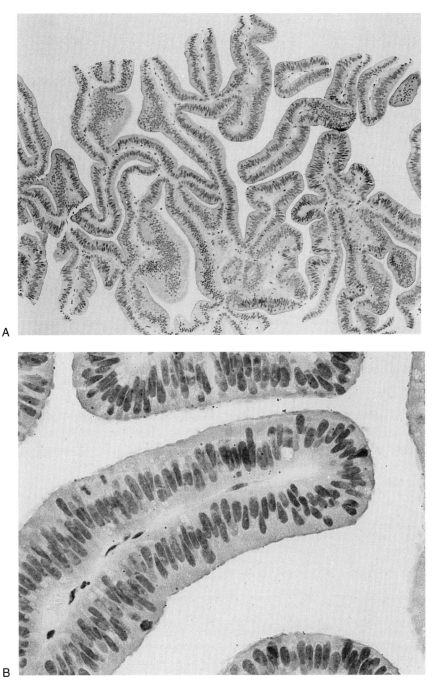

FIG. 11.15. (A) Prostatic duct adenocarcinoma on needle biopsy. **(B)** Papillary fronds lined by tall pseudostratified columnar cells with minimal cytological atypia.

who underwent radical prostatectomy had large tumors, advanced pathologic stage, and when compared to acinar carcinoma a shortened time to progression (9). The progression rate for ductal adenocarcinomas treated by radical prostatectomy is intermediate between that for Gleason score 7 and Gleason score 8–9 acinar tumors. What must also be factored in is that many ductal adenocarcinomas present with advanced clinical stage and are not even candidates for radical prostatectomy.

In cases where the urologist takes only a limited transurethral biopsy of the prostate, the entire specimen may consist of a small focus of prostatic duct adenocarcinoma. These tumor foci represent the "tip of the iceberg," where there is more extensive unsampled duct adenocarcinoma involving the underlying ductal system. Ductal adenocarcinomas, as they arise in ducts, may show residual staining for high molecular weight cytokeratin staining (efig 1340-1341) (see Chapter 5 for discussion on "intraductal carcinoma"). Regardless of whether the ductal adenocarcinomas consists of a small focus or there is basal cell staining, these tumors should be treated aggressively. The one exception to their treatment is the rare case when there is a good sampling of the prostate with a sizable transurethral resection, and there is only a small focus of ductal adenocarcinoma; the prognosis in this situation is unknown (efig 1342-1344).

Our study of ductal adenocarcinoma on needle biopsy implicitly challenges the definition of ductal adenocarcinoma of the prostate as an entity unique to the transition zone. We do not adhere to the belief that "clinical and pathological evidence of involvement of large periurethral prostatic ducts or urethra is required for definitive diagnosis." (12). A previous study of 15 radical prostatectomies with ductal adenocarcinoma found that ten involved both the peripheral and transition zones of the prostate, yet five involved only the peripheral zone (11). Prostate cancer may differentiate along ductal or acinar lines, analogous to ductal and lobular differentiation in breast cancer. The "ductal" morphology represents the more aggressive pattern.

REFERENCES

1. Bostwick DG, Kindrachuk RW, Rouse RV. Prostatic adenocarcinoma with endometrial features: clinical, pathological and ultrastructural findings. *Am J Surg Pathol* 1985;9:595–609.
2. Epstein JI, Woodruff J. Prostatic carcinomas with endometrioid features: a light microscopic and immunohistochemical study of 10 cases. *Cancer* 1986;57:111–119.
3. Green LF, Farrow GM, Ravits JM, et al. Prostatic adenocarcinoma of ductal origin. *J Urol* 1979; 121:303–305.
4. Melicow MM, Pachter MR. Endometrial carcinoma of prostatic utricle (uterus masculinus). *Cancer* 1967;20:1715–1722.
5. Melicow MM, Tannenbaum M. Endometrial carcinoma of uterus masculinus (prostatic utricle): Report of 6 cases. *J Urol* 1971;106:892–902.
6. Young BW, Lagios MD. Endometrial (papillary) carcinoma of the prostatic utricle–response to orchiectomy. A case report. *Cancer* 1973;32:1293–1300.
7. Ro JY, Ayala AG, Wishnow KI, et al. Prostatic duct adenocarcinoma with endometrioid features: immunohistochemical and electron microscopic features. *Semin Diagn Pathol* 1988;5:301–311.
8. Zaloudek C, Williams JW, Kempson, RL. "Endometrial" adenocarcinoma of the prostate–a distinctive tumor of probable prostatic duct origin. *Cancer* 1976;37:2255–2262.

9. Brinker DA, Potter SR, Epstein JI. Ductal adenocarcinoma of the prostate diagnosed on needle biopsy: correlation with clinical and radical prostatectomy findings and progression. *Am J Surg Pathol* 1999;23:1471–1479.
10. Millar EKA, Sharma NK, Lessells AM. Ductal (endometrioid) adenocarcinoma of the prostate: a clinicopathologic study of 16 cases. *Histopathology* 1996;29:11–19.
11. Christensen WN, Steinberg WN, Walsh PC, et al. Prostatic duct adenocarcinoma: Findings at radical prostatectomy. *Cancer* 1991;67:2118–2124.
12. Bostwick DG. Neoplasms of the Prostate. In: Bostwick DG, Eble JN, eds. *Urologic Surgical Pathology.* St. Louis, Mo: Mosby; 1997:366–368.

12

Neuroendocrine Differentiation in the Benign and Malignant Prostate

In 1971, Azzopardi and Evans recognized the presence of argentaffin cells within normal prostatic epithelium (1). Most of these neuroendocrine cells contain chromogranin and serotonin. A fewer number of cells contain calcitonin, and less commonly gastrin-releasing peptide, somatostatin, alpha–human chorionic gonadotropin (HCG), thyroid-stimulating hormone (TSH)-like peptide, parathyroid hormone-related protein, and cholecystokinin (2). Occasionally, these cells can be recognized on hematoxylin-and-eosin (H&E)-stained sections by their basally located deeply eosinophilic fine cytoplasmic granules. Coarser eosinophilic clumped granules located throughout the cytoplasm represent lipofuscin.

In histologically typical adenocarcinomas of the prostate and occasionally in high-grade prostatic intraepithelial neoplasia (PIN), similar-appearing eosinophilic cells can be identified that are chromogranin-positive and contain neurosecretory granules by electron microscopy (Color Plate 38, efig 1345;1346-1348;1349-1351;1352). These cells may react with antibodies to serotonin, adrenocorticotropic hormone (ACTH), calcitonin, HCG, neuron-specific enolase (NSE), somatostatin, leuenkephalin, or beta-endorphin (2). Even in ordinary adenocarcinomas of the prostate without light microscopic evidence of neuroendocrine differentiation, between 30% to 100% show neuroendocrine differentiation when evaluated with immunohistochemistry for multiple neuroendocrine markers. Most of these cases have no evidence of ectopic hormonal secretion clinically.

It is controversial whether neuroendocrine differentiation in typical adenocarcinomas worsens prognosis, with some studies suggesting a correlation, yet most others showing no effect of neuroendocrine differentiation on outcome (2). Even in our study where the extent of neuroendocrine differentiation was prognostic in radical prostatectomy specimens, the relationship was weak and not sufficient to be useful clinically (3). In the one study analyzing neuroendocrine differentiation in prostate cancer on needle biopsy, there was no relationship with prognosis (4).

Several cases have been reported where a "carcinoid" appearance of the tumor has been present either as the sole histologic pattern or admixed with more typical adenocarcinoma of the prostate (Fig. 12.1, efig 1353)(5–7). In none of these cases has a carcinoid syndrome been present. When studied, almost all such cases have been positive with antibodies for prostate-specific antigen (PSA) and prostate-specific acid phosphatase (PSAP) and have clinically behaved like ordinary prostate carcinomas. While most ordinary adenocarcinomas and "carcinoid-like" tumors showing neuroendocrine differentiation have not produced clinical symptoms, several cases have produced ACTH in sufficient quantity to result in Cushing's syndrome (7). A single case of a "mixed carcinoid-adenocarcinoma of the prostate with spindle cell carcinoid" features has also been reported (8). As "carcinoid tumors" of the prostate do not appear to be a distinct clinicopathologic entity, a more appropriate designation for these lesions would be "prostatic adenocarcinomas with neuroendocrine differentiation." A unique carcinoid tumor unrelated to prostate cancer was reported in a 7-year-old boy with multiple endocrine neoplasia IIb (9).

Small cell carcinomas of the prostate have a cytologic appearance similar to that found in small cell carcinomas of the lung (10,11) (Figs. 12.2 and 12.3, efig 1354-1356;1357-1358). In approximately 50% of the cases, the tumors are

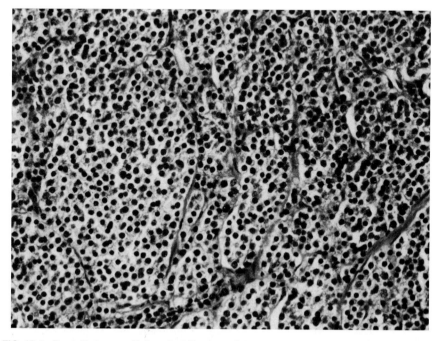

FIG. 12.1. Prostatic tumor with "carcinoid" pattern. Other areas showed typical prostatic adenocarcinoma. ×180.

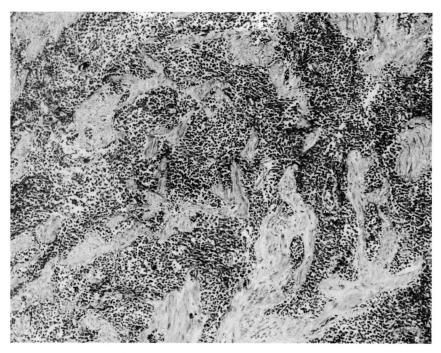

FIG. 12.2. Small cell carcinoma of the prostate. ×65.

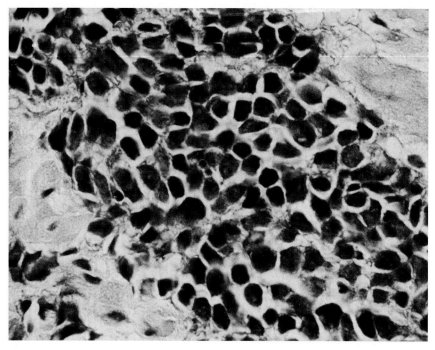

FIG. 12.3. Small cell carcinoma of the prostate showing features identical to those seen within small cell carcinoma in other sites. ×700.

mixed small cell carcinoma and adenocarcinoma of the prostate (Fig. 12.4, efig 1359-1360;1361-1363). As with other unusual subtypes of prostate cancer, we do not assign a Gleason score to small cell carcinoma, but only to the conventional adenocarcinoma component, if present. Neurosecretory granules have been demonstrated within several prostatic small cell carcinomas. Using immunohistochemical techniques, the small cell component may be positive for NSE and negative for PSA and PSAP, positive for PSA and PSAP with negative immunoreactivity for NSE, or negative for all three antigens. In our experience, it is typically negative for prostate markers. In order to distinguish primary small cell carcinoma of the prostate from a metastasis from the lung, Ordonez reported that thyroid transcription factor-1 (TTF-1) was positive in 96% of small cell carcinomas of the lung and negative in all three prostate small cell cancers (12). In a conflicting study, Agoff found that all four prostate small cell cancers reacted with antibodies to TTF-1 (13).

While most small cell carcinomas of the prostate lack clinically evident hormone production, they account for the majority of prostatic tumors with clinically evident ACTH or antidiuretic hormone production. The average survival of patients with small cell carcinoma of the prostate is less than a year. There is no difference in prognosis between patients with pure small cell carcinomas and those with mixed

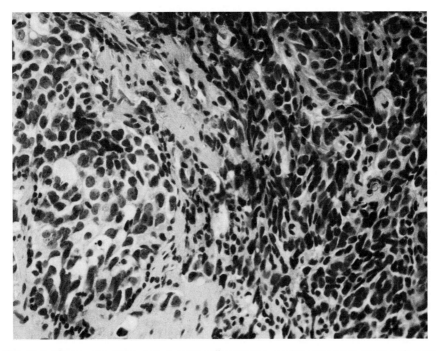

FIG. 12.4. Biopsy showing areas of small cell carcinoma *(right)* adjacent to areas with more abundant cytoplasm and visible nucleoli that are more consistent with poorly differentiated adenocarcinoma of non-small cell type *(left)*. ×275.

glandular and small cell carcinomas. Similarly, the pattern of immunostaining does not affect survival. The appearance of a small cell component within the course of adenocarcinoma of the prostate usually indicates an aggressive terminal phase of the disease. The heterogeneity of prostatic small cell carcinomas suggests that they arise from multipotential prostatic epithelial cells that may express divergent differentiation. In a review of the literature of genitourinary small cell carcinoma, whereas cisplatin chemotherapy was beneficial for bladder tumors, only surgery was prognostic for prostate small cell carcinomas (14). While this study concluded that hormonal manipulation and systemic chemotherapy had little effect on the natural history of disease in the prostate, the number of patients were small and others suggest to treat small cell carcinoma of the prostate with the same combination chemotherapy used to treat small cell carcinomas in other sites (15,16).

A couple of case reports of pheochromocytomas originating in the prostate have also been reported, including one in a child (17,18).

REFERENCES

1. Azzopardi JG, Evans DJ. Argentaffin cells in prostatic carcinoma: differentiation from lipofuscin and melanin in prostatic epithelium. *J Pathol* 1971;104:247–251.
2. Abrahamsson PA. Neuroendocrine differentiation in prostatic carcinoma. *Prostate* 1999;39:135–148.
3. Weinstein MH, Partin AW, Veltri RW, et al. Neuroendocrine differentiation in prostate cancer. Enhanced prediction of progression following radical prostatectomy. *Hum Pathol* 1996;27:683–687.
4. Casella R, Bubendorf L, Sauter G, et al. Focal neuroendocrine differentiation lacks prognostic significance in prostate core needle biopsies. *J Urol* 1998;160:406–410.
5. Almargro UA. Argyrophilic prostatic carcinoma: case report with literature review on prostatic carcinoid and "carcinoid-like" prostatic carcinoma. *Cancer* 1985;55:608–614.
6. Azumi N, Shibuya H, Ishikura M. Primary prostatic carcinoid tumor with intracytoplasmic prostatic acid phosphatase and prostate-specific antigen. *Am J Surg Pathol* 1984;8:545–550.
7. Ghali VS, Garcia RL. Prostatic adenocarcinoma with carcinoidal features producing adrenocorticotrophic syndrome: immunohistochemical study and review of the literature. *Cancer* 1984;54:1043–1048.
8. Egan AJM, Youngskin TP, Bostwick DG. Mixed carcinoid-adenocarcinoma of the prostate with spindle cell carcinoid: the spectrum of neuroendocrine differentiation in prostatic neoplasia. *Pathol Case Rev* 1996;1:65–69.
9. Whelan T, Gatfield CT, Robertson S. Primary carcinoid of the prostate in conjunction with multiple endocrine neoplasia IIb in a child. *J Urol* 1995;153:1080–1082.
10. Ro JY, Tetu B, Ayala AG, et al. Small cell carcinoma of the prostate: immunohistochemical and electron microscopic studies of 18 cases. *Cancer* 1987;59:977–982.
11. Tetu B, Ro JY, Ayala AG, et al. Small cell carcinoma of prostate Part 1: a clinicopathologic study of 20 cases. *Cancer* 1987;59:1803–1809.
12. Ordonez NG. Value of thyroid transcription factor-1 immunostaining in distinguishing small cell lung carcinomas from other small cell carcinomas. *Am J Surg Pathol* 2000;24:1217–1223.
13. Agoff SN, Lamps LW, Philip AT, et al. Thyroid transcription factor-1 is expressed in extrapulmonary small cell carcinomas but not in other extrapulmonary neuroendocrine tumors. *Mod Pathol* 2000;13:238–242.
14. Mackey JR, Au HJ, Hugh J, et al. Genitourinary small cell carcinoma: determination of clinical and therapeutic factors associated with survival. *J Urol* 1998;159:1624–1629.
15. Amato RJ, Logothetis CJ, Hallinan R, et al. Chemotherapy for small cell carcinoma of prostatic origin. *J Urol* 1992;147:935–937.
16. Rubenstein JH, Katin MJ, Mangano MM, et al. Small cell anaplastic carcinoma of the prostate: seven new cases, review of the literature, and discussion of a therapeutic strategy. *Am J Clin Oncol* 1997;20:376–380.
17. Voges GE, Wippermann F, Duber C, et al. Pheochromocytoma in the pediatric age group: the prostate—an unusual location. *J Urol* 1990;144:1219–1221.
18. Dennis PJ, Lewandowski AE, Rohner TJ, et al. Pheochromocytoma of the prostate: An unusual location. *J Urol* 1989;141:130–132.

13

Mucinous Differentiation in the Benign and Malignant Prostate

Benign secretory cells of the prostate contain scant neutral mucin (1). Although initial reports claimed that benign prostatic glands lacked acid mucin, we have demonstrated that adenosis and occasional atrophic glands can also express acid mucin (2).

Another form of mucin differentiation in benign prostate is mucous gland metaplasia, which is found in approximately 1% of prostates (3,4). The lesion consists of tall mucin-filled goblet cells with tiny, dark, basal nuclei (Fig. 13.1, efig 1364-1365;1366-1367;1368-1369;1370,1371-1375). The cells are positive for prostate-specific antigen (PSA) and are diastase resistant as well as positive for mucicarmine and alcian blue. The cells are negative for PSA and prostate-specific acid phosphatase (PSAP). These may occur as randomly scattered individual cells or in groups of five to ten cells. Most foci are small, very rarely measuring over 1 square mm. Mucous gland metaplasia may be found in normal and hyperplastic prostate glands and in areas of transitional cell metaplasia, basal cell hyperplasia (efig 1376-1379), or atrophy (efig 1380-1382). Rarely, it may be seen in high-grade prostatic intraepithelial neoplasia (PIN) (efig 1383-1384). Although it may mimic cancer, it does not appear to be related to cancer or inflammation.

Mucinous (colloid) adenocarcinoma of the prostate gland is one of the least common morphologic variants of prostatic carcinoma (5,6,7). A lack of precision in the definition of these mucinous neoplasms has resulted in reports that have overstated the incidence of this lesion. Much of the confusion in the terminology of this entity arises from the lack of recognition that between 60% and 90% of prostatic adenocarcinomas secrete mucosubstances, depending on the histochemical technique used (1,8–10). Only when extracellular mucin is secreted in sufficient quantity to result in pools of mucin should the term "mucinous" be employed. If the mucinous area occupies only a small portion of the tumor, it should not be called a "mucinous prostatic carcinoma" but rather a "prostatic adenocarcinoma with focal mucinous areas" (efig 1385;1386-1387).

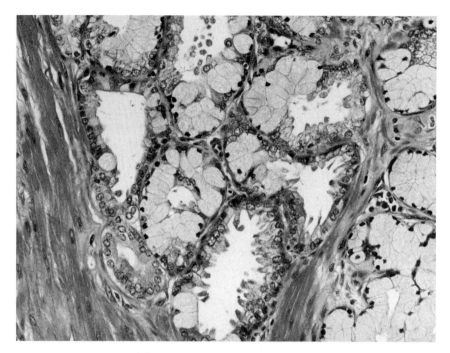

FIG. 13.1. Mucinous gland metaplasia.

Using criteria developed for mucinous carcinomas of other organs, the diagnosis of mucinous adenocarcinoma of the prostate gland should be made when at least 25% of the tumor resected contains lakes of extracellular mucin (6). Histologically, mucinous adenocarcinomas of the prostate are predominantly intermediate-grade tumors. A cribriform pattern tends to predominate in the mucinous areas (Figs. 13.2–13.5, efig 1388;1389-1390;1391-1393;1394-1395;1396-1398;1399;1400;1401). As with other unusual subtypes of prostate cancer, we do not assign a Gleason score to mucinous adenocarcinoma, but only to the conventional adenocarcinoma component if present. In contrast to bladder adenocarcinomas, mucinous adenocarcinoma of the prostate rarely contains mucin positive signet cells. Some carcinomas of the prostate will have a signet-ring cell appearance, yet the vacuoles do not contain intracytoplasmic mucin (efig 1402;1403-1404;1405-1407;1408-1409;1410)(11). Only a few cases of prostate cancer have been reported with mucin-positive signet cells (12,13). In one of these cases, the signet cell carcinoma appeared to arise from intestinal metaplasia of the overlying urothelium (14).

We have seen five cases, two of which have been reported, of in situ and infiltrating mucinous adenocarcinoma arising from glandular metaplasia of the prostatic urethra with invasion into the prostate (efig 1411-1415)(15). The histologic growth pattern found in these tumors were identical to mucinous

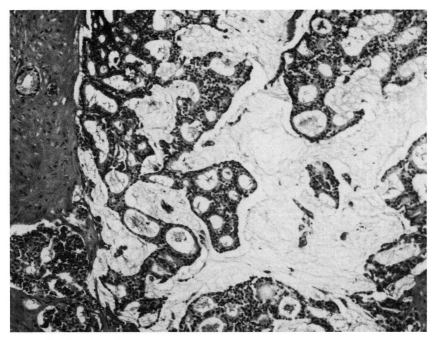

FIG. 13.2. Colloid carcinoma of the prostate with cribriform formation. ×100.

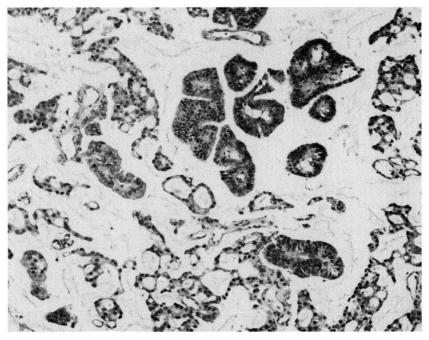

FIG. 13.3. Mucinous carcinoma of the prostate with tubules, cribriform formation, and papillary fronds. ×150.

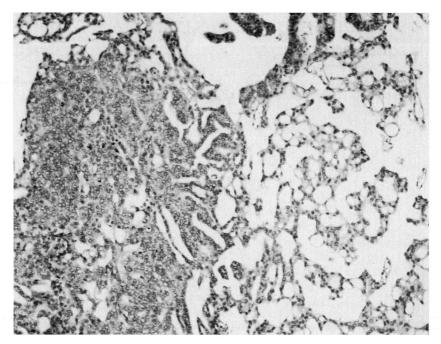

FIG. 13.4. Colloid carcinoma of the prostate showing, in addition, areas of solid tumor. ×100.

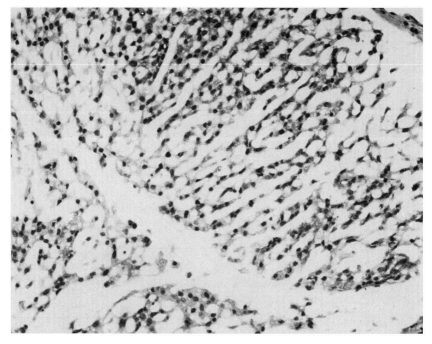

FIG. 13.5. Mucinous carcinoma of the prostate with tumor cells showing a filigree pattern. ×245.

adenocarcinoma of the bladder consisting of lakes of mucin lined by tall columnar epithelium with goblet cells showing varying degrees of nuclear atypia. In some of these cases, mucin-containing signet cells were also identified within the mucinous lakes. These tumors have been negative immunohistochemically for PSA and PSAP. Ductal adenocarcinomas of the prostate may cytologically resemble these tumors; however, prostatic ductal adenocarcinoma lacks extracellular mucin and is immunohistochemically uniformly positive for PSA and PSAP.

Bladder adenocarcinomas, either when the sole component or when admixed with transitional cell elements, in a minority of cases may show cross-reactive staining with antibodies to PSAP (16). While we have not seen bladder adenocarcinomas labeled with PSA, others have reported that this may also occur (17,18). Although most bladder adenocarcinomas with PSA or PSAP positivity are focally positive as contrasted to the diffuse reactivity in prostate adenocarcinomas, careful consideration of the light microscopic appearance of the tumor is necessary to distinguish between an adenocarcinoma of the bladder and prostate. CEA staining is of limited use in differentiating between prostate and bladder adenocarcinomas, since 20% to 25% of prostate adenocarcinomas express this substance.

Mucinous prostate adenocarcinomas behave aggressively (5–7). In the largest reported series, seven of 12 patients died of tumor (mean 5 years) and five were alive with disease (mean 3 years). Although these tumors are not as hormonally responsive as their nonmucinous counterparts, some respond to androgen withdrawal. Mucinous prostate adenocarcinomas have a propensity to develop bone metastases and increased serum PSA levels with advanced disease.

REFERENCES

1. Levine AJ, Foster EA. The relation of mucicarmine-staining properties of carcinomas of the prostate to differentiation, metastasis, and prognosis. *Cancer* 1964;17:21–25.
2. Epstein JI, Fynheer J. Acidic mucin in the prostate: can it differentiate adenosis from adenocarcinoma? *Human Pathol* 1992;23:1321–1325.
3. Shiraishi T, Kusano I, Watanabe M, et al. Mucous gland metaplasia of the prostate. *Am J Surg Pathol* 1993;17:618–622.
4. Grignon DJ, O'Malley FP. Mucinous metaplasia in the prostate gland. *Am J Surg Pathol* 1993; 17:287–290.
5. Epstein JI, Lieberman PH. Mucinous adenocarcinoma of the prostate: mucinous adenocarcinomas of the prostate gland. *Am J Surg Pathol* 1985;9:299–307.
6. Ro JY, Grignon J, Ayala AG, et al. Mucinous adenocarcinoma of the prostate: histochemical and immunohistochemical studies. *Hum Pathol* 1990;21:593–600.
7. Saito S, Iwaki H. Mucin-producing carcinoma of the prostate: review of 88 cases. *Urology* 1999; 54:141–144.
8. Foster EA, Levine AJ. Mucin production in metastatic carcinomas. *Cancer* 1963;16:506–509.
9. Franks LM, O'Shea JD, Thomson AER. Mucin in the prostate: a histochemical study in normal glands, latent, clinical, and colloid cancers. *Cancer* 1964;17:983–991.
10. Hukill PB, Vidone RA. Histochemistry of mucus and other polysaccharides in tumors: carcinoma of the prostate. *Lab Invest* 1967;16:395–406.
11. Ro JY, Naggar A, Ayala AG, et al. Signet-ring cell carcinoma of the prostate. *Am J Surg Pathol* 1988; 12:453–460.

12. Hejka AG, England DM. Signet ring cell carcinoma of prostate: immunohistochemical and ultra-structural study of a case. *Urology* 1989;34:155–158.
13. Uchijima Y, Ito H, Takahashi M, et al. Prostate mucinous adenocarcinoma with signet ring cell. *Urology* 1991;36:267–268.
14. Skordas G, Wang J, Kragel PJ. Primary prostatic signet-ring cell carcinoma. *Urology* 1993;42: 338–342.
15. Tran KP, Epstein JI. Mucinous adenocarcinoma of urinary bladder type arising from the prostatic urethra. *Am J Surg Pathol* 1996;20:1346–1350.
16. Epstein JI, Kuhajda FP, Lieberman PH. Prostate specific acid phosphatase immunoreactivity in adenocarcinomas of the urinary bladder. *Hum Pathol* 1986;17:939–942.
17. Heyderman E, Brown VE, Richardson TC. Epithelial markers in prostatic, bladder and colo-rectal cancer: an immunoperoxidase study of epithelial membrane antigen, carcinoembryonic antigen, and prostatic acid phosphatase. *J Clin Pathol* 1984;37:1363–1369.
18. Minkowitz G, Peterson P, Godwin TA. A histochemical and immunohistochemical study of adenocarcinomas involving urinary bladder. *Mod Pathol* 1990;3:68A.

14

Benign and Malignant Prostate Following Treatment

ANTIANDROGEN THERAPY

There are several different forms of antiandrogen therapy, some used for treating benign prostatic hyperplasia (BPH) and other more potent ones used for treating prostate cancer. In the prostate, testosterone is converted to the more potent androgen dihydrotestosterone (DHT) by type-2 5 alpha-reductase. Finasteride (Proscar) inhibits type-2 5 alpha-reductase. By blocking the production of DHT, finasteride leads to a shrinkage of the prostate in some men, and improves their urinary obstructive symptoms. As testosterone is still present, this therapy does not result in total androgen withdrawal. We have demonstrated that finasteride does not alter the histology of either benign or malignant tissue (1). It also does not appear that the parameters of tissue composition on needle biopsy (percentage of epithelium, epithelial volume, and stromal/epithelial ratio) can predict a favorable response to hormonal treatment of BPH (2).

The more potent hormonal therapy used to treat prostate cancer consists of a luteinizing hormone-releasing hormone (LHRH) agonist (Lupron) typically in association with the antiandrogen flutamide. Some urologists use this regimen prior to radical prostatectomy (neoadjuvant hormone therapy), as it has been demonstrated that it results in less frequent positive margins at radical prostatectomy (3). Other urologists use this therapy if there is going to be a delay of several months between the diagnosis of cancer and radical surgery, so as to allay any concerns that patients may have not received immediate treatment for their tumor. Despite the less frequently positive margins, this combination endocrine therapy has not been demonstrated to improve the prognosis and has fallen somewhat out of favor (3). Typically, pathologists encounter combination endocrine treated radical prostatectomy specimens, although occasionally needle biopsies or transurethral resections of the prostate (TURP) may be performed following this therapy.

TABLE 14.1. *Changes in the prostate following hormonal therapy*

Benign prostate tissue
Diffuse squamous metaplasia
Diffuse transitional cell metaplasia
Diffuse basal cell hyperplasia
Glandular atrophy
Stromal fibrosis
Malignant prostate tissue
Atrophic cancer
Glands with xanthomatous cytoplasm and pyknotic nuclei
Individual tumor cells resembling xanthomatous histiocytes
Individual tumor cells in fibrotic and inflamed stroma

The histology of both the normal and neoplastic tissue may be significantly altered with this therapy, making the assessment of these specimens difficult (4–9) (Table 14.1). Within the nonneoplastic prostate, antiandrogen therapy results in squamous metaplasia in both the overlying urethra as well as diffusely throughout the prostate (Fig. 14.1, efig 1416-1417;1418-1420;1421-1422). In areas, the altered glands have the appearance of transitional cell metaplasia and

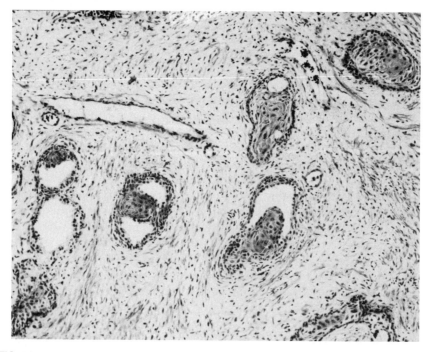

FIG. 14.1. Extensive squamous metaplasia diffusely present within acini resulting from antiandrogen therapy. ×100.

basal cell hyperplasia. There is less abundant squamous differentiation than in patients who have been treated in the past with estrogen therapy. Other situations where one may see squamous metaplasia within the urethra is following transurethral resection. The diffuse nature of squamous metaplasia with antiandrogen therapy is characteristic, since the only other situation in which squamous metaplasia occurs within the prostate is when it is localized to the immediate vicinity of prostatic infarcts. Other changes with antiandrogen therapy seen in the nonneoplastic tissue include atrophy of the glandular epithelium with some stromal fibrosis.

Therapy with LHRH agonists and flutamide may result in three different histologic patterns in prostate cancer. The neoplastic acini may become atrophic (Fig. 14.2, efig 1423-1425;1426-1428;1429-1430) (5–9). At higher power, these neoplastic glands are identical to benign atrophic glands. Only their crowded infiltrative appearance or location outside of the prostate is diagnostic of adenocarcinoma. Furthermore, there may be other areas of the tumor that do not show as prominent response to hormonal therapy and are more recognizable as carcinoma. The second pattern is when the atrophic neoplastic glands develop pyknotic nuclei and abundant xanthomatous cytoplasm (Figs. 14.3 and 14.4). These cells then desquamate into the lumen of the malignant glands where they resemble histiocytes and lymphocytes (Color

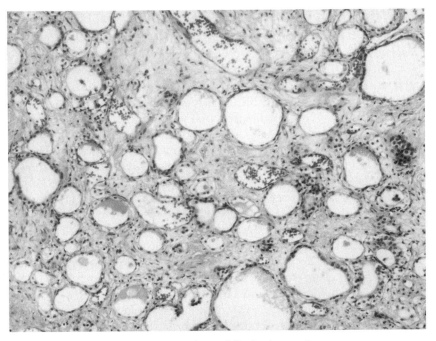

FIG. 14.2. Adenocarcinoma following Lupron therapy.

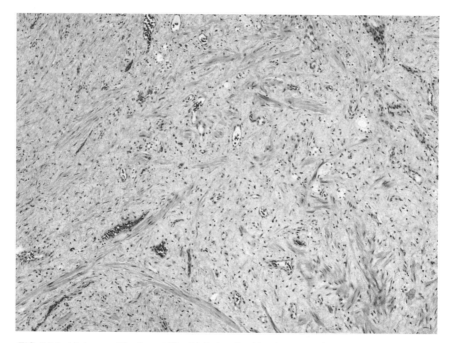

FIG. 14.3. High magnification of Fig. 14.3 showing bland tumor cells with clear cytoplasm.

Plate 39, efig 1431-1433). The fact that they are still identifiable as glandular structures is helpful in establishing the diagnosis. There may be areas where only scattered cells resembling foamy histiocytes with pyknotic nuclei and xanthomatous cytoplasm are visible. These cells, however, are pancytokeratin-positive demonstrating their epithelial nature. The third pattern is when there are individual tumor cells resembling inflammatory cells. At low power, these areas may be difficult to identify, and often the only clue to areas of hormon-ally treated carcinoma is a fibrotic background with scattered cells (Fig. 14.3). At higher magnification, individual tumor cells should be looked for (Fig. 14.5, efig 1434-1435). Immunohistochemistry for prostate-specific antigen (PSA) or pancytokeratin can aid in the diagnosis of carcinoma in these cases by identifying the individual cells as epithelial cells of prostatic origin (Fig. 14.6). Cancer cells following hormonal therapy demonstrate a lack of high molecular weight cytokeratin staining, identical to untreated prostate cancer. Following hormonal therapy, there may be a decrease in immunoreactivity with PSA and prostate-specific acid phosphatase (PSAP), but most tumors maintain some labeling with these antibodies (10,11). Following a response to combination endocrine therapy, the grade of the tumor appears artifactually higher, when compared to the grade of the pretreated tumor (7,12). While some authors propose that one can still assign an accurate grade to cancers

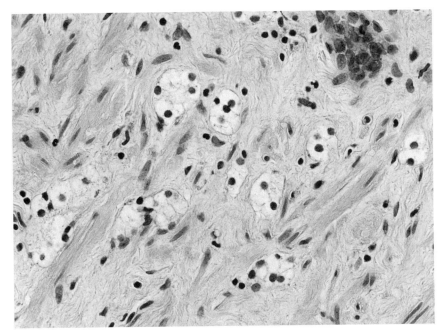

FIG. 14.4. Adenocarcinoma following antiandrogen therapy.

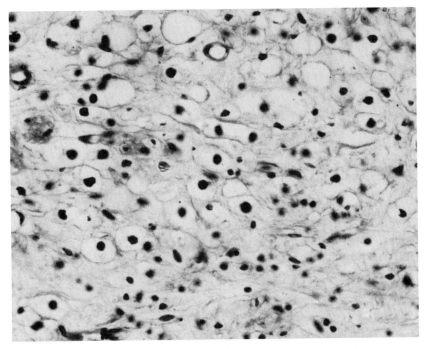

FIG. 14.5. Prominent estrogen effect within individually infiltrating cells of adenocarcinoma of the prostate. ×340.

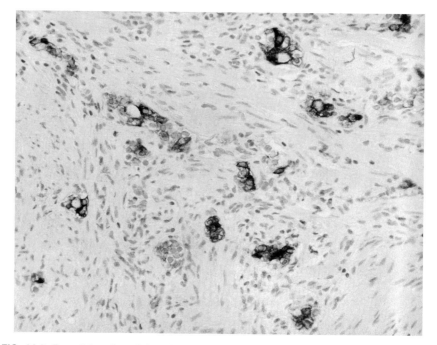

FIG. 14.6. Pancytokeratin staining of tumor shown in Fig. 14.3 demonstrating scattered neoplastic epithelial cells.

showing hormonal effect, the majority of experts do not grade cancers showing treatment effect.

Several studies have demonstrated that the extent and prevalence of high-grade prostatic intraepithelial neoplasia (PIN) is substantially decreased in prostates that have been treated with androgen deprivation for 3 months prior to radical prostatectomy (9,13). High-grade PIN may still persist following androgen blockade therapy, although tufted PIN may be replaced by flat high-grade PIN (14).

Treatment with estrogen, such as diethylstilbestrol (DES), is no longer widely used. The typical changes following DES include widespread fully developed squamous metaplasia in the benign prostate, and tumor cells with strikingly clear cytoplasm and small pyknotic nuclei (15). Following estrogen therapy, the prostate may also develop squamous metaplasia in some of the neoplastic glands as well, resulting in adenosquamous carcinomas (Fig. 14.7, efig 1436-1438) (16). The metastases may be adenosquamous carcinoma or pure squamous carcinoma. There have also been reports of adenosquamous carcinoma of the prostate in which there was no previous estrogen therapy (17,18). In some cases of adenosquamous carcinoma, the squamous components have been reported to be positive for PSA or PSAP (16).

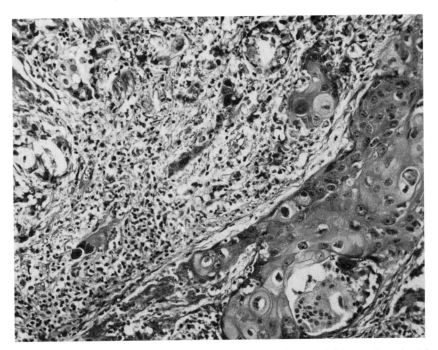

FIG. 14.7. Prostatic tumor showing squamous differentiation *(bottom right)* as well as glandular differentiation *(upper left).* ×240.

RADIATION

The use of radiotherapy as a primary treatment for clinically localized prostate cancer has been increasing. In particular, the use of brachytherapy (seed implantation) has become more popular in recent years. Typically, following radiotherapy the serum PSA level will decrease to a nadir level. In some men, the PSA will then subsequently rise; a consecutive rise of three serial PSA measurements is the most widely accepted definition of radiotherapy failure. It is controversial whether it is necessary to perform a biopsy to histologically demonstrate carcinoma if the serum PSA is rising after radiotherapy. Some experts argue that one can document that tumor is recurring following radiotherapy solely based on the rising serial PSA measurements and treat the patients, for example, with hormone therapy. Other oncologists feel more comfortable histologically documenting progression of cancer before initiating therapy. For more definitive therapy of postradiotherapy failures (i.e., salvage prostatectomy), where associated morbidity is higher, histological documentation of recurrent cancer is mandatory. Often pathologists will not get a history of prior irradiation, such that it is necessary for them to recognize the histologic features of radiation atypia in benign glands so as to avoid a misdiagnosis of cancer.

TABLE 14.2. *Distinction between radiated benign and malignant prostate glands*

Radiated benign	Radiated malignant
Lobular	Infiltrative
Glands separated by stroma	Back-to-back
Multilayering	Single cell layer
Atrophic cytoplasm	Abundant cytoplasm
Scattered markedly atypical nuclei in glands	Gland-forming tumors lack prominent atypia
Nuclear atypia appears degenerative	Detailed nuclear features with prominent nucleoli

Within the nonneoplastic prostatic glands, radiation results in glandular atrophy, squamous metaplasia, and cytologic atypia (19) (efig 1439-1440;1441; 1442-1444;1445-1446;1447-1449;1450-1453). Though one may find vascular radiation changes, the stromal atypia characteristic of radiation in other organs is not usually seen.

The distinction between irradiated nonneoplastic prostatic glands and carcinoma is best made on the low magnification architectural pattern of the glands (Table 14.2). Within the radiated normal prostate, glands maintain their normal architectural lobular configuration (Fig. 14.8). In contrast to car-

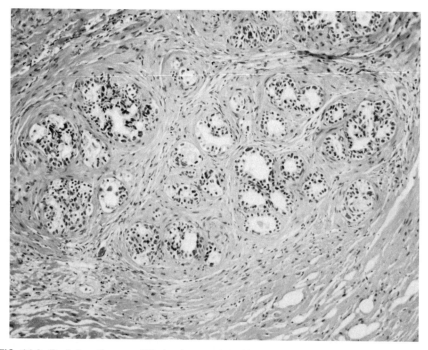

FIG. 14.8. Radiation change within benign prostate. Note retention of lobular configuration of normal prostate glands separated by a modest amount of stroma. ×110.

cinoma, the nonneoplastic glands are separated by a modest amount of prostatic stroma. On higher magnification, whereas glands of prostatic carcinoma are lined by a single cell layer, there is piling up of the nuclei within irradiated normal prostate as well as an occasional recognizable basal cell layer (Fig. 14.9). This piling up of the cells in radiated benign glands frequently appears slightly spindled resembling transitional cell metaplasia (Fig. 14.10). The finding of scattered markedly atypical nuclei within well-formed acini is typical of radiated benign glands and rare in prostate carcinoma (Fig. 14.11). Prostate carcinomas that are sufficiently differentiated to form glands rarely manifest the degree of atypia seen with radiation, and if present would be more uniformly present in all cells. Radiated nuclei also have a degenerative, hyperchromatic smudgy appearance as opposed to malignant prostatic nuclei that usually contain prominent nucleoli. Irradiated nonneoplastic glands often are atrophic (Fig. 14.12), in contrast to gland-forming prostatic adenocarcinomas that typically have abundant cytoplasm. It has been demonstrated that high molecular weight cytokeratin immunohistochemistry can aid in the diagnosis of irradiated prostate by identifying basal cells within benign radiated glands (20).

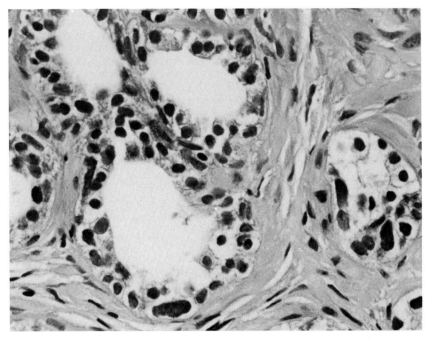

FIG. 14.9. Higher magnification of Fig 14.8 showing scattered atypical hyperchromatic nuclei within radiated normal glands. As opposed to glands of infiltrating carcinoma, the benign radiated glands have a multilayering of their epithelium. ×480.

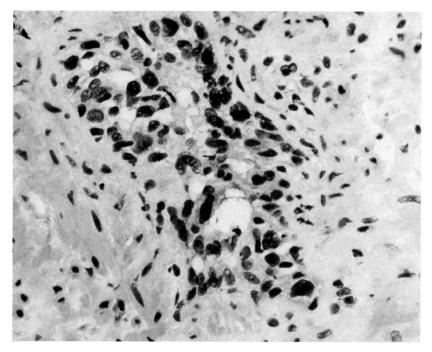

FIG. 14.10. Adenocarcinoma following radiation with multilayered nuclei and scattered atypical cells.

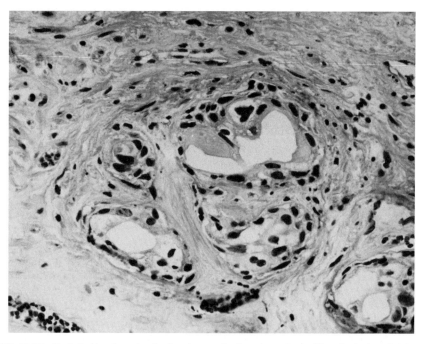

FIG. 14.11. Radiated benign glands showing marked nuclear atypia. The atypical nuclei, however, have a somewhat degenerative, hyperchromatic, smudgy appearance as opposed to prostatic adenocarcinoma cells. ×310.

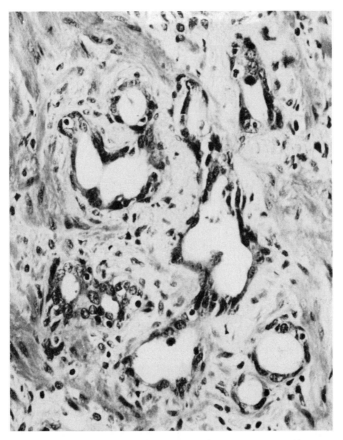

FIG. 14.12. Radiated benign glands showing an atrophic appearance with scattered atypical nuclei. ×340.

Although it may be difficult to diagnose high-grade PIN following radiation therapy, this diagnosis may occasionally be made in this setting (21). The typical nuclear changes of high-grade PIN characterized by prominent nucleoli are present, which differ from the degenerative smudgy chromatin seen with radiation atypia.

Radiated adenocarcinoma of the prostate may show either no recognizable difference from nonradiated cancer or the effects of radiation damage. In order to diagnose either pattern of cancer, the key feature is that architecturally the findings are inconsistent with benign glands. The presence of closely packed glands with a haphazard infiltrative growth pattern is typical of adenocarcinoma and cannot be attributed to radiation change (Fig. 14.13). Similarly, the presence of infiltrating individual epithelial cells is diagnostic of carcinoma (Fig. 14.14). Cancers not showing any treatment effect have typical prostate cancer nuclei

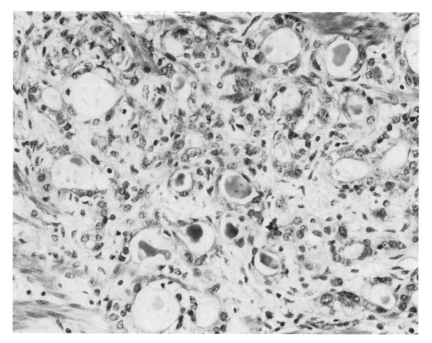

FIG. 14.13. Radiated adenocarcinoma of the prostate showing retention of abnormal growth pattern diagnostic of carcinoma. ×240.

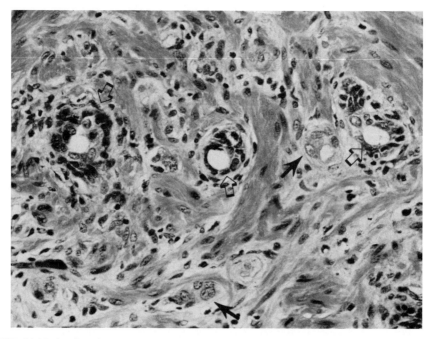

FIG. 14.14. Irradiated prostate showing individual neoplastic infiltrating cells *(arrows)* as well as irradiated benign glands with multilayering of their epithelium *(open arrows)*. ×270.

with prominent nucleoli and glands with a modest amount of cytoplasm (efig 1454-1457). Cancers with radiation effect demonstrate either glands or individual cells with abundant vacuolated cytoplasm or single cells with indistinct cytoplasm (efig 1454-1457;1458-1459;1460-1461;1462-1463;1464-1465;1466-1468;1469-1471;1472-1474). Nuclei lack apparent nucleoli and are either large with bizarre shapes or pyknotic with smudged chromatin (22).

The largest study to evaluate the significance of histological findings on postradiotherapy prostate biopsy is that by Crook et al. (23). In order to evaluate the time course of histologic resolution of prostate cancer following radiotherapy, men undergoing sequential biopsies were studied. Postradiotherapy biopsies were classified into three groups: positive, negative, or indeterminate (cancer with treatment effect). Biopsy pathology predicted prognosis with positive biopsies having a worse outcome than negative biopsies and cancers with treatment effect having an intermediate prognosis. As 30% of the men with a positive biopsy at 12 months after radiotherapy eventually showed delayed tumor regression with no evidence of disease at 30 months, it was recommended that biopsies should be performed at 30 to 36 months following radiotherapy in order for a positive biopsy to have true meaning. There were also problems with false/negative biopsies in that 19% of the biopsies that were initially negative became positive at 43 months. Patients with biopsies containing cancer with treatment effect had variable outcomes. Thirty percent eventually showed no evidence of disease at 32 months. However, 18% progressed to local failure at 38 months. Thirty four percent remained biopsy failures yet otherwise showed no evidence of disease. The remaining men demonstrated distant failure. In contrast to earlier studies published by the same authors, grading the degree of radiotherapy effect was not predictive of outcome. When signing out postradiotherapy biopsies, we diagnose them as "benign," "cancer without treatment effect" (a Gleason grade is assigned), or "cancer showing treatment effect" (no Gleason grade assigned). The expression of proliferation markers (PCNA/MIB-1) in postradiated cancer can also help predict clinical failure (23). Relatively few studies have been done on the immunohistochemistry of radiated prostate, with most cases showing retention of their PSAP positivity (11,24).

POSTRADICAL PROSTATECTOMY BIOPSIES

Following radical prostatectomy, a needle biopsy of the prostatic fossa may be performed to detect recurrence. There are no uniform guidelines as to when postradical prostatectomy biopsies are performed to document postoperative failure. Practices range from routine biopsies in men with rising postoperative serum PSA levels to reliance on clinical findings to establish a diagnosis of recurrent prostate cancer. Several investigators have demonstrated the difficulty in diagnosing recurrent adenocarcinoma on biopsy, sometimes requiring the patient to have several needle biopsies over time (25–27). We have demonstrated that recurrent cancer on needle biopsy may be focal and difficult to diagnose, in part due to the limited extent of cancer seen on biopsy (Fig. 14.15, efig 1475-1476;1477-1478;1479-1480)(28). Another factor that leads to diagnostic difficulties is that the usual clues for the diagnosis of prostate cancer are often not present. We believe that there should be a lower histologic threshold for diagnosing recurrent prostate cancer in men who have had a prior radical prostatectomy. First, these men have a history of prostate cancer, where rare malignant-appearing glands may be consistent with recurrent cancer, yet insufficient to establish a primary diagnosis. Secondly, the prostate has been removed, such that the finding of a few atypical glands in soft tissue without surrounding benign prostate tissue is not expected and indicates recurrent cancer. Although in 14% of our postoperative biopsies we found benign prostate tissue, these glands were histologically bland and typically away from the recurrent cancer. Consequently, the presence of a few atypical glands is often diagnostic of recurrent prostate cancer, although those same glands sampled on a needle biopsy of the intact prostate might be called suspicious but not diagnostic of cancer. One cannot rely on the clinical, radiological, or prior radical prostatectomy data to establish a diagnosis of locally recurrent prostate cancer. The diagnosis of locally recurrent cancer must be based on a constellation of the histologic findings along with the history of prior surgery.

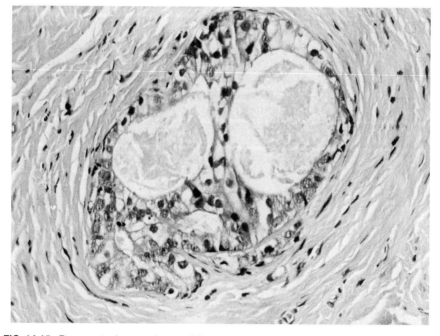

FIG. 14.15. Recurrent adenocarcinoma of the prostate following radical prostatectomy. This was the only gland present in the biopsy of the prostatic fossa following surgery. The gland was present only on deeper sections into the paraffin block.

Several prior studies have noted the presence of benign glands in biopsies following radical prostatectomy. Foster reported on eight patients with benign glands on biopsy following radical prostatectomy (29). Of six patients who underwent repeat biopsies, four were eventually shown to have, in addition, recurrent adenocarcinoma of the prostate. Fowler describes six patients who had benign prostate glands on biopsy following radical prostatectomy (26). The only patient who underwent repeat biopsy was also found to have carcinoma. Benign glands on biopsy after radical prostatectomy imply that the prostate was not removed in its entirety. It remains unknown whether and how frequently the presence of only benign prostate glands left after radical prostatectomy can give rise to an elevated postoperative serum PSA level and the false impression of recurrent prostate cancer.

POSTCRYOSURGICAL PROSTATIC BIOPSIES

A less popular alternative to surgery or radiotherapy for localized prostate cancer is cryosurgery. The histologic findings in postcryosurgical prostatic biopsies include residual cancer (which is identical to precryosurgical cancer), necrosis, hyalinization, fibrosis, granulomatous inflammation, foci of calcification, squamous and transitional cell metaplasia, hemosiderin deposition, and hemorrhage (efig 1481;1482-1483) (30).

HYPERTHERMIA

Hyperthermia is used to treat BPH. This therapy results in areas of hemorrhagic coagulative necrosis and occasionally reactive changes (efig 1484-1486) (31).

PHYTOTHERAPY

The use of alternative medicines, such as various plant extracts, to treat prostatic diseases have gained widespread popularity in recent years. One of the most frequently used is that of saw palmetto. We have demonstrated that this therapy does not significantly alter the histology of benign prostate tissue (32). Sabal, another plant extract which is in widespread use for treating BPH in Germany, similarly does not alter the histology of benign or neoplastic epithelium (33).

POST-TEFLON INJECTION GRANULOMAS

Teflon is injected into the periurethral tissues and submucosa of the bladder for the treatment of incontinence. On occasion, the foreign material may migrate into the prostate. Teflon has a very basophilic appearance, is birefringent, and induces a marked granulomatous reaction (34).

POSTNEEDLE BIOPSY CHANGES

Needle biopsy tracts of the prostate in radical prostatectomy specimens manifest differently depending on the plane of section and location in the prostate. At the edge of the prostate, hemosiderin, recent hemorrhage, and fibrosis are noted in the periprostatic tissue. Within the prostate one can visualize an irregular stellate defect surrounded by fibrosis or a linear fibrous tract (efig 1487;1488). Although there is literature on the tracking of cancer into the periprostatic tissue with larger core needle biopsies, there is no evidence that contemporary thin-gauge needle biopsy instruments result in local cancer seeding (35,36).

REFERENCES

1. Yang XJ, Lecksell K, Short K, et al. Does long-term finasteride therapy affect the histologic features of benign prostatic tissue and prostate cancer on needle biopsy? *Urology* 1999;53:696–700.
2. Eri LM, Svinland A. Can prostate epithelial content predict response to hormonal treatment of patients with benign prostatic hyperplasia? *Urology* 2000;56:261–265.
3. Van Poppel H, De Ridder D, Elgamal AA, et al. Neoadjuvant hormonal therapy before radical prostatectomy decreased the number of positive surgical margins in stage T2 prostate cancer: interim results of a prospective randomized trial. *J Urol* 1995;154:429–434.
4. Balaji KC, Rabbani F, Tsai H, et al. Effect of neoadjuvant hormonal therapy on prostatic intraepithelial neoplasia and its prognostic significance. *J Urol* 1999;162:753–757.
5. Tetu B, Srigley JR, Boivin J, et al. Effect of combination endocrine therapy (LHRH agonist and flutamide) on normal prostate and prostatic adenocarcinoma. *Am J Surg Pathol* 1991;15:111–120.
6. Murphy WM, Soloway MS, Barrows GH. Pathologic changes associated with androgen deprivation therapy for prostate cancer. *Cancer* 1991;68:821–828.
7. Smith DM, Murphy WM. Histologic changes in prostate carcinomas treated with leuprolide (luteinizing hormone-releasing hormone effect). *Cancer* 1991;73:1472–1477.
8. Armas OA, Aprikian AG, Melamed J, et al. Clinical and pathobiological effects of neoadjuvant total androgen ablation therapy on clinically localized prostatic adenocarcinoma. *Am J Surg Pathol* 1994; 18:979–991.
9. Vaillancourt L, Têtu B, Fradet Y, et al. Effect of neoadjuvant endocrine therapy (combined androgen blockade) on normal prostate and prostatic carcinoma. A randomized study. *Am J Surg Pathol* 1996; 20:86–93.
10. Grignon D, Troster M. Changes in immunohistochemical staining in prostatic adenocarcinoma following diethylstilbestrol therapy. *Prostate* 1985;7:195–202.
11. Vernon SE, Williams WD. Pre-treatment and post-treatment evaluation of prostatic adenocarcinoma for prostatic-specific acid phosphatase and prostatic-specific antigen by immunohistochemistry. *J Urol* 1983;130:95–98.
12. Smith DM, Murphy WM. Histologic changes in prostate carcinomas treated with Leuprolide (luteinizing hormone-releasing hormone effect): distinction from poor tumor differentiation. *Cancer* 1994;73:1472–1477.
13. Ferguson J, Zincke H, Ellison E, et al. Decrease of prostatic intraepithelial neoplasia following androgen deprivation therapy in patients with stage T3 carcinoma treated by radical prostatectomy. *Urology* 1994;44:91–95.
14. Van der Kwast TH, Labrie F, Tetu B. Persistence of high-grade prostatic intra-epithelial neoplasia under combined androgen blockade therapy. *Hum Pathol* 1999;30:1503–1507.
15. Franks LM. Estrogen-treated prostatic cancer: the variation in responsiveness of tumor cells. *Cancer* 1960;13;490–501.
16. Accetta PA, Gardner WA. Squamous metastases from prostatic adenocarcinoma. *Prostate* 1982;3: 515–521.
17. Accetta PA, Gardner WA Jr. Adenosquamous carcinoma of prostate. *Urology* 1983;22:73–75.
18. Bassler TJ Jr, Orozco R, Bassler IC, et al. Adenosquamous carcinoma of the prostate: case report with DNA analysis, immunohistochemistry, and literature review. *Urology* 1999; 53:832–834.

19. Bostwick DG, Egbert BM, Fajardo LF. Radiation injury of the normal and neoplastic prostate. *Am J Surg Pathol* 1982;6:501–551.
20. Brawer MK, Nagle RB, Pitts W, et.al. Keratin immunoreactivity as an aid to the diagnosis of persistent adenocarcinoma following prostatic irradiation. *Cancer* 1989;63:454–460.
21. Arkawa A, Song S, Scardino PT, et al. High-grade prostatic intraepithelial neoplasia in prostates following irradiation failure in the treatment of prostatic adenocarcinoma. *Pathol Res Pract* 1995;191: 868–872.
22. Crook JM, Bahadur YA, Robertson SJ, et al. Evaluation of radiation effect, tumor differentiation, and prostate specific antigen staining in sequential prostate biopsies after external beam radiotherapy for patients with prostate carcinoma. *Cancer* 1997; 79:81–89.
23. Crook J, Malone S, Perry G, et al. Postradiotherapy prostate biopsies: what do they really mean? Results for 498 patients. *Int J Rad Onc Biol Phys* 2000;48:355–367.
24. Mahan DE, Bruce AW, Manley PN, et al. Immunohistochemical evaluation of prostatic carcinoma before and after radiotherapy. *J Urol* 1980;124:488–491.
25. Connolly JA, Shinohara K, Presti JC Jr, et al. Local recurrence after radical prostatectomy: characterization in size, location, and relationship to prostate-specific antigen and surgical margins. *Urology* 1986;41:225–231.
26. Fowler JE Jr, Brooks J, Pandey P, et al. Variable histology of anastomotic biopsies with detectable prostate specific antigen after radical prostatectomy. *J Urol* 1995;153:1011–1014.
27. Saleem MD, Sanders H, El Naser MA, et al. Factors predicting cancer detection in biopsy of the prostatic fossa after radical prostatectomy. *Urology* 1998;51:283–286.
28. Ripple MG, Potter SR, Partin AW, et al. Needle biopsy of recurrent adenocarcinoma of the prostate after radical prostatectomy. *Mod Pathol* 2000;13:521–527.
29. Foster LS, Jajodia P, Fournier G Jr, et al. The value of prostate specific antigen and transrectal ultrasound guided biopsy in detecting prostatic fossa recurrences following prostatectomy. *J Urol* 1993; 149:1024–1028.
30. Borkowski P, Robinson MJ, Poppiti RJ, et al. Histologic findings in postcryosurgical prostatic biopsies. *Mod Pathol* 1996;9:807–811.
31. Orihuela E, Motamedi M, Pow-Sang M, et al. Histopathological evaluation of laser thermocoagulation in the human prostate: optimization of laser irradiation for benign prostatic hyperplasia. *J Urol* 1995; 153: 1531–1536.
32. Marks LS, Partin AW, Epstein JI, et al. Effects of saw palmetto herbal blend in men with symptomatic benign prostatic hyperplasia. *J Urol* 2000;163:1451–1456.
33. Helpap B, Oehler U, Weisser H, et al. Morphology of benign prostatic hyperplasia after treatment with Sabal Extract IDS89 or placebo: results of a prospective, randomized, double-blind trial. *J Urol Path* 1995;3:175–182.
34. Orozco RE, Peters RL. Teflon granuloma of the prostate mimicking adenocarcinoma: report of two cases. *J Urol Path* 1995;3:365–368.
35. Bastacky SS, Walsh PC, Epstein JI. Needle biopsy associated tumor tracking of adenocarcinoma of the prostate. *J Urol* 1991;145:1003–1007.
36. Bostwick DG, Vonk J, Picado A. Pathologic changes in the prostate following contemporary 18-gauge needle biopsy: no apparent risk of local cancer seeding. *J Urol Path* 1994;2:203–212.

15

Transitional Cell Carcinoma

Prostatic transitional cell (urothelial) carcinoma seen in association with bladder urothelial neoplasia may be invasive via direct stromal extension from the bladder, purely intraductal, or intraductal and invasive.

DISTINCTION OF HIGH-GRADE PROSTATIC ADENOCARCINOMA FROM TRANSITIONAL CELL CARCINOMA

Prostatic involvement by transitional cell carcinoma in a patient with bladder urothelial neoplasia may result from direct invasion of an infiltrating bladder cancer into the stroma of the prostate (1,2). In this situation the prognosis of the transitional cell carcinoma of the bladder worsens dramatically and is equivalent in survival to cases of bladder carcinoma with regional lymph node metastases.

In these cases, a common diagnostic problem is in differentiating on transurethral resection of the prostate (TURP) between a poorly differentiated transitional cell carcinoma of the bladder and a poorly differentiated prostatic adenocarcinoma. The differences in therapy between these two diseases differ significantly, making the distinction between these two entities crucial. Even in poorly differentiated prostatic carcinomas, there is relatively little pleomorphism or mitotic activity compared to poorly differentiated transitional cell carcinoma (Figs. 15.1 and 15.2). Poorly differentiated prostate cancers may have enlarged nuclei and prominent nucleoli, yet there is little variability in nuclear shape or size from one nucleus to another. High-grade transitional cell carcinomas often reveal marked pleomorphism with tumor giant cells (efig 1489-1492). A subtler finding is that the cytoplasm of prostatic adenocarcinoma is often very foamy and pale imparting a "soft" appearance. In contrast, transitional cell carcinomas may demonstrate hard glassy eosinophilic cytoplasm or more prominent squamous differentiation (Color Plate 40, efig 1493). The findings of infiltrating cords of cells (Fig. 15.3) or focal cribriform glandular differentiation (Fig. 15.4) are other features more typical of prostatic adenocarcinoma than transitional cell carcinoma (efig 1494-1496). Transitional cell cancer tends to grow in nests, even when poorly differentiated.

Within poorly differentiated prostatic adenocarcinomas, 70% of the cases in Svanholm's study (3) and 35% of the cases in Ellis's study (4) showed <25% of the

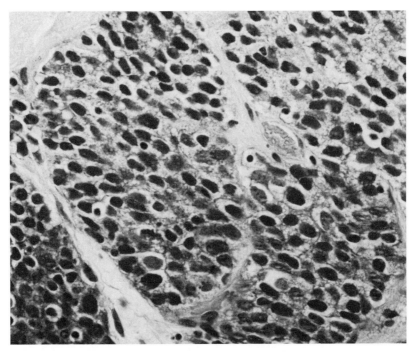

FIG. 15.1. Poorly differentiated (high-grade) prostatic adenocarcinoma with relatively little anaplasia, as opposed to poorly differentiated transitional-cell carcinoma. Note paucity of mitotic figures despite the tumor's poor differentiation. ×420.

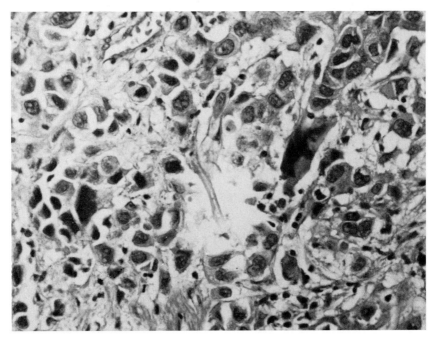

FIG. 15.2. Infiltrating, poorly differentiated transitional-cell carcinoma within the prostate showing marked nuclear atypia. ×360.

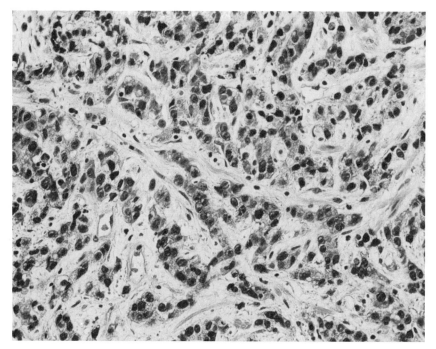

FIG. 15.3. Infiltrating cords of cells more typical of prostatic adenocarcinoma versus transitional-cell carcinoma. ×263.

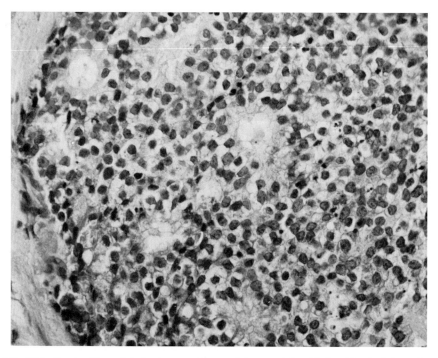

FIG. 15.4. Poorly differentiated adenocarcinoma of the prostate with focal luminal formation, favoring adenocarcinoma of the prostate versus transitional-cell carcinoma. ×325.

tumor staining with prostate-specific acid phosphatase (PSAP). Fifty-eight percent, 25%, and 50% of the cases had <25% of the cells showing immunoreactivity in the studies of Svanholm, Ellis, and Ford (5), respectively. The significance of these figures is that given a limited amount of tissue, almost 50% of the cases may be interpreted as negative with immunohistochemistry to prostate-specific antigen (PSA) or PSAP, owing to only focal positivity that may not be sampled. Within the same series, 5% to 6% of the high-grade tumors were entirely negative for PSA, and 10% to 13% of the high-grade tumors were entirely nonreactive for PSAP. While some studies claim superiority of PSA over PSAP in staining prostatic carcinoma (3,5), other articles have demonstrated poorly differentiated prostatic carcinomas that lacked PSA staining but still maintained their immunoreactivity with antibodies to PSAP (6,7). In our own hands, PSAP has in general been more sensitive. Because in some cases antibodies to PSA are more sensitive in identifying prostatic tumors, while PSAP antibodies give superior results in other cases, both antibodies should be used in establishing if the tumor is of prostatic origin. Even when both PSA and PSAP are employed, the lack of immunoreactivity in a poorly differentiated tumor within the prostate, especially if present in limited amount, does not exclude the diagnosis of a poorly differentiated prostatic adenocarcinoma. Monoclonal antibodies to PSAP have lower sensitivities than their polyclonal counterparts (8). In general, various cytokeratins (CK7, CK20, 34βE12) show strong positivity in cases of urothelial carcinoma involving the prostate. Both CK7 and CK20 are more frequently seen in urothelial carcinoma as compared to adenocarcinoma of the prostate, although they may be positive in adenocarcinoma of the prostate as well (9). The more specific marker 34βE12 is only extremely rarely expressed in adenocarcinoma of the prostate; it is positive in approximately 60% of urothelial carcinomas (efig 1497-1498). Newer markers that appear specific for urothelial carcinoma include uroplakin and thrombonodulin.

With only a few exceptions, immunoperoxidase staining for PSA and PSAP is very specific for prostatic tissue. Situations that can cause diagnostic difficulty include PSA and PSAP within periurethral glands, as well as cystitis cystica and cystitis glandularis in both men and women (10–12). Other examples of cross-reactive staining include anal glands in men (PSA, PSAP) and urachal remnants (PSA) (13,14).

Some intestinal carcinoids and pancreatic islet cell tumors are strongly reactive with antibodies to PSAP, yet are negative with antibodies to PSA (15). Periurethral gland carcinomas in women and various salivary gland tumors may also be PSA and PSAP positive (16,17). Weak false–positive staining for PSAP has been reported in several breast and renal cell carcinomas, and we have seen some cases where PSA was focally and weakly positive though the patient was subsequently shown to have a nonprostatic tumor. This suggests that weak focal positive staining for either antigen should be interpreted with caution.

Although adenocarcinomas of the bladder, whether as a pure tumor or with mixed transitional cell carcinoma, have also been reported positive for PSA or PSAP (18,19), there has yet to be a case reported positive for both. In assessing an adenocarcinoma involving the prostate and bladder where only one marker is positive, the tumor must be diagnosed on the histological differences between

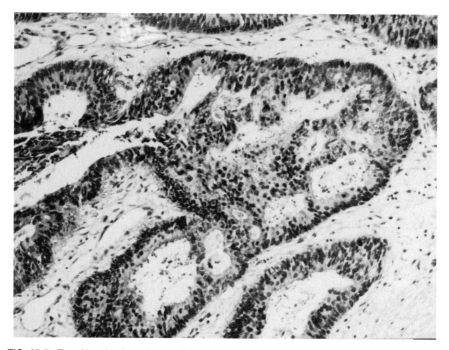

FIG. 15.5. Transitional-cell carcinoma of the prostate with areas of glandular differentiation. ×165.

bladder and prostate adenocarcinoma. In general, adenocarcinomas of the bladder resemble adenocarcinomas of the intestine (Fig. 15.5). In a poorly differentiated tumor occurring in the bladder and the prostate where the differential diagnosis is between a high-grade prostatic adenocarcinoma and a transitional cell carcinoma, focal strong staining for either marker can be used reliably to make the diagnosis of prostatic adenocarcinoma, since PSAP and PSA false positivity have not been convincingly described in transitional cell carcinomas (8,20,21).

Almost 50% of cystoprostatectomy specimens performed for transitional cell carcinoma also contain adenocarcinoma of the prostate (1,22,23). Therefore, the finding in a TURP of a small focus of well-differentiated adenocarcinoma of the prostate should not necessarily influence whether a separate focus of poorly differentiated tumor is transitional cell carcinoma or adenocarcinoma of the prostate.

INTRADUCTAL TRANSITIONAL CELL CARCINOMA INVOLVING THE PROSTATE

Most commonly, transitional cell carcinoma involves the prostate in a setting of a patient with bladder transitional cell carcinoma. Since topical chemotherapy and immunotherapy for superficial bladder carcinomas appear to act by direct contact with neoplastic epithelium, it has become critical to identify those cases of bladder transitional cell carcinomas with prostatic involvement, since conservative management will not treat these cases effectively. Currently, biopsies of the prostatic

urethra and suburethral prostate tissue are often recommended as a staging procedure in patients undergoing conservative treatment for superficial bladder tumors.
It is also important to evaluate the urothelium in routine TURP specimens, as we
have seen several cases of carcinoma in situ (CIS) where no history of bladder cancer was present. Several studies have shown that by examining random sections of
the prostate at the time of cystectomy for transitional cell carcinoma of the bladder,
between 12% to 20% of the cases will be shown to have prostatic involvement by
transitional cell carcinoma. If serial sections of the prostate in cystoprostatectomy
specimens with bladder transitional cell carcinoma are performed, involvement of
the prostate by transitional cell carcinoma may be found in 37% to 45% of the
cases. (1,22–24). If intraductal transitional cell carcinoma is identified on TURP or
transurethral biopsy, patients usually will be recommended for radical cystoprostatectomy. The finding of intraductal transitional cell carcinoma also has been
demonstrated to increase the risk of urethral recurrence following cystoprostatectomy, such that its identification may also result in prophylactic total urethrectomy.

Intraductal transitional cell carcinoma of the prostate is usually accompanied by CIS of the prostatic urethra (22). Involvement of the prostate appears
to be by direct extension from the overlying urethra, since in the majority of
cases the more centrally located prostatic ducts are involved by transitional
cell neoplasia to a greater extent than the peripheral ducts and acini (Fig. 15.6).

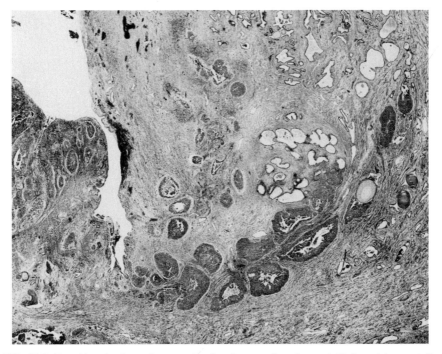

FIG. 15.6. Transitional-cell carcinoma extending from urethra *(upper left)* down into prostatic
ducts, resulting in filling and expansion of the ducts by transitional-cell carcinoma. ×13.

Intraductal transitional cell carcinoma of the prostatic ducts initially consists of malignant transitional cells insinuating themselves between the basal cell layer and the columnar to cuboidal luminal epithelium of the prostatic ducts (Fig. 15.7). More peripherally, transitional cell carcinoma spreads in a pagetoid fashion within the ducts (Fig. 15.8). Similar to that seen in the breast, large tumor cells with clear cytoplasm are seen in the midst of otherwise normal urothelium. With more extensive involvement, transitional cell carcinoma fills and expands ducts and often develops central comedonecrosis (Fig. 15.9, efig 1499;1500-1503;1504-1506;1507-1508). Intraductal transitional cell carcinoma of the prostatic ducts without prostatic stromal invasion tends to be seen in lower stage bladder transitional cell carcinomas. Once resected by cystoprostatectomy, the noninvasive involvement of the prostate by transitional cell carcinoma does not adversely effect survival; the prognosis is determined by the stage of the bladder tumor (1,2,25).

In prostates with intraductal transitional cell carcinoma and stromal invasion, the associated bladder tumors tend to be high-stage, in which case the already poor prognosis is not affected by the prostatic involvement (1). However, intraductal and infiltrating prostatic transitional cell carcinoma may also be associated with low-stage bladder tumors. The significance of prostatic

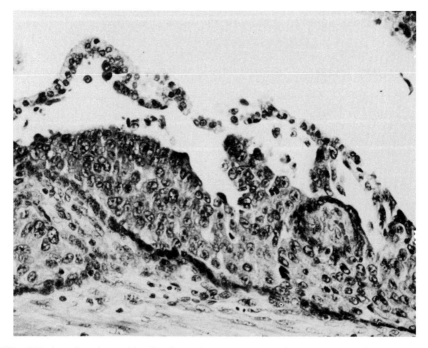

FIG. 15.7. Intraductal transitional-cell carcinoma extending beneath pale-staining cuboidal secretory prostatic epithelium. Note preserved basal cell layer.

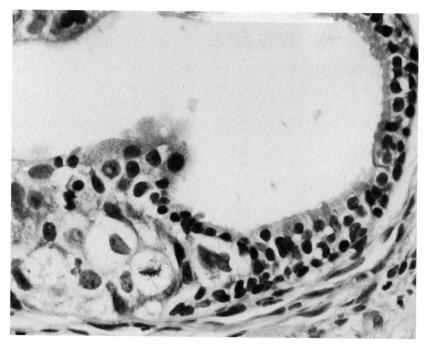

FIG. 15.8. Pagetoid spread of transitional-cell carcinoma within prostatic acini and ducts. ×540.

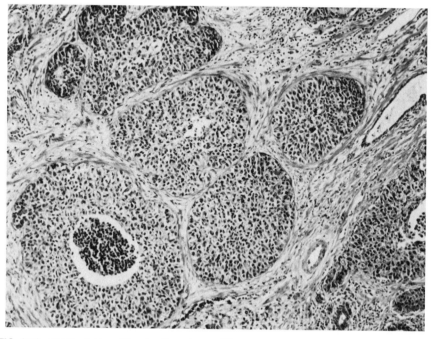

FIG. 15.9. Intraductal transitional-cell carcinoma filling up and expanding several prostatic ducts and acini with areas of central necrosis.

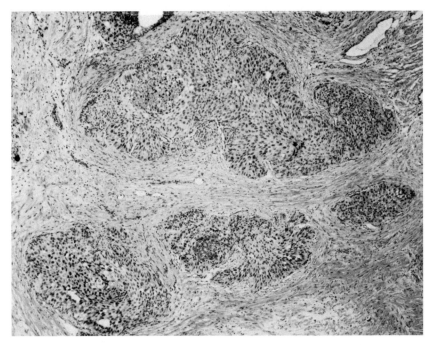

FIG. 15.10. Intraductal transitional-cell carcinoma. Note lack of desmoplastic response surrounding these nests. This is a helpful feature in excluding infiltrating transitional-cell carcinoma.

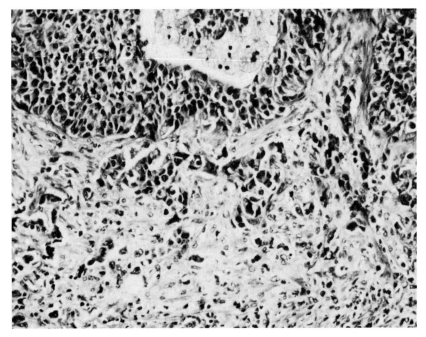

FIG. 15.11. Intraductal transitional-cell carcinoma *(top)* associated with infiltrating cords and single cells of transitional-cell carcinoma inducing the desmoplastic response.

stromal invasion in these cases is controversial, with most studies showing a worse prognosis (24,25).

The differentiation between extensive intraductal transitional cell carcinoma from intraductal and invasive transitional cell carcinoma may be difficult. With intraductal transitional cell carcinoma of the prostate, nests of transitional cell carcinoma have the contours and distribution of prostatic ducts and acini. The nests are circumscribed with a smooth discrete edge between the epithelium and the adjacent stroma, and the stroma lacks a desmoplastic response (Fig. 15.10). Infiltrating transitional cell carcinoma is characterized by small cords, nests, or individual cells eliciting a desmoplastic stromal response (Figs. 15.11–15.13, efig 1509-1511;1512-1513;1514-1515). In some instances numerous closely packed irregular large nests and small nests are diagnosable as infiltrating transitional cell carcinoma, since this architectural pattern is not consistent with intraductal growth of transitional cell carcinoma (Fig. 15.14). It is important not to overdiagnose transitional cell carcinoma involving von Brunn's nests as intraductal or invasive transitional cell carcinoma (Fig. 15.15).

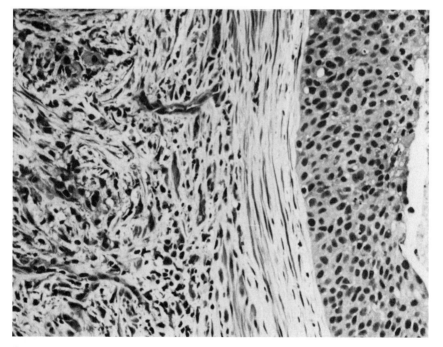

FIG. 15.12. Intraductal transitional-cell carcinoma *(right)*. Note that the stroma immediately adjacent to intraductal transitional-cell carcinoma lacks the desmoplastic response. Toward the left of the field, infiltrating transitional-cell carcinoma is associated with an inflammatory and desmoplastic stromal response.

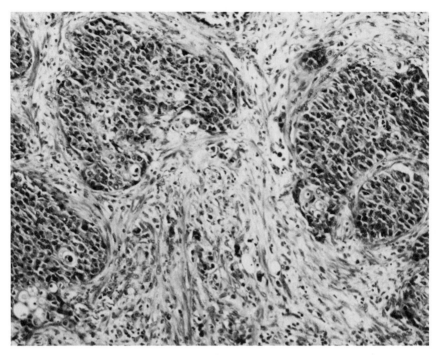

FIG. 15.13. Infiltrating nests of transitional-cell carcinoma with a desmoplastic stromal response and irregular borders in the infiltrating tumor nests. ×280.

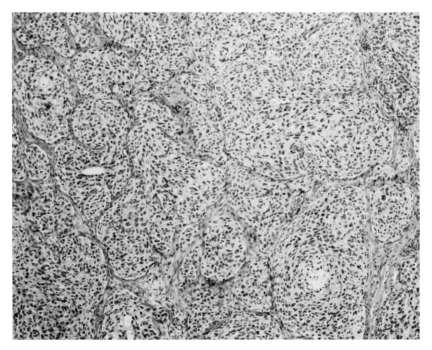

FIG. 15.14. Numerous closely packed nests of infiltrating transitional-cell carcinoma. ×75.

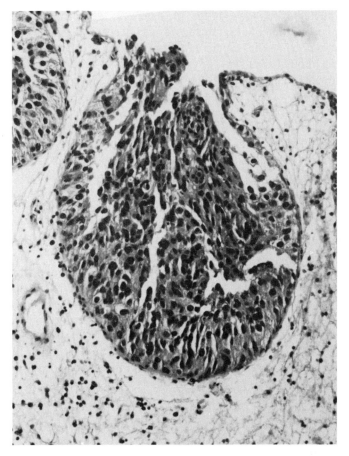

FIG. 15.15. Transitional-cell carcinoma in situ within cystitis cystica. ×205.

TRANSITIONAL CELL CARCINOMA SEEN ON NEEDLE BIOPSY

The diagnosis of urothelial carcinoma on prostate needle biopsy is especially difficult for several reasons (efig 1489-1493;1504-1506;1507-1508;1514-1515). First, urothelial carcinoma on prostate biopsy is rare, especially relative to the frequency with which adenocarcinoma of the prostate is diagnosed on needle biopsy. Secondly, we have shown that urothelial carcinoma involving the prostate clinically can mimic prostatic adenocarcinoma in terms of findings on digital rectal exam and ultrasound, along with the potential for an elevated serum PSA level (26). Thirdly, there may be no prior or concurrent history of urothelial carcinoma in the bladder (47% of our cases).

Histologic features and immunohistochemical studies are therefore essential to establish the correct diagnosis. Urothelial carcinoma involving the prostate differs from adenocarcinoma of the prostate both architecturally and cytologically. Urothelial carcinoma in the prostate typically forms nests of tumor, whereas poorly differentiated prostate cancer tends to form sheets, individual cells, or cords. Urothelial carcinoma involving the prostate in our study contained areas of necrosis in 43% of cases. Necrosis is an unusual finding in even high-grade adenocarcinoma of the prostate. The presence of an intraductal growth where preexisting benign prostate glands are filled with solid nests of tumor also differs from high-grade prostatic intraepithelial neoplasia, which is composed of flat, tufting, papillary, or cribriform patterns. The presence of squamous differentiation seen in 14% of our cases would also be unusual for adenocarcinoma of the prostate. Cytologically, transitional cell carcinomas involving the prostate tend to show greater nuclear pleomorphism, variably prominent nucleoli, and increased mitotic activity compared to even poorly differentiated prostate adenocarcinoma. In high-grade adenocarcinomas of the prostate, nuclei tend to be more uniform from one to another with centrally located prominent eosinophilic nucleoli. Mitotic figures in high-grade prostate cancer are typically not as frequent compared to what is seen in transitional cell carcinoma on biopsy. Finally, the presence of stromal inflammation, seen in 76% of our cases of transitional cell carcinoma on biopsy, differs from the typical lack of associated inflammation seen with ordinary adenocarcinoma of the prostate.

The overall prognosis of urothelial cell carcinoma diagnosed on prostatic needle biopsy is poor, even in cases without histologic evidence of stromal invasion on biopsy (26). In these cases with intraductal cancer on biopsy, most likely invasive cancer is present elsewhere in the prostate that was not sampled. Although the prognosis is poor, even with only apparent intraductal involvement, histologic recognition is essential, as the only opportunity for improved outcome is early and aggressive therapy.

PRIMARY TRANSITIONAL CELL CARCINOMA

Primary transitional cell carcinoma of the prostate without bladder involvement is a rare lesion (27–31). Primary transitional cell carcinoma of the prostate should not be called periurethral prostatic duct carcinoma, as sometimes reported in the literature, since this term may be confused with prostatic duct adenocarcinomas. Histologically, primary transitional cell carcinoma of the prostate is characterized by intraductal transitional cell carcinoma, almost always accompanied by infiltration. A continuum from transitional cell hyperplasia without atypia to atypical transitional cell hyperplasia to carcinoma in situ can also be identified (32). Rarely, transitional cell carcinoma in situ may be papillary within enlarged dilated prostatic ducts (27). Though Greene claims that one-third of the cases of primary transitional cell carcinoma of the prostate have areas of adenocarcinoma, this number is probably overstated (27). This study predated the use of immunohistochemistry for PSA and PSAP, and these cases may have been adenocarcinomas of the prostate with areas of poor differentiation, resembling transitional cell carcinoma.

Primary transitional cell carcinomas of the prostate tend to infiltrate the bladder neck and surrounding soft tissue such that over 50% of the patients present with tumors extending out of the prostate. Twenty percent of the patients present with distant metastases, bone and liver being the most common sites. In contrast to adenocarcinoma of the prostate, bone metastases are usually osteolytic. Rubenstein and Rubnitz described ten cases of urothelial cell carcinoma arising within the large periurethral prostatic ducts. These patients all died within 2 years of diagnosis, with eight (80%) dying within 1 year (30). Greene et al. reported a series of 39 patients with primary urothelial cell carcinoma of the prostate. Again, the prognosis was poor with 34 (87%) patients dying within 5 years (27). Average survival was only 17 months (27). In their review of three additional cases, Nicolaisen and Williams emphasized clinical presentation (obstructive symptoms in younger patients), an aggressive course with a propensity for local invasion, and stressed radical surgery as the only hope for survival (29).

REFERENCES

1. Schellhammer PF, Bean MA, Whitmore WF Jr. Prostatic involvement by transitional cell carcinoma: pathogenesis, patterns and prognosis. *J Urol* 1977;118:399–403.
2. Chibber PJ, McIntyre MA, Hindmarsh JR, et al. Transitional cell carcinoma involving the prostate. *Br J Urol* 1981;53:605–609.
3. Svanholm H. Evaluation of commercial immunoperoxidase kits for prostate specific antigen and prostate specific acid phosphatase. *Acta Pathol Microbiol Immunol Scand* [A] 1986;94:7–12.
4. Ellis DW, Leffers S, Davies JS, et al. Multiple immunoperoxidase markers in benign hyperplasia and adenocarcinoma of the prostate. *Am J Clin Pathol* 1984;81:279–284.
5. Ford TF, Butcher DN, Masters JRW, et al. Immunocytochemical localization of prostate-specific antigen: Specificity and application to clinical practice. *Br J Urol* 1985;57:50–55.
6. Feiner HD, Gonzales R. Carcinoma of the prostate with atypical immunohistochemical features: Clinical and histologic correlates. *Am J Surg Pathol* 1986;10:765–770.
7. Keillor JS, Aterman K. The response of poorly differentiated prostatic tumors to staining for prostate specific antigen and prostatic acid phosphatase: a comparative study. *J Urol* 1987;137:894–896.
8. Epstein JI. PSAP and PSA as immunohistochemical markers. *Urol Clin North Am* 1993; 20:757–770.
9. Genega EM, Hutchinson B, Reuter VE, et al. Immunophenotype of high grade prostatic adenocarcinoma and urothelial carcinoma. *Mod Pathol* 2000;13:1186–1191.
10. Nowels K, Kent E, Rinsho K, et al. Prostate-specific antigen and acid phosphatase-reactive cells in cystitis cystica and glandularis. *Arch Pathol Lab Med* 1988;112:734–737.
11. Pollen JJ, Dreilinger A. Immunohistochemical identification of prostatic acid phosphatase and prostate-specific antigen in female periurethral glands. *Urology* 1984;23:303–304.
12. Tepper SL, Jagirdar J, Heath D, et al. Homology between the female paraurethral (Skene's) glands and the prostate. *Arch Pathol Lab Med* 1984;108:423–425.
13. Kamoshida S, Tsutsumi Y. Extraprostatic localization of prostatic acid phosphatase and prostate-specific antigen: distribution in cloacogenic glandular epithelium and sex-dependent expression in human anal gland. *Hum Pathol* 1990;21:1108–1111.
14. Golz R, Schubert GE. Prostatic specific antigen: immunoreactivity in urachal remnants. *J Urol* 1989; 141:1480–1482.
15. Sobin LH, Hjermstad BM, Sesterhenn IA, et al. Prostatic acid phosphatase activity in carcinoid tumors. *Cancer* 1986;58:136–138.
16. Van Krieken JHM. Prostate marker immunoreactivity in salivary gland neoplasms: a rare pitfall in immunohistochemistry. *Am J Surg Pathol* 1993;17:410–414.
17. Spencer JR, Brodin AG, Ignatoff JM. Clear cell adenocarcinoma of the urethra: evidence for origin within paraurethral ducts. *J Urol* 1990;143:122–125.

18. Epstein JI, Kuhajda FP, Lieberman PH. Prostate-specific acid phosphatase immunoreactivity in ade-nocarcinomas of the urinary bladder. *Hum Pathol* 1986;17:939–942.
19. Grignon D, Ro J, Ayala A, et al. Primary adenocarcinoma of the urinary bladder. A clinicopathologic analysis of 72 cases. *Cancer* 1991;67:2165–2172.
20. Heyderman E, Brown BME, Richardson TC. Epithelial markers in prostatic, bladder, and colorectal cancer: an immunoperoxidase study of epithelial membrane antigen, carcinoembryonic antigen, and prostatic acid phosphatase. *J Clin Pathol* 1984;37:1363–1369.
21. Nadji M, Tabei SZ, Castro A, et.al. Prostatic-specific antigen: An immunohistologic marker for pro-static neoplasms. *Cancer* 1991;48:1229–1232.
22. Mahadevia PS, Koss LG, Tar IJ. Prostatic involvement in bladder cancer: prostatic mapping in 20 cystoprostatectomy specimens. *Cancer* 1986;58:2096–2102.
23. Wood DP Jr, Montie JE, Pontes JE, et al. Transitional cell carcinoma of the prostate in cystoprosta-tectomy specimens removed for bladder cancer. *J Urol* 1989;141:346–349.
24. Esrig D, Freeman JA, Elmajian DA, et al. Transitional cell carcinoma involving the prostate with a proposed staging classification for stromal invasion. *J Urol* 1996;156:1071–1076.
25. Wishnow KI, Ro JY. Importance of early treatment of transitional cell carcinoma of prostatic ducts. *Urology* 1988;32:11–12.
26. Oliai BR, Kahane H, Epstein JI. A clinicopathologic analysis of urothelial carcinomas diagnosed on prostate needle biopsy. *Am J Surg Pathol* 2001;25:794–801.
27. Greene LF, O'Dea MJ, Dockerty MB. Primary transitional cell carcinoma of the prostate. *J Urol* 1976;116:761–763.
28. Goebbels R, Amberger L, Wernert N, et al. Urothelial carcinoma of the prostate. *Appl Pathol* 1985;3: 242–254.
29. Nicolaisen GS, Williams RD. Primary transitional cell carcinoma of prostate. *Urology* 1984;24: 544–549.
30. Rubenstein AB, Rubnitz ME. Transitional cell carcinoma of the prostate. *Cancer* 1969;24:543–546.
31. Sawczuk I, Tannenbaum M, Olsson CA, et al. Primary transitional cell carcinoma of prostatic peri-urethral ducts. *Urology* 1985;25:339–343.
32. Ullmann AS, Ross OA. Hyperplasia, atypism, and carcinoma in-situ in prostatic periurethral glands. *Am J Clin Pathol* 1967;47:497–504.

16

Mesenchymal Tumors and Tumor-Like Conditions

TUMORS OF SPECIALIZED PROSTATIC STROMA

Sarcomas and related proliferative lesions of specialized prostatic stroma are rare. In a large series of 22 cases, lesions were classified into prostatic stromal proliferations of uncertain malignant potential (STUMP) and prostatic stromal sarcoma based on the degree of stromal cellularity, presence of mitotic figures, necrosis, and stromal overgrowth (1).

There are several different patterns of stromal proliferations of uncertain malignant potential, including those that resemble benign phyllodes tumor seen in the breast; these may be specifically designated "benign phyllodes tumor of the prostate" (efig 1516-1518;1519-1520). Other patterns included: (a) hypercellular stroma with scattered atypical cells associated with benign glands (Figs. 16.1–16.3, efig 1521-1523;1524-1526;1527-1528;1529-1531;1532-1534;1535-1536); (b) hypercellular stroma with minimal cytologic atypia associated with benign glands (efig 1537-1539); and (c) hypercellular stroma without atypia and without glands (efig 1540-1541;1542-1544;1545-1546)(1). Small incidentally discovered prostatic lesions with the morphology of fibroadenomas have also been described (2) (efig 1547-1548). The nature of STUMPs has been controversial. Some have considered certain STUMPs pseudosarcomatous or hyperplastic lesions, whereas others have considered them neoplastic. We believe that many STUMPs are neoplastic, based on the observations that they may diffusely infiltrate the prostate gland and extend into adjacent tissues, and often recur. Although most cases of STUMP do not behave in an aggressive fashion, occasional cases have been documented to recur rapidly after resection and some have progressed to stromal sarcoma (1,3). We also recognize and concede that STUMPs encompass a broad spectrum of lesions, a subset of which is focal, neither recurs nor progresses, and thus, could be construed as nonneoplastic. In cases diagnosed during transurethral resection of the prostate (TURP) or enucleation in which the lesion appears small and focal, it may be appropriate to use terminology such as glandular-stromal or stromal nodule with atypia. However,

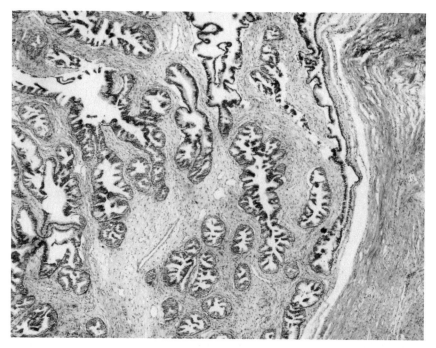

FIG. 16.1. Well-circumscribed glandular stromal nodule of benign prostatic hyperplasia with stromal atypia.

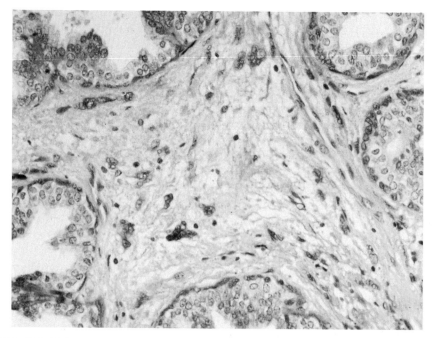

FIG. 16.2. High magnification of Fig. 16.1 showing scattered stromal cells with degenerative atypia.

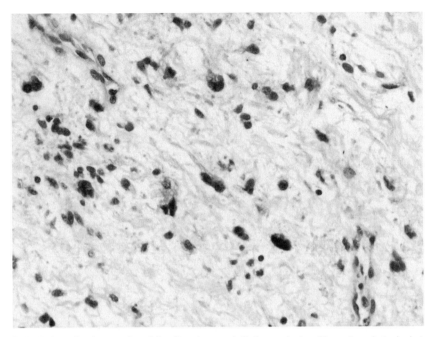

FIG. 16.3. Localized stromal nodule of benign prostatic hyperplasia with scattered atypical stromal cells. Atypical cells are scattered, lack mitotic figures, and have degenerative-appearing atypia.

when these lesions are more extensive or sampled during needle biopsy and the extent is not known, we recommend using the term "STUMP". In cases where we have seen focal STUMP on needle biopsy in a younger man, we have recommended repeat biopsy. If the repeat biopsy shows STUMP, implying that the lesion is more than an incidental finding, definitive therapy may be considered.

Stromal sarcomas may have the overall glandular growth pattern of a phyllodes tumor with obviously malignant stroma with increased cellularity, mitotic figures, and pleomorphism (Fig. 16.4, efig 1549-1552). Stromal sarcomas may also manifest as malignant hypercellular stroma surrounding normal prostate glands (efig 1553-1555). Other stromal sarcomas consist of sheets of hypercellular atypical stroma without the fascicular growth pattern of leiomyosarcomas (efig 1556-1557). The behavior of stromal sarcomas is not well understood due to their rarity, although some cases have gone on to metastasize to distant sites. Rare cases of adenocarcinoma of the prostate involving a phyllodes tumor have been identified (4) (efig 1558-1565).

The immunohistochemical results show that STUMP and stromal sarcomas both are typically positive for CD34. These results indicate that CD34 may be a useful immunohistochemical marker of prostatic stroma, STUMP, and stromal sarcomas, and may help distinguish the latter two from other prostatic mesenchymal

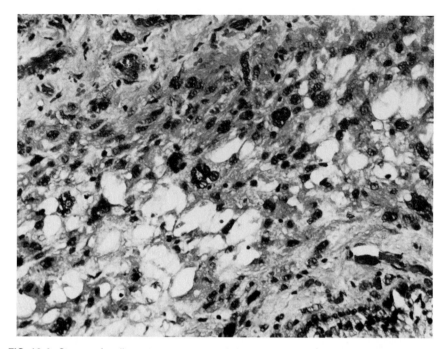

FIG. 16.4. Stroma of malignant cystosarcoma phyllodes showing marked pleomorphism. ×115.

neoplasms, such as rhabdomyosarcoma and leiomyosarcoma. Both STUMP and stromal sarcomas characteristically express progesterone receptors (PR) and uncommonly express estrogen receptors (ER). This staining pattern is consistent with previous studies that have examined the distribution of PR and ER in non-neoplastic prostatic stroma and is similar to the distribution of PR and ER in cystosarcoma phyllodes of the mammary gland (5–7). These results also support the concept that STUMP and stromal sarcomas are lesions involving hormonally responsive prostatic mesenchymal cells, the specialized prostatic stroma.

STUMPS typically react positively with desmin and actin, whereas prostatic stromal sarcomas react negatively, suggesting that the expression of muscle markers in these lesions is a function of differentiation. Importantly, prostatic stromal sarcomas appear to have an immunohistochemical profile that is distinct from leiomyosarcoma and rhabdomyosarcoma.

LEIOMYOMA

Benign soft tissue tumors of the prostate are rare, the most common being leiomyomas (8). The problem with diagnosing a leiomyoma of the prostate is that small stromal nodules with the histologic appearance of a leiomyoma may

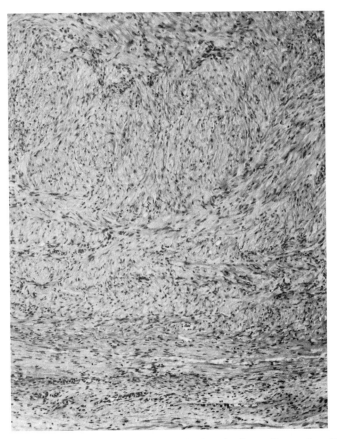

FIG. 16.5. Stromal nodule composed predominantly of smooth muscle. ×100.

often be found as incidental findings in prostates with benign prostatic hyperplasia (9) (Fig. 16.5, efig 1566-1567). These stromal nodules, though they contain abundant smooth muscle, lack the well-organized fascicles of a leiomyoma and do not have the other degenerative features commonly seen in leiomyomas such a hyalinization and calcification (Fig. 16.6). Large single leiomyomas that are symptomatic are rare.

POSTOPERATIVE SPINDLE CELL NODULE

A benign reactive spindle cell lesion, which can simulate a leiomyosarcoma, may rarely occur following recent transurethral resection (TUR) for benign prostatic hypertrophy (10,11). Histologically, these lesions appear infiltrative, replacing collagenous stroma and destroying smooth muscle. They are com-

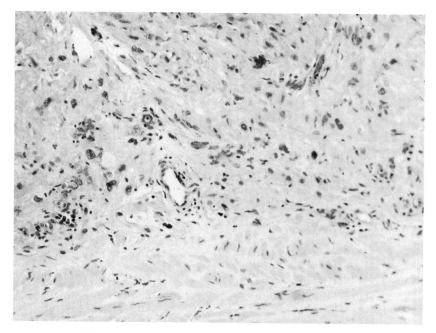

FIG. 16.6. Localized smooth-muscle nodule with degenerative atypia.

posed of intersecting fascicles of spindle cells (Fig. 16.7, efig 1568-1570;1571-1574) with a delicate network of small blood vessels. The spindle cells have abundant eosinophilic to amphophilic long tapering cytoplasm. Cells resemble reactive fibroblasts with uniform elongated nuclei containing delicate chromatin patterns and one or two distinct nucleoli. Mitotic figures may be numerous varying in cases from one to 25 per ten high power fields (Fig. 16.8). Some features seen within postoperative spindle cell nodules that favor a reactive process are the scattering of chronic inflammatory cells throughout the lesion (Fig. 16.9), and the presence of prominent dilated capillaries similar to that seen in granulation tissue (Fig. 16.10) (Table 16.1). The lesions lack significant nuclear pleomorphism and bizarre mitotic figures. Most importantly, is that these lesions are small and develop shortly after operation for benign disease, in which the lesion was not present in the initial TUR. Immunohistochemically they are positive for vimentin, desmin, and muscle-specific actin, and variably positive for cytokeratin (12). Use of immunohistochemical results to differentiate these tumors from a leiomyosarcoma are not helpful, since it has been reported that leiomyosarcoma of the prostate may show keratin immunoreactivity as well (13). Although follow-up of the patients with postoperative spindle cell nodules within the prostate are limited and some patients have been treated aggressively by radical prostatectomy, histologically similar lesions in other sites have remained free of tumor with fairly long-term follow-up after conservative therapy.

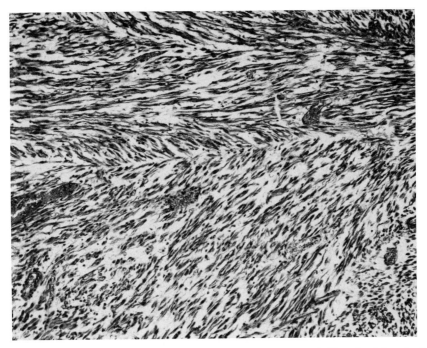

FIG. 16.7. Postoperative spindle-cell nodule of the prostate composed of long fascicles of spindle cells resembling a sarcoma. ×100.

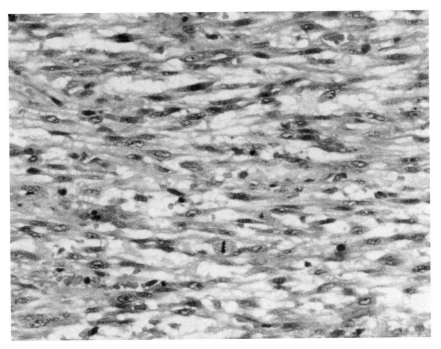

FIG. 16.8. Postoperative spindle-cell nodule with frequent mitotic figures.

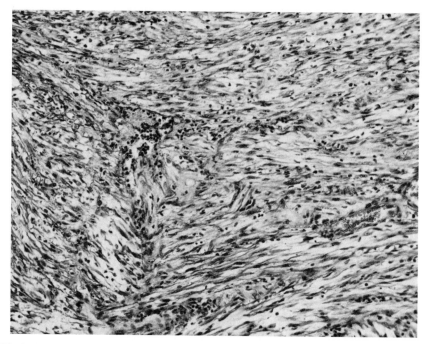

FIG. 16.9. Postoperative spindle-cell nodule of the prostate with areas showing a more inflammatory reactive appearance. ×135.

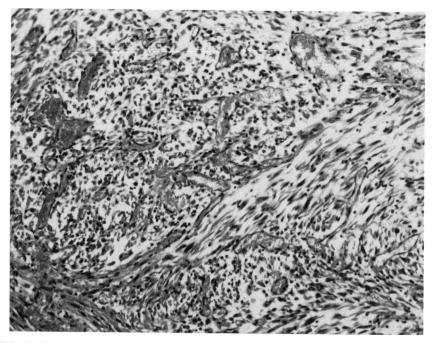

FIG. 16.10. Postoperative spindle-cell nodule of the prostate with a myxoid appearance containing numerous granulation tissue–type vessels. ×155.

TABLE 16.1. *Pseudosarcomas and sarcomas of the prostate*

Postoperative spindle cell nodule	Pseudosarcomatous fibromyxoid tumor	Leiomyosarcoma
Onset following surgery (2–15 mo, median 3 mo)	No history of prior surgery	No history of prior surgery
Usually <1.0 cm	Wide size range up to 9 cm	Typically large
Intersecting long fascicles	Haphazard growth pattern	Intersecting long fascicles
Transition to granulation tissue	Transition to granulation tissue	Not associated with granulation tissue
Uniform cytology, resembles fibroblasts	Although some pleomorphism, cells resemble reactive tissue-culture fibroblasts	Pleomorphic
Myxoid areas	Myxoid areas	Rarely myxoid
Frequent mitoses, none atypical	Usually <3 mitoses per 10 HPF, none atypical	Mitoses common, may be atypical
Prominent vascularity	Areas with increased vascularity	No increase in vascularity
Extravasated red blood cells and stromal lymphocytes	Extravasated red blood cells and stromal lymphocytes	Typically lacks inflammation and extravasated red blood cells

HPF, high-power field.

PSEUDOSARCOMATOUS FIBROMYXOID TUMORS

Another spindle cell tumor occurs in this region and arises without a prior history of surgery. Although this lesion shares many features with postoperative spindle cell nodule and the two lesions may be related, several distinct clinical and pathologic features warrant their classification as unique entities. These lesions have been reported under a multitude of names, most commonly pseudosarcomatous fibromyxoid tumor, inflammatory myofibroblastic tumor, myofibroblastoma, nodular fasciitis of bladder, pseudosarcomatous myofibroblastic proliferation, and inflammatory pseudotumor (14–17) (efig 1575-1576;1577-1578;1579-1583;1584-1590). These lesions occur within a wide age range from 2 to 73 years with a median age of 28 years. There is a two to one female predominance. Most cases have been described within the bladder with an occasional case found within the prostate. These lesions range from 1.5 to 9 cm. Histologically, these tumors resemble granulation tissue with variable cellularity. Cells are more haphazard in their distribution than postoperative spindle cell nodules. Lesions often show a densely cellular spindle cell pattern admixed with a very myxoid component (Fig. 16.11). Cells resemble those seen in nodular fasciitis with a tissue culture appearance. Occasionally, there may be prominent nucleoli with occasional moderately pleomorphic and hyperchromatic cells (Fig. 16.12). In contrast to sarcomas, these lesions have relatively few mitoses with typically at most three per ten high power fields, although we have seen a classic example of this entity with frequent mitotic figures. Atypical mitotic figures are not seen. As with postoperative spindle cell nodules, they may be deeply

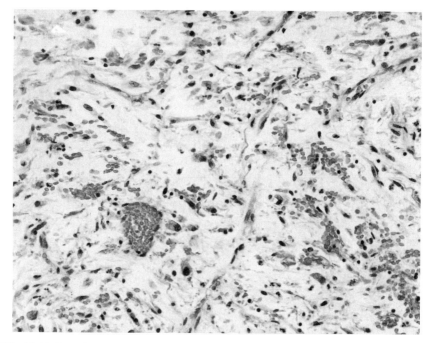

FIG. 16.11. Pseudosarcomatous fibromyxoid tumor with myxoid appearance, inflammatory cells, and disorganized spindle cells.

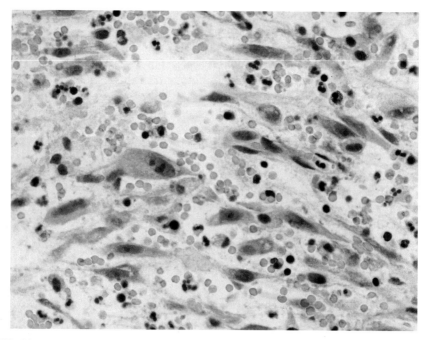

FIG. 16.12. Pseudosarcomatous fibromyxoid tumor with tissue culture–like fibroblasts, inflammatory cells, myxoid background, and scattered pleomorphic cells.

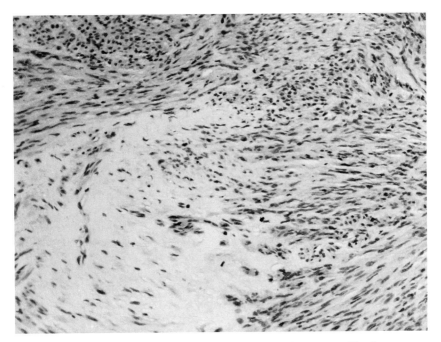

FIG. 16.13. Myxoid leiomyosarcoma on needle biopsy. While focally myxoid, other areas are more cellular (see Fig. 16.14).

invasive. Immunohistochemically, these lesions show myofibroblastic differentiation with expression of smooth muscle markers and occasional keratin positivity. In a limited sampling, this lesion may be difficult to distinguish from a sarcoma or a sarcomatoid carcinoma. Although the diagnosis of pseudosarcomatous fibromyxoid tumors can be suggested on small biopsy, additional tissue should be sampled to more definitively establish a diagnosis.

Pseudosarcomatous fibromyxoid tumors are distinguished from sarcomas and sarcomatoid carcinomas by less pleomorphism, fewer mitotic figures, and areas of the lesion resembling granulation tissue (Table 16.1). Prominent myxoid change in sarcomas arising within the prostate is also unusual (Fig. 16.13). Ultrastructural examination of sarcomatoid carcinomas and myosarcomas show epithelial and well-developed smooth muscle differentiation, respectively, neither of which are seen in pseudosarcomatous lesions.

Pseudosarcomatous fibromyxoid tumors are benign with only a rare recurrence following incomplete excision.

LEIOMYOSARCOMAS

Sarcomas of the prostate account for 0.1% to 0.2% of all malignant prostatic tumors. Leiomyosarcomas are the most common sarcomas involving the prostate in adults (13) (efig 1591-1593;1594-1595;1596-1597). The majority of patients are between 40 and 70 years of age, though in some series up to 20% of leiomyosarcomas have occurred in young adults. Leiomyosarcomas range in size between 2 cm and 24 cm with a median size of 5 cm. Following either local excision or resection of prostatic leiomyosarcomas, the clinical course tends to be characterized by multiple recurrences. Metastases, when present, are usually found in the lung. The average survival with leiomyosarcoma of the prostate is between 3 and 4 years. Histologically, leiomyosarcomas range from smooth muscle tumors showing moderate atypia to highly pleomorphic sarcomas (Fig. 16.14). As with leiomyosarcomas found elsewhere, these tumors immunohistochemically express keratin in addition to muscle markers. There have been several well circumscribed lesions with a variable amount of nuclear atypia and scattered mitotic activity which have been referred to as atypical leiomyoma of the prostate (18), giant leiomyoma of the prostate (19), or circumscribed leiomyosarcoma of the prostate (20) (efig 1598-1600). Because smooth muscle tumors of the prostate are rare, the criteria for distinguishing between leiomyosarcoma and leiomyoma with borderline features have not been elucidated. Although most "atypical leiomyomas" have shown no evidence of disease with short follow-up, a few have recurred.

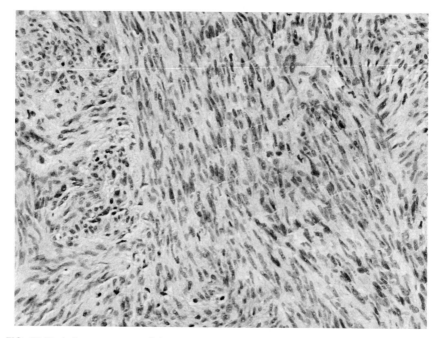

FIG. 16.14. Leiomyosarcoma of the prostate on needle biopsy (same case as shown in Fig. 16.13) with cellular fascicles typical of leiomyosarcoma.

RHABDOMYOSARCOMA

Rhabdomyosarcoma is the most frequent mesenchymal tumor within the prostate and is seen almost exclusively in childhood (21). Rhabdomyosarcomas of the prostate occur from infancy to early adulthood with an average age at diagnosis of 5 years. Most present with stage 3 disease, in which there is gross residual disease following incomplete resection or biopsy. A smaller, but significant proportion of patients present with distant metastases. Localized tumor that may be completely resected is only rarely present. Because of their large size at the time of diagnosis, distinction between rhabdomyosarcoma originating in the bladder and that originating in the prostate may be difficult. Following the development of effective chemotherapy for rhabdomyosarcomas, those few patients with localized disease (stage 1) or microscopic regional disease (stage 2) stand an excellent chance of being cured. While the majority of patients with gross residual disease (stage 3) have remained without evidence of disease for a long period of time, approximately 15% to 20% die of their tumor. The prognosis for patients with metastatic tumor (stage 4) is more dismal, with most patients dying of their tumor. The usual therapy for localized disease is to biopsy or partially excise the tumor, followed by intensive chemotherapy and radiotherapy. If tumor persists despite several courses of this therapy, then radical surgery is performed.

Histologically, most prostate rhabdomyosarcomas are of the embryonal subtype and are considered to be of favorable histology (efig 1601-1605). Embryonal rhabdomyosarcomas of the prostate are similar to those seen in other organs and may assume a wide variety of histologic patterns. Embryonal rhabdomyosarcoma cells may vary from primitive cells with scant cytoplasm to more well-differentiated tumors with abundant eosinophilic cytoplasm in which cross striations may be seen by light microscopy (Fig. 16.15). Embryonal rhabdomyosarcomas may also assume a cellular spindle cell appearance with a tendency to encircle preserved prostatic glands (Fig. 16.16) or a myxoid growth pattern (Fig. 16.17). The use of immunohistochemical, ultrastructural, and molecular techniques may be useful in the diagnosis of embryonal rhabdomyosarcoma involving the prostate. It is important to identify those rare cases of alveolar rhabdomyosarcoma involving the prostate, since this histologic subtype is unfavorable and necessitates more aggressive chemotherapy.

MISCELLANEOUS

Other rare mesenchymal lesions of the prostate are hemangioma (22), chondroma (23), cartilaginous metaplasia (24), hemangiopericytoma (25), malignant peripheral nerve sheath tumor (26), angiosarcoma (27), malignant fibrous histiocytoma (28), chondrosarcoma (29), synovial sarcoma (30), solitary fibrous tumor (efig 1606-1607) (31), and granular cell tumor (32).

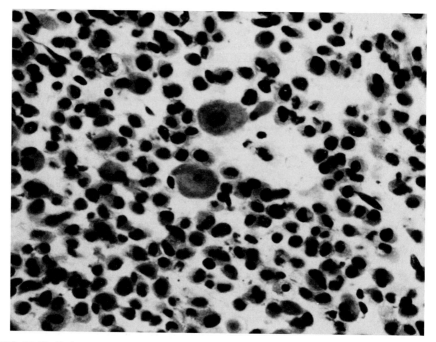

FIG. 16.15. Embryonal rhabdomyosarcoma showing a spectrum of differentiation from primitive cells with scant cytoplasm to cells with abundant eosinophilic cytoplasm that is typical of more well-differentiated rhabdomyoblasts. ×525.

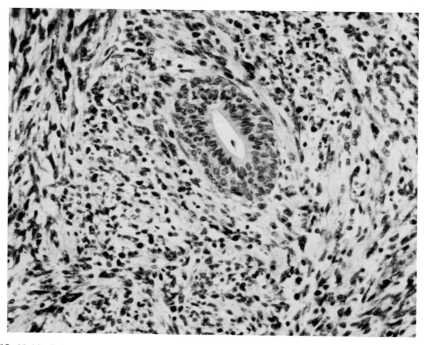

FIG. 16.16. Primitive embryonal rhabdomyosarcoma showing a spindle-cell pattern with preservation of prostatic acini. ×265.

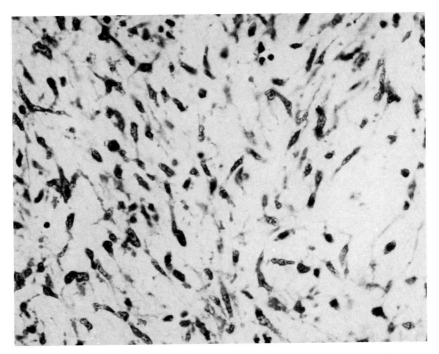

FIG. 16.17. Myxoid variant of primitive embryonal rhabdomyosarcoma. ×350.

REFERENCES

1. Gaudin PG, Rosai J, Epstein JI. Sarcomas and related proliferative lesions of specialized prostatic stroma: A clinicopathologic study of 22 cases. *Am J Surg Pathol* 1998;22:148–162.
2. Kafandaris PM, Polyzonis MB. Fibroadenoma-like foci in human prostatic nodular hyperplasia. *Prostate* 1983;4:33–36.
3. Yum M, Miller JC, Agrawal BL. Leiomyosarcoma arising in atypical fibromuscular hyperplasia (phyllodes tumor) of the prostate with distant metastases. *Cancer* 1991;68:910–915.
4. Kerley SW, Pierce P, Thomas J. Giant cystosarcoma phyllodes of the prostate associated with adenocarcinoma. *Arch Pathol Lab Med* 1992;116:195–197.
5. Brolin J, Skoog L, Ekman P. Immunohistochemistry and biochemistry in detection of androgen, progesterone, and estrogen receptors in benign and malignant human prostatic tissue. *Prostate* 1992;20:281–295.
6. Hiramatsu M, Maehara I, Orikasa S, et al. Immunolocalization of oestrogen and progesterone receptors in prostatic hyperplasia and carcinoma. *Histopathology* 1996;28:163–168.
7. Rao BR, Meyer JS, Fry CG. Most cystosarcoma phyllodes and fibroadenomas have progesterone receptor but lack estrogen receptor: stromal localization f progesterone receptor. *Cancer* 1981;47:2016–2021.
8. Michaels MM, Brown HE, Favino CJ. Leiomyoma of prostate. *Urology* 1974;3:617–620.
9. Moore RA. Benign hypertrophy of the prostate: a morphologic study. *J Urol* 1943;50:680–710.
10. Huang WL, Grignon DJ, Swanson D, et al. Postoperative spindle cell nodule of the prostate and bladder. *J Urol* 1990;143:824–826.
11. Proppe KH, Scully RE, Rosai J. Postoperative spindle cell nodules of genitourinary tract resembling sarcomas. A report of eight cases. *Am J Surg Pathol* 1984;8:101–108.
12. Wick MR, Brown BA, Young RH, et al. Spindle-cell proliferations of the urinary tract: an immunohistochemical study. *Am J Surg Pathol* 1988;12:379–389.

13. Cheville JC, Dundore PA, Nascimento AG, et al. Leiomyosarcoma of the prostate. *Cancer* 1995; 76:1422–1427.
14. Ro JY, El-Naggar AK, Amin MB, et al. Pseudosarcomatous fibromyxoid tumor of the urinary bladder and prostate: immunohistochemical, ultrastructural, and DNA flow cytometric analyses of nine cases. *Hum Pathol* 1993;24:1203–1210.
15. Saavedra JA, Manivel JC, Essenfeld H, et al. Pseudosarcomatous myofibroblastic proliferations in the urinary bladder of children. *Cancer* 1990;66:1234–1241.
16. Lamovec J, Zidar A, Trsinar B, et al. Sclerosing inflammatory pseudotumor of the urinary bladder in a child. *Am J Surg Pathol* 1992;12:1233–1238.
17. Jones ED, Clement PB, Young RH. Inflammatory pseudotumor of the urinary bladder. A clinicopathological, immunohistochemical, ultrastructural, and flow cytometric study of 13 cases. *Am J Surg Pathol* 1993;13:264–274.
18. Rosen Y, Ambiavagar PC, Vuletin JC, et al. Atypical leiomyoma of prostate. *Urology* 1980;15: 183–185.
19. Regan JB, Barrett DM, Wold LE. Giant leiomyoma of the prostate. *Arch Pathol Lab Med* 1987;111: 381–382.
20. Stenram U, Holby L. A case of circumscribed myosarcoma of the prostate. *Cancer* 1969;24:803–806.
21. Lobe TE, Wiener E, Andrassy RJ, et al. The argument for conservative, delayed surgery in the management of prostatic rhabdomyosarcoma. *J Pediatr Surg* 1997;31:1084–1087.
22. Sundarasivarao D, Banerjea S, Nageswararao A, et al. Hemangioma of the prostate: a case report. *J Urol* 1973;110:708–709.
23. Sloan SE, Rapoport JM. Prostatic chondroma. *Urology* 1985;25:319–321.
24. Bedrosian SA. Heterotopic cartilage in prostate. *Urology* 1983;1:536–537.
25. Reyes JW, Shinozuka H, Garry P, et al. A light and electron microscopy study of a hemangiopericytoma of the prostate with local extension. *Cancer* 1977;40:1122–1126.
26. Rames RA, Smith MT. Malignant peripheral nerve sheath tumor of the prostate: a rare manifestation of neurofibromatosis type 1. *J Urol* 1999;162:165–166.
27. Smith DM, Manivel C, Kappa D, et al. Angiosarcoma of the prostate: a report of 2 cases and review of the literature. *J Urol* 1986;135:382–384.
28. Chin W, Fay R, Ortega P. Malignant fibrous histiocytoma of prostate. *Urology* 1986;27:363–365.
29. Dogra PN, Aron M, Rajeev TS, et al. Primary chondrosarcoma of the prostate. *BJU Int* 1999;83: 150–151.
30. Fritsch M, Epstein JI, Perlman EJ, et al. Molecularly confirmed primary prostatic synovial sarcoma. *Hum Pathol* 2000;31:246–250.
31. Westra WH, Grenko RT, Epstein JI. Solitary fibrous tumor of the lower urogenital tract: a report of five cases involving the seminal vesicles, urinary bladder, and prostate. *Hum Pathol* 2000;31:63–68.
32. Furihata M, Sonobe H, Iwata J, et al. Granular cell tumor expressing myogenic markers in the prostate. *Pathol Int* 1996;46:298–300.

17

Miscellaneous Benign and Malignant Lesions

BENIGN LESIONS

Prostatic Cysts

Prostatic cysts may be subdivided in utricle cysts and retention cysts (1,2). Utricle cysts usually lie outside the prostate between the bladder and rectum with the orifice located at the prostatic utricle. The average age of patients with utricle cysts is 26 years. In approximately 25% of cases there may be abnormalities of the external genitalia and in 10% of cases there is unilateral renal dysgenesis or agenesis. Histologically, the cyst walls may lack an epithelial lining or be composed of columnar, cuboidal, transitional or less frequently squamous epithelium. Retention cysts arise when prostatic acini become distended with clear fluid and are lined by flattened prostatic glandular or transitional epithelium. Because small asymptomatic dilated prostatic acini are frequently seen, the term "retention cyst" should only be used for symptomatic cysts. Defined accordingly, retention cysts range in size from 1 cm to 2 cm, are usually unilocular, and are located adjacent to the urethra. In approximately 10% of cases, the cysts contain calculi. Four cases of cystadenoma and isolated cases of squamous cell carcinoma and adenocarcinoma have been reported arising in prostatic cysts (1,2).

Multilocular Cysts of the Prostate (Multilocular Prostatic Cystadenoma)

Several reports have described large multilocular cystic lesions between the bladder and the rectum (3–6). They may either be separate from the prostate or attached to the prostate by a pedicle. These masses have weighed up to 6,500 grams, ranging from 7.5 cm to 20 cm in diameter. On cross section, they are well-circumscribed and resemble nodular hyperplasia with multiple cysts, ranging from microscopic to several centimeters in diameter. Atrophic prostatic epithelium, reactive with antibodies to prostate-specific antigen (PSA) and prostate-specific acid phosphatase (PSAP), line the cysts. We have seen one case involved by high-grade prostatic intraepithelial neoplasia (PIN) (6). There also have been several reports of similar lesions within the prostate. The distinction of intraprostatic multilocular cysts from cystic nodular hyperplasia may be difficult. The diagnosis of intraprostatic cystadenoma should be restricted to cases where one-half of the prostate resembles normal prostate tissue and the remaining prostate is enlarged by a solitary encapsulated nodule composed of epithelium and/or cysts (7,8). Prostatic cystadenomas may recur if incompletely excised and may require extensive surgery because of their large size and impingement on surrounding structures.

Melanotic Lesions

Melanotic lesions of the prostate consist of cases with only stromal melanin, only glandular melanin, or both stromal and glandular melanin (9–14). The term "melanosis," if not otherwise specified, usually refers to melanin found in any location within the prostate. Blue nevus is used to describe stromal melanin deposition, and glandular melanosis denotes the presence of melanin within epithelial cells. Microscopically, blue nevi are characterized by deeply pigmented melanin-filled spindle cells within the fibromuscular stroma (Fig. 17.1,

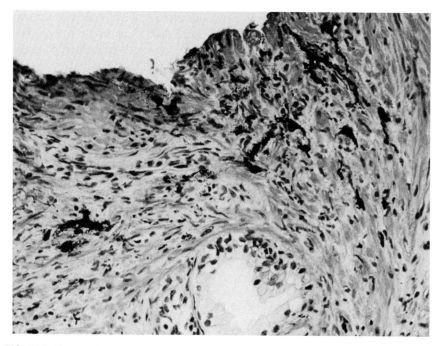

FIG. 17.1. Fontana Masson stain showing numerous dendritic, heavily pigmented melanocytes within prostatic stroma. ×320.

efig 1608). In two cases, in addition to glandular and stromal melanosis, melanin was also seen in adjacent glands of adenocarcinoma of the prostate. Nonneoplastic and neoplastic prostatic epithelial cells with melanin contain only mature melanosomes, suggesting that epithelial melanin results from a transfer of pigment from the stromal melanocytes. The incidence of microscopic focal prostatic blue nevi or glandular melanosis is about 4% each. Cases with more prominent melanosis such as those with grossly visible pigment are much less common and have only been published as isolated case reports. Melanotic lesions of the prostate are incidental findings with no evidence of malignant transformation. There has only been one report of a malignant melanoma that presented in the prostate gland (15).

Amyloid

Vascular amyloid can be identified in 2% to 10% of prostates removed for hyperplasia or carcinoma (16–19). Patients with multiple myeloma, primary amyloidosis of the kidney or chronic debilitating diseases have a higher incidence of prostatic amyloidosis. In these cases, amyloid is located in subepithelial areas as well as in vessels. Usually, amyloid within the prostate is an incidental finding, although rarely it may mimic carcinoma on rectal examination (19). Corpora amylacea often stain nonspecifically for amyloid (20).

Calculi and Calcification

Prostatic calculi are found within the tissues or acini of the gland, in contrast to urinary calculi that are found within the prostatic urethra (21,22). Prostatic calculi are present in 70% to 100% of the glands studied at autopsy, most commonly in men over 50 years of age. Generally, prostatic calculi are multiple and small with an average diameter of less than 5 mm. Histologically, calculi are composed of concentric layers resembling calcified corpora amylacea. They form by the consolidation and calcification of corpora amylacea or by calcification of precipitated prostatic secretions. Although prostatic calculi are common they are usually asymptomatic and are discovered incidentally. Abscesses may occur in patients who have urinary tract infections resistant to antimicrobial therapy in which the prostatic calculi are infected and provide a continual source of infection. Prostatic calculi are also significant in that they may be confused on rectal examination with carcinoma of the prostate.

Basal cell hyperplasia is the most common lesion containing laminated calcifications resembling psammoma bodies (Color Plate 29). This finding may be a diagnostic aid, since only rarely do carcinomas contain laminated calcifications. Calcifications within prostate cancers tend to be small stippled granular calcifications in areas of central necrosis, most commonly seen in high-grade carcinomas and ductal adenocarcinomas.

Infarcts

In between 20% to 25% of specimens removed for benign prostatic hypertrophy, prostatic infarcts ranging in size from a few millimeters to 5 cm may be found (23–26). Patients with acute prostatic infarcts have prostate glands that are twice as large as those without infarcts. Also, patients with infarcts are more prone to acute urinary retention and gross hematuria than those without infarcts. These symptoms, however, may not be due to the infarcts but rather may be due to the larger size of the gland containing them, since the infarcts are often small and not close to the urethra. Acute prostatic infarcts are discrete lesions with a characteristic histologic zonation (efig 1609-1611;1612-1613;1614-1615;1616-1621;1622-1623;1624-1626;1627-1628;1629-1630;1631-1632). The center of the infarct is characterized by acute coagulative necrosis and some recent hemorrhage. Immediately adjacent to the infarcted tissue, reactive epithelial nests with prominent nucleoli, some pleomorphism and even atypical mitotic figures can be seen (Fig. 17.2). Progressing away from the center of the infarct, more mature squamous metaplasia is seen (26) (Fig. 17.3). Another finding seen within prostatic infarcts are squamous islands with central cystic formation containing cellular debris. Remote infarcts may also be recognized by finding local areas of densely fibrotic stroma admixed with small glands containing immature

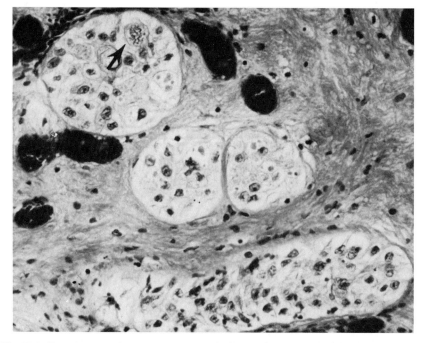

FIG. 17.2. Reactive squamous epithelium immediately adjacent to prostatic infarct showing some nuclear atypia and mitotic activity *(arrow).* ×275.

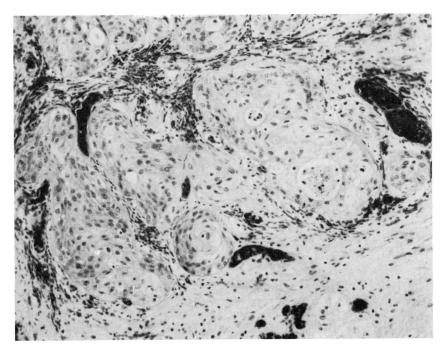

FIG. 17.3. Squamous metaplasia adjacent to recent prostatic infarct. ×145.

squamous metaplasia (efig 1633-1634). Prostatic infarcts may rarely be sampled on needle biopsy, where it may be more difficult to appreciate the zonation (26). If the infarct is not recognized, the reactive squamous metaplasia cases may be misdiagnosed as transitional cell carcinoma.

Miscellaneous

In a study of prostates from a medical examiner's office, 9% of prostates contained sperm (efig 1635-1636)(27). Rare cases of prostatic endometriosis, hair glanuloma, and lymphagiolipomatosis have been diagnosed (28–30). Vasculitis involving the prostate may occur, including polyarteritis nodosa, Wegener's granulomatosis, and giant cell arteritis (31–33) (efig 1637-1638). Extramedullary hematopoiesis, ganglioneuroma, and ectopic salivary gland tissue have been described in the prostate (34–36). A form of metaplasia has been designated "paneth cell-like metaplasia" or "paneth cell-like change" (37–39). Histologically, it is characterized by bright eosinophilic granules filling the apical cytoplasm, identical to neuroendocrine differentiation (see Color Plate 38). Electron microscopy reveals electron-dense variably-sized lysosome-like or exocrine-like granules, and the cells do not react with antibodies

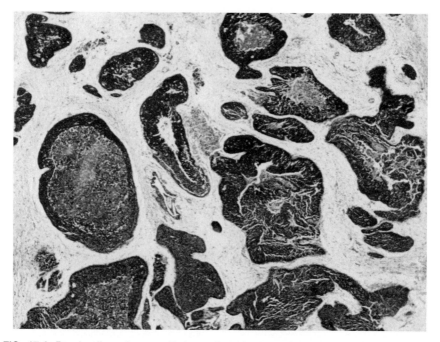

FIG. 17.4. Basal cell carcinoma with large, irregular basaloid nests and extensive central comedo-like necrosis. ×45. (Courtesy of Dr. V. Reuter, New York, NY.)

to neuroendocrine markers. Some authorities question whether paneth cell-like change is distinct from neuroendocrine differentiation (40). Another form of cytoplasmic change that occasionally occurs is eosinophilic metaplasia (efig 1639-1640).

Rarely, the ejaculatory duct may be a site of pathology. Cases of an adenofibroma and an adenomatoid tumor involving this structure have been reported (41,42). Amyloidosis, which involves the seminal vesicles in about 10% of radical prostatectomy specimens, can also extend into the ejaculatory duct (efigs 1641-1643)(43).

MALIGNANT LESIONS

Basaloid Carcinomas

At the other end of the spectrum of basal cell hyperplasia (Chapter 7) of the prostate is basaloid carcinoma (44–46). The histologic variability of basaloid carcinomas of the prostate is greater than that of basal cell hyperplasia. They may resemble basal cell carcinomas of the skin with large basaloid nests,

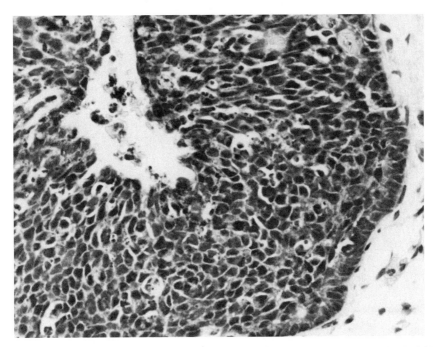

FIG. 17.5. Higher magnification of basal cell carcinoma with basaloid nests containing individual cell necrosis and peripheral palisading of the basal cell layer. ×480.

peripheral palisading, and necrosis (Figs. 17.4 and 17.5, efig 1644-1646). Other basaloid carcinomas resemble the adenoid basal cell pattern of basal cell hyperplasia, and have been referred to by some as adenoid cystic carcinoma of the prostate (Fig. 17.6, efig 1647-1650;1651-1653;1654-1656;1657-1659). Diagnostic criteria for malignancy in lesions resembling the adenoid basal form of basal cell hyperplasia are either: (a) extensive infiltration in between normal prostate glands (Fig. 17.7); (b) extension out of the prostate (Fig. 17.8); (c) perineural invasion; or (d) necrosis. The presence of a dense stromal response is more likely to be associated with basaloid carcinoma, as compared to the adenoid basal cell pattern of basal cell hyperplasia (Fig. 17.9, efig 1660-1662). Finally, there are isolated examples of basaloid carcinomas that appear identical to the ordinary glandular pattern of basal cell hyperplasia, yet are recognizably malignant because of infiltration out of the prostate (Fig. 17.10, efig 1663-1664;1665-1666;1667-1669). The natural history of basaloid carcinomas is not well known, since most cases have been reported with short follow-up. Despite periprostatic extension, distant metastases from basaloid carcinomas of the prostate have not yet been reported. The distinction between basaloid carcinomas of the prostate and basal cell hyperplasia

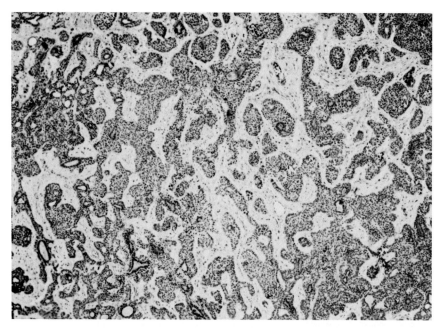

FIG. 17.6. Basal cell carcinoma resembling adenoid basal form of basal cell hyperplasia. Note extensive nature of the lesion as well as desmoplastic response of the stroma to the tumor. ×55.

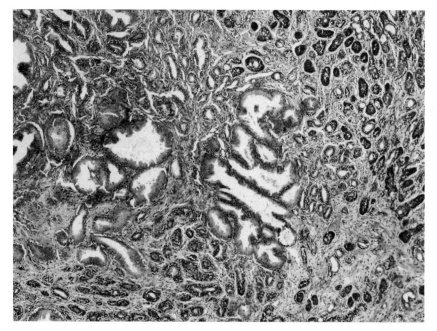

FIG. 17.7. Basaloid carcinoma with widespread infiltration between benign glands.

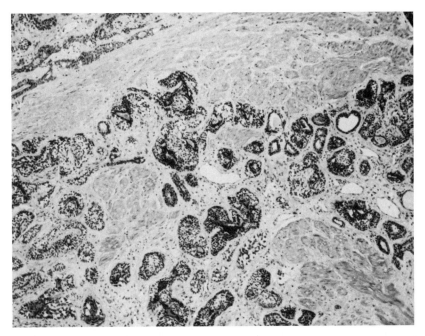

FIG. 17.8. Basal cell carcinoma infiltrating in and among smooth-muscle bundles of bladder neck. ×85.

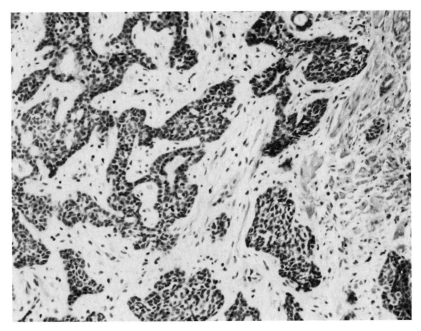

FIG. 17.9. Higher magnification of basal cell carcinoma showing desmoplastic response induced by tumor. Compare with normal prostatic stroma *(upper right corner).* ×140.

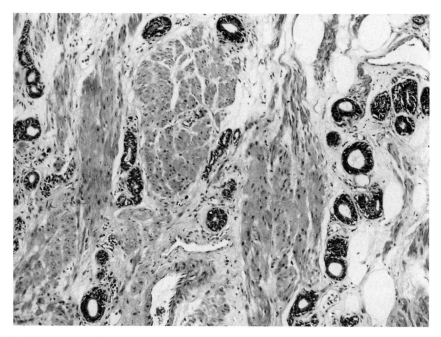

FIG. 17.10. Basal cell carcinoma (same case as shown in Fig. 17.7). Despite the benign histology, the glands infiltrated out of the prostate into periprostatic adipose tissue and thick smooth-muscle bundles of bladder neck. (From Epstein JI, Armas OA. Atypical basal cell hyperplasia of the prostate. *Am J Surg Pathol* 1992;16:1205-1214, with permission.)

must be performed by light microscopy since both lesions demonstrate a basal cell immunophenotype with antibodies to high molecular weight cytokeratin. Using immunohistochemistry for BCL-2 and KI-67 may aid in their distinction (46).

Carcinomas with Squamous Differentiation

Pure squamous cell carcinomas develop osteolytic metastases, do not respond to estrogen therapy, and do not develop elevated serum acid phosphatase levels with metastatic disease (47) (Fig. 17.11). In two cases studied, men had normal serum PSA levels. Primary prostatic squamous cell carcinomas must be distinguished on clinical grounds from secondary involvement of the gland by bladder or urethral squamous carcinomas. Squamous cell carcinoma of the prostate must also be differentiated from squamous metaplasia adjacent to a prostatic infarct (see earlier in Chapter 17). Primary prostatic squamous cell carcinomas have a poor prognosis, with radical cystoprostatectomy as the only chance of cure. Adenosquamous carcinomas may also be seen in the prostate with and without a prior history of endocrine therapy (efig 1670-1671;1672-1674;1675-1677) (48).

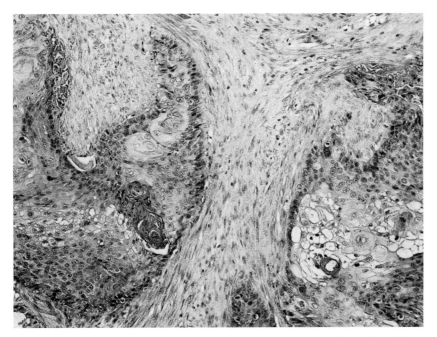

FIG. 17.11. Squamous cell carcinoma of the prostate. ×155. (Courtesy of Dr. I. Ansell, Nottingham, England.)

Carcinosarcoma

Carcinosarcomas of the prostate are rare with only a few series reported (49,50) (efig 1678-1680;1681-1683). The epithelial component of carcinosarcoma is either moderately or poorly differentiated adenocarcinoma. The spindle cell component commonly is undifferentiated, or shows chondroid or osteoid differentiation (Fig. 17.12). Less commonly, the spindle component has differentiated towards rhabdomyosarcoma, leiomyosarcoma, or angiosarcoma. Typically, the spindle component is negative for PSA and PSAP, although it may react with antibodies to keratin (51). Electron microscopy of the sarcomatoid areas in several cases revealed desmosomes. Some authors restrict the term "carcinosarcoma" for tumors with specific mesenchymal differentiation (i.e., cartilage or osteoid), and designate tumors with only a nonspecific spindle cell pattern as "metaplastic carcinomas." Given the similar prognosis between the two entities and the finding of epithelial differentiation in the spindle component of some "carcinosarcomas," we prefer to consider these lesions as one entity. A more appropriate term for all these neoplasms might be "prostatic carcinomas with spindle cell differentiation."

In most cases, patients present with adenocarcinoma. The sarcomatous component develops a mean of 33.5 months later. Although some patients have

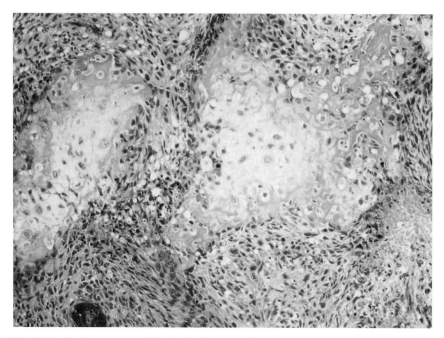

FIG. 17.12. Carcinosarcoma with chondroid areas. Other areas showed glandular differentiation.

developed the sarcomatous component after hormone or radiation therapy, others have arisen without these treatments. Carcinosarcomas have a dismal prognosis. Metastatic lesions may be purely glandular, mixed carcinosarcomatous, or purely sarcomatous.

Hematopoietic Tumors

Lymphomas of the prostate typically present in older men with urinary obstructive symptoms, urinary tract infections, or hematuria. Systemic symptoms are unusual. Primary prostatic lymphoma without lymph node involvement appears to be much less common than secondary infiltration of the prostate (52). Most reported lymphomas have been of the large cell and small cleaved cell types with a diffuse pattern (Fig. 17.13, efig 1684-1686;1687-1690;1691-1694). Poorly differentiated carcinomas can also mimic large cell lymphomas (efig 1695-1697). Lymphomas with a nodular pattern involving the prostate are seen infrequently (efig 1698-1699). The entire spectrum of malignant lymphomas seen in other sites may become manifest in the prostate. These include undifferentiated lymphomas, angiotropic lymphoma, Hodgkin's disease, myeloma, and T-cell lymphomas, as well as a case of pseudolymphoma (efig 1700-1703;1704-1705) (52–57). Malignant lymphoma involving the prostate is associated with a

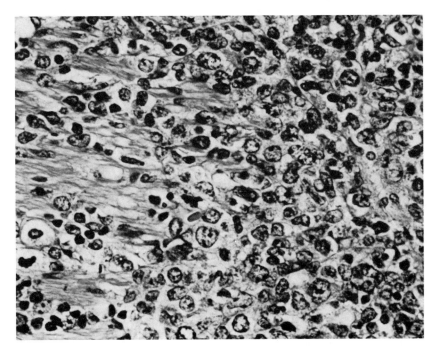

FIG. 17.13. Large cell lymphoma infiltrating prostatic stroma. ×320.

poor prognosis regardless of patient age, stage of presentation, histologic classification, or treatment regimen. The poor prognosis of prostatic lymphoma is related to the generalized disease that eventually results rather than to the prostatic involvement. The distinction between large cell lymphoma and poorly differentiated prostatic adenocarcinoma can readily be accomplished immunohistochemically with antibodies to PSA, PSAP, and lymphoid markers.

The most common form of leukemic involvement of the prostate is that of chronic lymphocytic leukemia (58) (efig 1706-1707). We have seen several cases where the patient was not known to be leukemic. Upon examination of tissue removed for presumed benign prostatic hyperplasia (BPH), there was a dense infiltrate of small mature round lymphocytes extensively infiltrating the prostatic stroma with preservation of prostatic glands (Figs. 17.14 and 17.15). These lesions differed from chronic prostatitis, where the inflammation tends to remain periglandular, is less dense, and often contains an admixture of plasma cells (Fig. 17.16). After raising the possibility of a leukemic infiltrate within the prostate, these patients, upon subsequent workup were demonstrated to have chronic lymphocytic leukemia. Most patients, however, with leukemic involvement of the prostate are known leukemics or have their diagnosis established at the time of workup for urinary symptoms. It is often unclear whether the prostatic leukemic infiltrate in chronic lymphocytic leukemia is an incidental finding

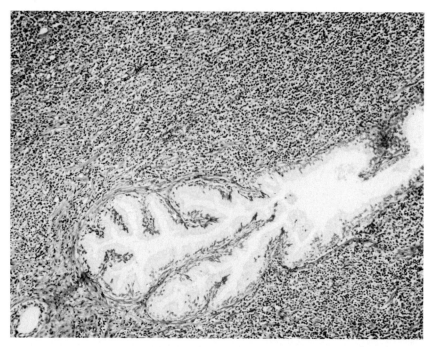

FIG. 17.14. Chronic lymphocytic leukemia infiltrating prostate with preservation of prostatic glands. ×90.

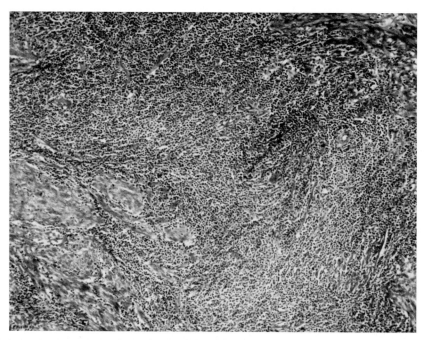

FIG. 17.15. Dense stromal infiltrate of small, mature, round lymphocytes seen with involvement of the prostate by chronic lymphocytic leukemia. ×90.

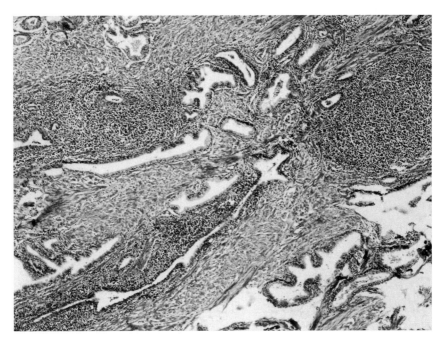

FIG. 17.16. Prostate with periglandular chronic inflammation.

in patients with BPH or the cause of their obstructive symptoms. Other forms of leukemia that have been described in the prostate include monocytic, granulocytic, and lymphoblastic leukemias.

Miscellaneous Primary Tumors

Other malignant tumors of the prostate include reports of a malignant mixed tumor resembling that seen in the salivary gland (59), endodermal sinus tumor (yolk sac tumor) (60), malignant mixed germ cell tumor (61), rhabdoid tumor (62), seminoma (63), papillary cystadenocarcinoma (64), tubulocystic clear cell adenocarcinoma as seen in the female genital tract (65), and ectomesenchymoma with rhabdomyosarcoma and ganglioneuroma (66). Prostate adenocarcinomas have also been described with lymphoepithelioma-like (67) and oncocytic features (68).

Involvement of the Prostate by Secondary Tumors

The most common tumor to secondarily infiltrate the prostate is transitional cell carcinoma of the bladder. Colorectal adenocarcinomas may also directly invade the prostate. Usually colorectal adenocarcinomas that invade the prostate are not occult. Adenocarcinoma of the rectum infiltrating the prostate may

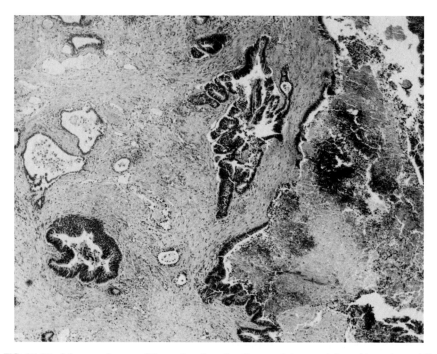

FIG. 17.17. Adenocarcinoma of the rectum invading the prostate, consisting of large basophilic glands with central extensive necrosis. ×55

resemble one of the patterns of prostatic duct adenocarcinomas (Fig. 17.17, efig 1708-1710) (see Chapter 11). Excluding hematopoietic neoplasms, the prostate is rarely involved by metastatic tumor. Metastases from malignant melanoma and carcinoma of the lung predominate (69).

REFERENCES

1. Magri J. Cysts of the prostate gland. *Br J Urol* 1960;32:295–301.
2. Schuhrke TD, Kaplan GW. Prostatic utricle cysts (müllerian duct cysts). *J Urol* 1978;119:765–767.
3. Lin DJ, Hayden RT, Murad T, et al. Multilocular prostatic cystadenoma presenting as a large complex pelvic cystic mass. *J Urol* 1993;139:856–859.
4. Yasukawa S, Aoshi H, Pakamatsu M. Ectopic adenoma in retrovesicle space. *J Urol* 1987;37: 998–999.
5. Maluf HM, King ME, DeLuca FR, et al. Giant multilocular prostatic cystadenoma: a distinctive lesion of the retroperitoneum in men. A report of 2 cases. *Am J Surg Pathol* 1991;15:131–135.
6. Allen EA, Brinker DA, Coppola D, et al. Multilocular prostatic cystadenoma with focal high-grade prostatic intraepithelial neoplasia: a case report and review of the literature. *Hum Pathol* (in press).
7. Kirkland JL, Bale PM. A cystic adenoma of the prostate. *J Urol* 1967;97:324–327.
8. Melen DR. Multilocular cysts of the prostate. *J Urol* 1932;27:343–349.
9. Aguilar M, Gaffney EF, Finnerty DP. Prostatic melanosis with involvement of benign and malignant epithelium. *J Urol* 1982;128:825–827.
10. Botticelli AR, DiGregorio C, Losi L, et al. Melanosis (pigmented melanocytosis) of the prostate gland. *Eur Urol* 1989;16:229–232.

11. Jao W, Fretzin DF, Christ NL, et al. Blue nevus of the prostate gland. *Arch Pathol* 1971;91:187–191.
12. Ro JY, Grignon DJ, Ayala AG, et al. Blue nevus and melanosis of the prostate. Electron-microscopic and immunohistochemical studies. *Am J Clin Pathol* 1988;90:530–535.
13. Ryan J, Crow J. Melanin in the prostate gland. *Br J Urol* 1988;61:455–456.
14. Martinez MCJ, Garcia GR, Castaneda CAL. Blue nevus of the prostate: report of two new cases with immunohistochemical and electron microscopic studies. *Eur Urol* 1992;22:339–342.
15. Berry NE, Reese L. Malignant melanoma which had its first clinical manifestations in the prostate gland. *J Urol* 1953; 69:286–290.
16. Mattocks MS, Molyneux AJ, Doyle P. Localised amyloidosis of the prostate. *Br J Urol* 19993; 72: 655–656.
17. Lupovitch A. The prostate and amyloidosis. *J Urol* 1972;108:301–302.
18. Wilson SK, Buchanan RD, Stone WJ, et al. Amyloid deposition in the prostate. *J Urol* 1973;110: 322–323.
19. Carris CK, McLaughlin AP III, Gittes RF. Amyloidosis of the lower genitourinary tract. *J Urol* 1976; 115:423–426.
20. Cross PA, Bartley CJ, McClure J. Amyloid in prostatic corpora amylacea. *J Clin Pathol* 1992;45: 894–897.
21. Hassler O. Calcifications in the prostate gland and adjacent tissues: A combined biophysical and histologic study. *Pathol Microbiol (Basel)* 1968;31:97–107.
22. Drach GW. Urinary lithiasis: etiology, diagnosis and medical management, In: Walsh PC, Retik AB, Stamey TA, Baugham ED Jr, eds. *Campbell's Urology*. 6th ed. Philadelphia, Pa: WB Saunders; 1992: 2142–2144.
23. Moore RA. Benign hypertrophy of the prostate: a morphologic study. *J Urol* 1943;50:680–710.
24. Baird HH, McKay HW, Kimmelstiel P. Ischemic infarction of the prostate gland. *South Med J* 1950;43:234–240.
25. Mostofi FK, Morse WH. Epithelial metaplasia in "prostatic infarction." *Arch Pathol* 1951;51: 340–345.
26. Milord RA, Kahane H, Epstein JI. Infarct of the prostate gland: experience on needle biopsy specimens. *Am J Surg Pathol* 2000;24:1378–1384.
27. Nelson G, Delberson DE, Gardner WA, Jr. Intraprostatic spermatozoa. *Hum Pathol* 1988;19: 541–544.
28. Beckman EN, Leonard GL, Pintado SO, et al. Endometriosis of the prostate. *Am J Surg Pathol* 1985; 9:374–379.
29. Day DS, Carpenter HD, Allsbrook WC Jr. Hair granuloma of the prostate. *Hum Pathol* 1996;27: 196–197.
30. Blitz BF, Kramer CE. Lymphangiolipomatosis: a new pathological entity. *J Urol* 1997;157: 1364–1365.
31. Lopez-Beltran A. Vasculitis involving the prostate: report of two cases. *Pathol Case Rev* 1996;1: 70–73.
32. Khattak, Nair M, Haqqani MT, et al. Wegener's granulomatosis: prostatic involvement and recurrent urinary tract infections. *BJU Int.* 1999;84:531–532.
33. Bretal-Laranga M, Insua-Vilarino S, Blanco-Rodriguez J, et al. Giant cell arteritis limited to the prostate. *J Rheumatol* 1995;22:566–568.
34. Humphrey PA, Vollmer RT. Extramedullary hematopoiesis in the prostate. *Am J Surg Pathol* 1991; 15:486–490.
35. Dickman SH, Toker C. Seromucinous gland ectopia within the prostatic stroma. *J Urol* 1973;109: 852–854.
36. Nassiri M, Ghazi C, Stivers JR, et al. Ganglioneuroma of the prostate: a novel finding in neurofibromatosis. *Arch Pathol Lab Med* 1994;118:938–939.
37. Frydman CP, Bleiweiss IJ, Unger PD, et al. Paneth cell-like metaplasia of the prostate gland. *Arch Pathol Lab Med* 1992;116:274–276.
38. Weaver MG, Abdul-Karim FW, Srigley J, et al. Paneth cell-like changes of the prostate gland: a histological, immunohistochemical, and electron microscopic study. *Am J Surg Pathol* 1992;16:62–68.
39. Weaver MG, Abdul-Karim FW. Paneth cell-like change of the prostate. *Arch Pathol Lab Med* 1992; 116:1101–1102.
40. Adlakha H, Bostwick DG. Paneth cell-like change in prostatic adenocarcinoma represents neuroendocrine differentiation: report of 30 cases. *Hum Pathol* 1994;25:135–139.
41. Mai KT, Walley VM. Adenofibroma of the ejaculatory duct. *J Urol Path* 1994;2:301–305.
42. Fan K, Johnson DF. Adenomatoid tumor of the ejaculatory duct. *Urology* 1985;653–654.

43. Coyne JD, Kealy WF. Seminal vesicle amyloidosis: morphological, histochemical, and immunohistochemical observations. *Histopathology* 1993;22:173–176.
44. Denholm SW, Webb JN, Howard GCW, et.al. Basaloid carcinoma of the prostate gland: histogenesis and review of the literature. *Histopathology* 1992;20:151–155.
45. Frankel K, Craig JR. Adenoid cystic carcinoma of the prostate. *Am J Clin Pathol* 1974;62:639–645.
46. Yang XJ, McEntee M, Epstein JI. Distinction of basaloid carcinoma of the prostate from benign basal cell lesions by using immunohistochemistry for BCL-2 and KI-67. *Hum Pathol* 1998;29:1447–1450.
47. Little NA, Wiener JS, Walther PJ, et al. Squamous cell carcinoma of the prostate: 2 cases of a rare malignancy and review of the literature. *J Urol* 1993;149:137–139.
48. Bassler TJ Jr, Orozco R, Bassler IC, et al. Adenosquamous carcinoma of the prostate: case report with DNA analysis, immunohistochemistry, and literature review. *Urology* 1999; 53: 832–834.
49. Lauwers GY, Schevchuk M, Armenakas N, et al. Carcinosarcoma of the prostate. *Am J Surg Pathol* 1993;17:342–349.
50. Dundore PA, Nascimento AG, Cheville JC, et al. Carcinosarcoma of the prostate: report of 22 cases. *Cancer* 1995;76:1035–1042.
51. Shannnon RL, Grignon J, Ro JY, et al. Sarcomatoid carcinoma of the prostate: a clinicopathologic study of 12 patients. *Cancer* 1992;69:2676–2682.
52. Bostwick DG, Mann RB. Malignant lymphoma involving the prostate. A study of 13 cases. *Cancer* 1985;56:2932–2938.
53. Quien ET, Wallach B, Sandhaus L, et al. Primary extramedullary leukemia of the prostate: case report and review of the literature. *Am J Hematol* 1996;53:267–271.
54. Hollenberg GM. Extraosseous myeloma simulating primary prostatic neoplasm. *J Urol* 1978;119: 292–294.
55. Klotz LH, Herr HW. Hodgkin's disease of the prostate: a detailed case report. *J Urol* 1986;135: 1261–1262.
56. Peison B, Benisch B, Nicora B, et al. Acute urinary obstruction secondary to pseudolymphoma of prostate. *Urology* 1977;10:478–479.
57. Tomaru U, Ishikura H, Kon S, et al. Primary lymphoma of the prostate with features of low grade B-cell lymphoma of mucosa associated lymphoid tissue: a rare cause of urinary obstruction. *J Urol* 1999;162:496–497.
58. Dajani YF, Burke M. Leukemic infiltration of the prostate: a case study and clinicopathologic review. *Cancer* 1976;38:2442–2446.
59. Manrique JJ, Albores Saavedra J, Orantes A, et al. Malignant mixed tumor of the salivary gland type, primary in the prostate. *Am J Clin Pathol* 1978;70:932–937.
60. Tay HP, Bidair M, Gilbaugh JH 3rd, et al. Primary yolk sac tumor of the prostate in a patient with Klinefelter's syndrome. *J Urol* 1995;153:1066–1069.
61. Michel F, Gattegno B, Roland J, et al. Primary non-seminomatous germ cell tumor of the prostate. *J Urol* 1986;135:597–599.
62. Ekfors TO, Aho HJ, Kekomaki M. Malignant rhabdoid tumor of the prostate region: immunohistological and ultrastructural evidence for epithelial origin. *Virchows Arch A Pathol Anat Histopathol* 985;406:381–388.
63. Hayman R, Patel A, Fisher C, et al. Primary seminoma of the prostate. *Br J Urol* 1995;76:273–274.
64. Kojima K, Uehara H, Naruo S, et al. Papillary cystadenocarcinoma of the prostate. *Int J Urol* 1996;3: 511–513.
65. Pan CC, Chiang H, Chang YH, et al. Tubulocystic clear cell adenocarcinoma arising within the prostate. *Am J Surg Pathol* 2000;24:1433–1436.
66. Govender D, Hadley GP. Ectomesenchymoma of the prostate: histological diagnostic criteria. *Pediatr Surg Int* 1999;l5:68–70.
67. Bostwick DG, Adlakha K. Lymphoepithelioma-like carcinoma of the prostate. *J Urol Path* 1994;2: 319–325.
68. Pinto JA, Gonzalez JE, Granadillo MA. Primary carcinoma of the prostate with diffuse oncocytic changes. *Histopathology* 1994;25:286–288.
69. Johnson DE, Chalbaud R, Ayala AG. Secondary tumors of the prostate. *J Urol* 1974;112:507–508.

18

Prostatic Urethral Lesions

PROSTATIC URETHRAL POLYPS

Prostatic urethral polyps are usually single, polypoid lesions growing into the prostatic urethra in and around the verumontanum (1,2). These lesions typically present with gross and microscopic hematuria and frequently hemospermia, dysuria, and frequency. The lesions may occur over a wide age range, from adolescent to elderly males, with conflicting reports as to the most commonly involved age group. Several of these lesions have also been described within the bladder, usually around the trigone. Histologically, the submucosal component of the urethral polyps is composed of stroma and prostatic glands (Figs. 18.1 and 18.2, efig 1711-1712;1713). The glands may be closely packed and in some areas they may be cystically dilated at the periphery. The surface of urethral polyps is often papillary with broad papillae lined by transitional cells, prostatic epithelial cells, or a combination of both. Rarely, these polyps have broad finger-like villous projections lined by benign prostatic epithelium (efig 1714-1716). Prostatic urethral polyps are totally benign. Cases that have been reported as villous polyps of the urethra represent papillary prostatic duct adenocarcinomas (3). In lesions reported as villous polyps, the glandular epithelium resembles the cells in colonic villous adenomas. In contrast, the cells lining prostatic urethral polyps are indistinguishable from normal prostatic glandular epithelium (Fig. 18.3). Various proposals for the etiology of urethral polyps include: (a) acquired lesions following instrumentation (2); (b) persistent evagination of glandular epithelium which normally evaginates to form the prostate during embryonic development (1,4); (c) development from the subcervical glands of Albarran (5); (d) postpubertal hyperplasia due to hormonal stimulation (6); (e) extrinsic hyperplasia of the prostate (7); and (f) prolapse of the prostatic ducts in the posterior urethra (8).

MISCELLANEOUS URETHRAL POLYPS

A rare type of prostatic polyp arising in the prostatic urethra is fibroepithelial polyp (efig 1717-1720;1721-1722)(9). They are found at all ages, from the

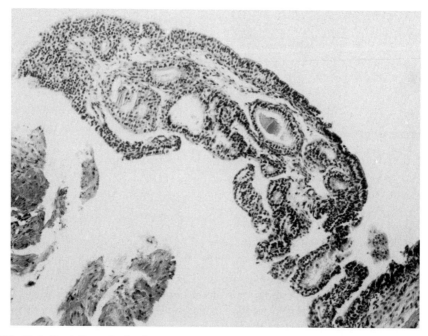

FIG. 18.1. Prostatic urethral polyp lined by transitional epithelium, with the core of the polyp containing prostatic glands and stroma. ×115.

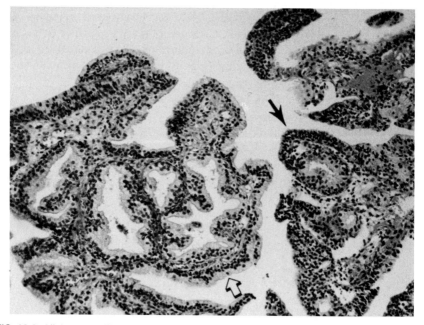

FIG. 18.2. Higher magnification of prostatic urethral polyp showing surface lining of both transitional-type epithelium *(arrow)* as well as prostatic glandular epithelium *(open arrow)*. ×115.

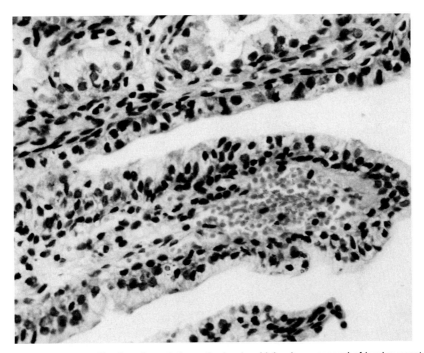

FIG. 18.3. High magnification of prostatic urethral polyp. Lining is composed of benign prostatic epithelial cells.

newborn to the elderly. The stroma within the polyps may have degenerative atypia as seen in similar lesions in the female genital tract. We have seen similar lesions in the female urethra, as well as in the bladder in both men and women.

Posterior urethral polyps are benign polypoid lesions arising from the verumontanum (10). Most commonly, patients complain of urinary obstruction, hematuria or complete urinary retention. These lesions almost exclusively occur in young boys under 10 years of age. Histologically, they are characterized by a polypoid lesion lined by normal urothelium. The lesion has a simple morphology without branching papillae and appears to be a polypoid lesion as a result of edematous stroma.

Reactive polypoid lesions may also result in the prostatic urethra. Identical to polypoid cystitis, these lesions are termed "polypoid urethritis" (efig 1723-1725;1726).

NEPHROGENIC ADENOMAS

Nephrogenic adenomas usually arise in the setting of prior urothelial injury, such as past surgery (60%), calculi (14%), or trauma (9%). Eight percent have a history of renal transplantation. These lesions are thought to represent a reaction to injury, and may also be designated as nephrogenic metaplasia. In one-third of patients, the lesion is found in patients less than 30 years of age.

Nephrogenic adenomas appear as papillary, polypoid, hyperplastic, fungating, friable, or velvety lesions. Typically found in the bladder, 12% are seen in the urethra. Most nephrogenic adenomas measure less than 1 cm, although they may attain dimensions as large as 7 cm. In 18% of cases, multiple lesions are identified. Lesions occurring in the prostatic urethra may be confused with adenocarcinoma of the prostate (11,12).

Nephrogenic adenomas have a broad histologic spectrum. Proliferations of small solid to hollow tubules, lined by low columnar to cuboidal epithelial cells with eosinophilic to clear cytoplasm, are identified in the majority of cases (Fig. 18.4, efig 1727-1730). Vascular-like structures with attenuated epithelium, with or without hobnail nuclei, are the second most common pattern (efig 1731-1735). Verification that these vascular-like structures are epithelial can be

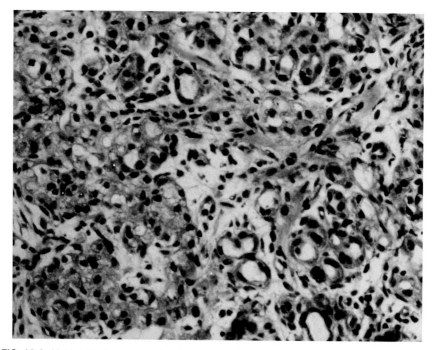

FIG. 18.4. Nephrogenic adenoma (nephrogenic metaplasia) involving prostatic urethra. Fused glands may resemble high-grade adenocarcinoma of the prostate. (From Epstein JI. *Differential Diagnoses in Pathology: Urologic Disorders.* New York: Igaku-Shoin; 1992:132–133, with permission.)

accomplished with immunohistochemistry for cytokeratin, which can help establish the correct diagnosis (Figs. 18.5–18.7). Cords and individual cells with cuboidal, eosinophilic to clear cytoplasm, polypoid or papillary configurations, and rare signet ring cell-like structures are identified in a decreasing percent of cases (Fig. 18.8, efig 1736;1737;1738-1741). A distinguishing feature of nephrogenic adenoma is the presence of a thickened hyaline sheath around some of the tubules, which may be enhanced with periodic acid Schiff (PAS) stains (efig 1729; 1742-1744;1745). Most cases of nephrogenic adenoma are composed of multiple histologic patterns, with a minority consisting of small tubules alone.

Nuclear atypia, when present, appears degenerative and mitoses are either absent or rare. Nuclei are enlarged and hyperchromatic, yet have a smudged indistinct chromatin pattern. These atypical nuclei often reside in cells with an endothelial or hobnail appearance lining vascular-like dilated tubules (Fig. 18.6, efig 1735). The presence of prominent nucleoli in many cases examined is also a source of possible confusion with prostate cancer (efig 1730;1743;1745).

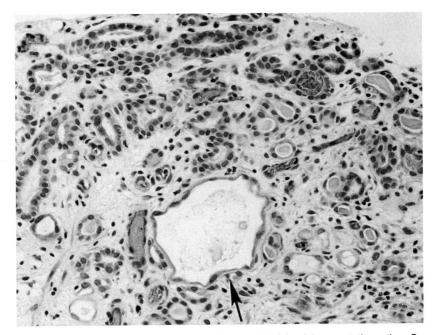

FIG. 18.5. Nephrogenic adenoma (nephrogenic metaplasia) involving prostatic urethra. Some glands are lined by cuboidal epithelium and others have an endothelial-like appearance (arrow). Many are filled with a colloid-like substance. (From Epstein JI. *Differential Diagnoses in Pathology: Urologic Disorders.* New York: Igaku-Shoin; 1992:132–133, with permission.)

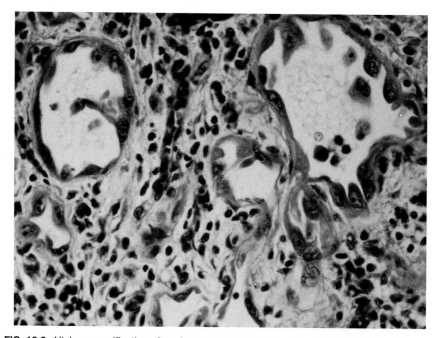

FIG. 18.6. Higher magnification of nephrogenic adenoma showing some tubules lined by atypical endothelial-like nuclei with prominent nucleoli. ×300.

However, prominent nucleoli are usually only focally present within a lesion, and often seen in association with degenerative nuclear atypia or with other features not commonly seen in prostate cancer, such as hobnail-like cells or peritubular hyaline sheaths.

Cystic tubules may contain thyroid-like eosinophilic secretions (efig 1746-1747;1748). A possible source of confusion with a malignant lesion of the prostate is the presence of blue-tinged mucinous secretions within tubular lumina. However, this "blue mucin" is seen in structures such as vascular-like tubules, or in lesions with other features more typical of nephrogenic adenoma than of prostate cancer. Nephrogenic adenomas may persist or recur in up to one-third of cases.

We have found that a majority of cases of nephrogenic adenoma arising from the prostatic urethra have some degree of muscle involvement, and in conjunction with a tubule or cord-like architectural pattern, is the most likely source of confusion with prostate cancer (11) (efig 1727-1728;1742;1746-1747;1749-1751). Features helpful to distinguish these cases of nephrogenic adenoma from prostate cancer include the presence of more typical nephrogenic adenoma architectural patterns in other areas of the lesion and that the lesion is located

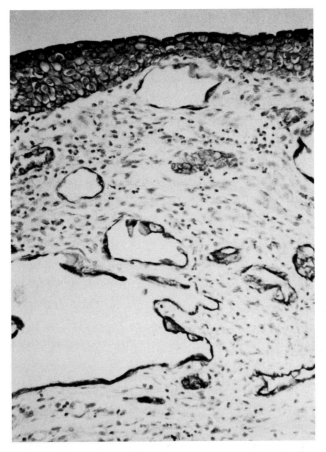

FIG. 18.7. Intense keratin immunoreactivity within tubules of nephrogenic adenoma, including those that resembled vascular channels. ×260.

immediately below the urothelial lining, a site unusual for prostate cancer (Fig. 18.9).

The presence of an acute and/or chronic inflammatory infiltrate within tubular lumina and in association with nephrogenic adenoma structures is seen in almost all nephrogenic adenomas (efig 1752). This intimate association of inflammation is not a feature of most prostate cancers.

As an adjunct to the histologic features of nephrogenic adenoma, immunohistochemical staining patterns that are helpful in identifying nephrogenic adenoma, and excluding prostate cancer, include cytoplasmic staining with the antibody clone directed against the high molecular weight cytokeratin, 34BE12.

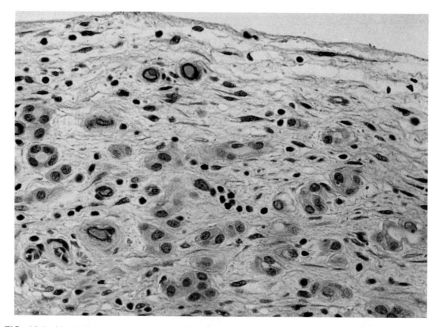

FIG. 18.8. Nephrogenic adenoma involving prostatic urethra composed of single cells. (From Epstein JI. *Differential Diagnoses in Pathology: Urologic Disorders.* New York: Igaku-Shoin; 1992:132–133, with permission.)

Cytoplasmic staining for 34BE12 is found in more than one half the cases of nephrogenic adenoma (efig 1753). Positive staining for 34BE12 may, therefore, help to establish the correct diagnosis of nephrogenic adenoma, but negative staining should not lead one to a misdiagnosis of prostate cancer.

Nephrogenic adenomas show diffuse cytokeratin 7 cytoplasmic localization (efig 1754-1755). Adjacent normal and metaplastic urothelium also shows cytoplasmic localization with cytokeratin 7, while adjacent benign prostate glands are uniformly negative. Localization of cytokeratin 7 is a sensitive method for identifying nephrogenic adenoma, but may lack specificity in that some prostate cancers may show staining with this antibody (13). Focal cytoplasmic staining and/or positive tubular secretions for PAS and prostate-specific acid phosphatase (PSAP) may be seen in almost half of nephrogenic adenomas (11) (efig 1756-1758). The presence of epitopes to PAS and PSAP in nephrogenic adenoma arising from the prostatic urethra may not be surprising in that the transitional urothelium which lines this portion of the male urethra and extends into the main prostatic ducts differs histologically, and perhaps embryologically, from that of the bladder and female urethra, and can elaborate both PAS and PSAP. In the absence of other diagnostic criteria, the presence of positive staining for PAS and/or PSAP in nephrogenic adenoma may lead to confusion with prostate can-

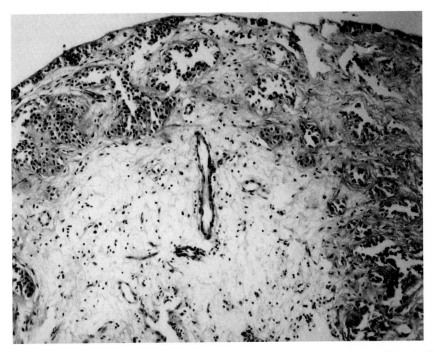

FIG. 18.9. Nephrogenic adenoma situated directly beneath prostatic urethra. (From Epstein Jl. *Differential Diagnoses in Pathology: Urologic Disorders.* New York: Igaku-Shoin; 1992:132–133, with permission.)

cer. However, absent staining for PAS and/or PSAP in well-formed tubular structures would be unusual for prostate cancer and should raise the possibility of nephrogenic adenoma.

In summary, isolated features of nephrogenic adenoma, taken out of context, may closely mimic prostate cancer. However, an assessment of the full constellation of histologic features, as well as the judicious interpretation of adjuvant immunohistochemical stains, should lead to the correct diagnosis in the majority of cases.

MISCELLANEOUS

We have seen rare cases of inverted papilloma in the prostatic urethra, although they are more frequent in the bladder (efig 1759-1760;1761-1762). These lesions have not been associated with an increased risk of urothelial cancer elsewhere in the urinary tract. Other lesions typically seen in the bladder can also involve the prostatic urethra, including urethral clear cell adenocarcinoma, primary amyloidosis, and paraganglioma (14–16).

REFERENCES

1. Butterick JD, Schnitzer B, Abell MR. Ectopic prostatic tissue in urethra: a clinico-pathological entity and a significant cause of hematuria. *J Urol* 1971;105:97–104.
2. Remick DG, Kumar NB. Benign polyps with prostatic-type epithelium of urethra and the urinary bladder. *Am J Surg Pathol* 1984;8:833–839.
3. Walker AN, Mills SE, Fechner RE, et al. "Endometrial" adenocarcinoma of the prostatic urethra arising in a villous polyp: a light microscopic and immunoperoxidase study. *Arch Pathol Lab Med* 1982; 106:624–627.
4. Nesbit RM. The genesis of benign polyps in the prostatic urethra. *J Urol* 1962;87:416–418.
5. Gutierrez J, Nesbit RM. Ectopic prostatic tissue in bladder. *J Urol* 1967;98:474–478.
6. Craig JR, Hart WR. Benign polyps with prostatic-type epithelium of urethra. *Am J Clin Pathol* 1975; 63:343–347.
7. Goldstein AMB, Bragin SD, Terry R, et al. Prostatic urethral polyps in adults: histopathologic variations and clinical presentations. *J Urol* 1981;126:129–131.
8. Hara S, Horie A. Prostatic caruncle: a urethral papillary tumor derived from prolapse of the prostatic duct. *J Urol* 1977;117:303–305.
9. Young RH. Non-neoplastic and tumor-like abnormalities. In: Young RH, ed. *Pathology of the Urinary Bladder*. New York, NY: Churchill Livingstone; 1989:36–37.
10. Foster RS, Garrett RA. Congenital posterior urethral polyps. *J Urol* 1986;136:670–672.
11. Allan CH, Epstein JI. Nephrogenic adenoma of the prostatic urethra: a mimicker of prostate adenocarcinoma. *Am J Surg Pathol* 2001; 25:802–808.
12. Malpica A, Ro JY, Troncoso P, et al. Nephrogenic adenoma of the prostatic urethra involving the prostate gland: a clinicopathologic and immunohistochemical study of eight cases. *Hum Pathol* 1994; 25:390–395.
13. Genega EM, Hutchinson B, Reuter VE, et al. Immunophenotype of high-grade prostatic adenocarcinoma and urothelial carcinoma. *Mod Pathol* 2000;13:1186–1191.
14. Young RH, Scully RE. Clear cell adenocarcinoma of the bladder and urethra. A report of 3 cases and review of the literature. *Am J Surg Pathol* 1985;9:816–826.
15. Vasudevan P, Stein AM, Pinn VW, et al. Primary amyloidosis of urethra. *Urology* 1981;17:181–183.
16. Badalament RA, Kenworthy P, Pellegrini A, et al. Paraganglioma of urethra. *Urology* 1991;38:76–78.

Appendix: Macros

As described in the text, the use of macros (canned text) has many advantages. Below are listed some of the macros that we most commonly use in our diagnoses. One may alter these macros to suit individual cases or one's individual preference.

BENIGN DIAGNOSES

/BPT: Benign prostatic tissue.
The macro "/BPT" is used for the diagnosis of benign tissue on prostate needle biopsy.
/BPH: Benign prostatic hyperplasia.
The macro "/BPH" is only used on transurethral resections of the prostate.
/SVED: Benign portion of seminal vesicle/ejaculatory duct.
/CROWDED: Prostate tissue with focus of benign crowded glands.
The macro "/CROWDED" is used for a small cluster of glands that is not sufficiently extensive to justify the diagnosis of adenosis.
/ADENOSIS: Benign prostate tissue with focus of adenosis. See note.
Note: This case is characterized by a fairly well-circumscribed collection of close-packed glands of different sizes. The diagnosis of adenosis rests on the nuclear and cytoplasmic similarity of the small, crowded glands to admixed larger and more recognizably benign glands. Although adenosis mimics infiltrating adenocarcinoma architecturally, it has not been shown to have any association to carcinoma. (See *Am J Surg Pathol* 18:863–870, 1994. *Am J Surg Pathol* 19:737–747, 1995.)

DIAGNOSES WITH ATYPIA OR PIN

/ATYP: Prostate tissue with small focus of atypical glands. See note.
Note: Although these findings are atypical and suspicious for adenocarcinoma, there is insufficient cytologic and/or architectural atypia to establish a definitive diagnosis. Repeat biopsy is recommended. (See *Urology* 52:803–807,

1998, for biopsy protocol to increase the likelihood of detecting prostate cancer after an initial atypical biopsy.)

In the macro "/ATYP," one may leave off the last two sentences concerning repeat biopsy. Some pathologists may not feel comfortable recommending the repeat biopsies. We also leave off these last two sentences in this macro when the patient is very elderly or when the patient has already had multiple biopsies in the past.

/ATYPNN: Prostate tissue with small focus of atypical glands.

We use the macro "/ATYPNN" in cases where there is carcinoma elsewhere in the diagnosis and we merely want to describe another focus of atypical glands.

/PINATYP: Focus of high-grade prostatic intraepithelial neoplasia (PIN) with adjacent small atypical glands. See note.

Note: Adjacent to glands of high-grade PIN, there are a few small adjacent atypical glands. While these small glands may represent a microscopic focus of infiltrating cancer, we cannot exclude that they represent a tangential section or outpouchings of the adjacent PIN glands. Repeat biopsy is recommended.

/PIN: High-grade prostatic intraepithelial neoplasia.

/LGPIN: Benign prostate tissue. See note.

Note: There are foci that may represent low-grade prostatic intraepithelial neoplasia (PIN). However, we do not diagnose low-grade PIN, since its recognition is subjective and it lacks clinical relevance.

We use the macro "/LGPIN" for cases were there is a focus that stands out at low magnification as suggestive of PIN, yet it fails to satisfy the criteria for high-grade PIN.

/CRIB: Atypical cribriform glands suspicious for cribriform adenocarcinoma; however, high-grade PIN cannot be excluded with certainty.

/NOCAAT: Due to atrophic features, a definitive diagnosis cannot be made.

/NOCAPIN: High-grade PIN cannot be excluded with certainty.

/NOCAINF: Due to the presence of inflammation, a definitive diagnosis cannot be made.

/NOCAAD: Adenosis cannot be excluded with certainty.

The macros beginning with "/NOCA..." can be used at the end of an atypical macro describing why a definitive cancer diagnosis was not made. (i.e., /ATYP/NOCAAT).

DIAGNOSES DESCRIBING HIGH MOLECULAR WEIGHT CYTOKERATIN STAINING

/HMWCK: Note: The diagnosis of carcinoma is supported by the failure of immunoperoxidase staining for high molecular weight cytokeratin to demonstrate basal cells in the atypical glands.

/NEGHMWCK: Note: By itself, negative staining for high molecular weight cytokeratin in a small focus is not diagnostic of cancer.

/POSHMWCK: Note: Stains for high molecular weight cytokeratin demonstrate positive staining for basal cells in the focus in question, ruling out carcinoma.

DIAGNOSES DESCRIBING TUMOR

We have separate macros for each Gleason score; for example: the macro "/336" comes out as "Adenocarcinoma of the prostate Gleason score 3+3=6."

/SKEL: The tumor is seen within skeletal muscle. The presence of tumor infiltrating skeletal muscle does not necessarily indicate extraprostatic extension.

/ATROPHIC: Note: The tumor has atrophic features (*Am J Surg Pathol* 21:289–295, 1997).

/PSEUDO: Note: This tumor has features of "pseudohyperplastic carcinoma" (*Am J Surg Pathol* 22:1239–1246, 1998).

/FOAMY: Note: The tumor in areas has the appearance of foamy gland carcinoma (*Am J Surg Pathol* 20:419–426, 1996).

/RTCA: The tumor in this case shows treatment effect in that there are individual cells with abundant vacuolated cytoplasm where the nuclei show smudged chromatin and absent nucleoli. Cancers that show radiation therapy effect have in some studies been associated with a better prognosis than tumor that appear unaltered by radiation (*Cancer* 79:81–89, 1997).

Subject Index